MORE
4U!

the d... ....

This Clin...

Here's what you get:

■ Full text of EVERY issue from 2002 to NOW

■ Figures, tables, drawings, references and more

■ Searchable: find what you need fast

Search | All Clinics ▼ | for [   ] | GO |

■ Linked to MEDLINE and Elsevier journals

■ E-alerts

INDIVIDUAL SUBSCRIBERS

LOG ON TODAY. IT'S FAST AND EASY.

Click **Register** and follow instructions

You'll need your account number

Your subscriber account number is on your mailing label

This is your copy of:

THE CLINICS OF NORTH AMERICA

CXXX **2296532-2** 2 Mar 05

J.H. DOE, MD
531 MAIN STREET
CENTER CITY, NY 10001-001

BOUGHT A SINGLE ISSUE? Sorry, you won't be able to access full text online. Please subscribe today to get complete content by contacting customer service at 800 645 2452 (US and Canada) or 407 345 4000 (outside US and Canada) or via email at elsols@elsevier.com.

NEW!

Now also available for INSTITUTIONS

ELSEVIER

Works/Integrates with MD Consult
Available in a variety of packages: Collections containing
14, 31 or 50 Clinics titles
Or Collection upgrade for existing MD Consult customers

Call today! 877-857-1047 or e-mail: mdc.groupinfo@elsevier.com

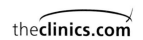

VETERINARY CLINICS

OF NORTH AMERICA

Small Animal Practice

Dentistry

GUEST EDITOR
Steven E. Holmstrom, DVM

July 2005 • Volume 35 • Number 4

SAUNDERS

An Imprint of Elsevier, Inc.
PHILADELPHIA   LONDON   TORONTO   MONTREAL   SYDNEY   TOKYO

W.B. SAUNDERS COMPANY
A Division of Elsevier Inc.

Elsevier, Inc., 1600 John F. Kennedy Blvd., Suite 1800, Philadelphia, PA 19103-2899

http://www.vetsmall.theclinics.com

VETERINARY CLINICS OF NORTH AMERICA: Volume 35, Number 4
SMALL ANIMAL PRACTICE   ISSN 0195-5616
July 2005   ISBN 1-4160-2846-3
Editor: John Vassallo

The ideas and opinions expressed in *Veterinary Clinics of North America: Small Animal Practice* do not necessarily reflect those of the Publisher. The Publisher does not assume any responsibility for any injury and/or damage to persons or property arising out of or related to any use of the material contained in this periodical. The reader is advised to check the appropriate medical literature and the product information currently provided by the manufacturer of each drug to be administered to verify the dosage, the method and duration of administration, or contraindications. It is the responsibility of the treating physician or other health care professional, relying on independent experience and knowledge of the patient, to determine drug dosages and the best treatment for the patient. Mention of any product in this issue should not be construed as endorsement by the contributors, editors, or the Publisher of the product or manufacturers' claims.

Veterinary Clinics of North America: Small Animal Practice (ISSN 0195-5616) is published bimonthly (For Post Office use only: volume 35 issue 4 of 6) by Elsevier, Inc. Corporate and editorial offices: Elsevier, Inc., 1600 John F. Kennedy Blvd., Suite 1800, Philadelphia, PA 19103-2899. Accounting and circulation offices: 6277 Sea Harbor Drive, Orlando, FL 32887-4800. Periodicals postage paid at Orlando, FL 32862, and additional mailing offices. Subscription prices are $170.00 per year for US individuals, $260.00 per year for US institutions, $85.00 per year for US students and residents, $215.00 per year for Canadian individuals, $325.00 per year for Canadian institutions, $225.00 per year for international individuals, $325.00 per year for international institutions and $113.00 per year for Canadian and foreign students/residents. To receive student/resident rate, orders must be accompanied by name of affiliated institution, date of term, and the *signature* of program/residency coordinator on institution letterhead. Orders will be billed at individual rate until proof of status is received. Foreign air speed delivery is included in all *Clinics* subscription prices. All prices are subject to change without notice. POSTMASTER: Send address changes to *Veterinary Clinics of North America: Small Animal Practice*, Elsevier, Customer Service Department, 6277 Sea Harbor Drive, Orlando, FL 32887-4800, USA; phone: (+1)(877) 839-7126 [toll free number for US customers], or (+1)(407) 345-4020 [customers outside US]; fax: (+1)(407) 363-1354; email: usjcs@elsevier.com

Veterinary Clinics of North America: Small Animal Practice is also published in Japanese by Gakusosha Company Ltd., 2-16-28 Nishikata, Bunkyo-ku, Tokyo 113, Japan.

Reprints. For copies of 100 or more, of articles in this publication, please contact the Commercial Reprints Department, Elsevier Inc., 360 Park Avenue South, New York, New York 10010-1710. Tel. (212) 633-3813 Fax: (212) 462-1935, email: reprints@elsevier.com

Veterinary Clinics of North America: Small Animal Practice is covered in *Current Contents/Agriculture, Biology and Environmental Sciences, Science Citation Index, ASCA, Index Medicus, Excerpta Medica, and BIOSIS.*

Printed in the United States of America.

GUEST EDITOR

STEVEN E. HOLMSTROM, DVM, Diplomate, American Veterinary Dental College; Animal Dental Clinic, San Carlos, California

CONTRIBUTORS

VANESSA G.G. CARVALHO, DVM, MS, Doctoral student, Department of Surgery, Comparative Dental Laboratory of the School of Veterinary Medicine, University of São Paulo, São Paulo, Brazil

BENJAMIN COLMERY III, DVM, Diplomate, American Veterinary Dental College; Vet Dentistry PLC, Ann Arbor, Michigan

LINDA J. DEBOWES, DVM, MS, Diplomate, American College of Veterinary Internal Medicine; Diplomate, American Veterinary Dental College; Shoreline Veterinary Dental Clinic, Seattle; Veterinary Dental Referral Service of Puget Sound, Tacoma, Washington

GREGG A. DUPONT, DVM, Fellow, Academy of Veterinary Dentistry; Diplomate, American Veterinary Dental College; Co-Owner, Shoreline Veterinary Dental Clinic, Seattle, Washington

MARCO A. GIOSO, DVM, DDS, PhD, Diplomate, American Veterinary Dental College; Professor of Surgery, Department of Surgery, School of Veterinary Medicine and Zootechny, University of São Paulo, São Paulo, Brazil

FRASER A. HALE, DVM, Fellow, Academy of Veterinary Dentistry; Diplomate, American Veterinary Dental College; Hale Veterinary Clinic, Guelph, Ontario, Canada

COLIN E. HARVEY, BVSc, FRCVS, Diplomate, American College of Veterinary Surgeons; Diplomate, American Veterinary Dental College; Professor of Surgery and Dentistry, School of Veterinary Medicine, University of Pennsylvania, Philadelphia, Pennsylvania

STEVEN E. HOLMSTROM, DVM, Diplomate, American Veterinary Dental College; Animal Dental Clinic, San Carlos, California

LOÏC LEGENDRE, DVM, Diplomate, American Veterinary Dental College; Northwest Veterinary Dental Services Ltd., North Vancouver, British Columbia, Canada

JOHN R. LEWIS, VMD, Fellow, Academy of Veterinary Dentistry; Diplomate, American Veterinary Dental College; Staff Veterinarian in Dentistry, Department of Clinical Studies, School of Veterinary Medicine, University of Pennsylvania, Philadelphia, Pennsylvania

KENNETH F. LYON, DVM, Fellow, Academy of Veterinary Dentistry; Diplomate, American Veterinary Dental College; Arizona Veterinary Dentistry and Oral Surgery, Gilbert, Arizona

BROOK A. NIEMIEC, DVM, Fellow, Academy of Veterinary Dentistry; Diplomate, American Veterinary Dental College; Chief of Staff, Southern California Veterinary Dental Specialties, San Diego, Murrieta, and Upland, California

AYAKO OKUDA, DVM, PhD, Diplomate, American Veterinary Dental College; Associate Lecturer, Department of Anatomy, School of Veterinary Medicine, Azabu University, Fuchinobe; Director of Vettec Dentistry, Tokyo, Japan

ALEXANDER M. REITER, Dipl Tzt, Dr Med Vet, Diplomate, American Veterinary Dental College; Diplomate, European Veterinary Dental College; Assistant Professor of Dentistry, Department of Clinical Studies, School of Veterinary Medicine, University of Pennsylvania, Philadelphia, Pennsylvania

JUDY ROCHETTE, DVM, Fellow, Academy of Veterinary Dentistry; Diplomate, American Veterinary Dental College; Private Practice, Burnaby, British Columbia, Canada

THOULTON W. SURGEON, DVM, Fellow, Academy of Veterinary Dentistry; Diplomate, American Veterinary Dental College; ANC Veterinary Center Dental and Surgical Services, New Rochelle, New York

FRANK J.M. VERSTRAETE, DrMedVet, MMedVet, Diplomate, American Veterinary Dental College; Diplomate, European College of Veterinary Surgeons; Diplomate, European Veterinary Dental College; Professor of Dentistry and Oral Surgery, Department of Surgical and Radiological Sciences, School of Veterinary Medicine, University of California, Davis, California

CONTENTS

For the others, being aware of the potential problems, recognizing them early, and instituting appropriate care in a timely manner can improve the quality of life immediately and avoid more serious problems in the long term.

Periodontal disease is the most common disease occurring in domestic dogs and cats, and local severity and the impact on the rest of the body are reasons why all companion animal patients should receive an oral examination every time they are seen. This article provides the background information on how an effective periodontal management program can be tailored for each patient.

Endodontic disease is a highly prevalent (>10% of all dogs) and insidiously painful process that can have significant local and systemic effects. The root canal system is a delicate organ and is prone to inflammation, infection, and partial and complete necrosis. Vital pulp therapy must be performed quickly, gently, and meticulously if it is to be effective. The relatively high rate of failure in direct pulp capping makes regular follow-up radiographs of critical importance to ensure patient health. Once a tooth is dead, there are often no obvious clinical signs; therefore, clinicians must be educated in the diagnosis of the disease processes. Once properly educated, the practitioner must remain vigilant for subtle signs of the disease process. Standard root canal therapy is an effective method of removing the inflammation, infection, and associated discomfort of the endodontically diseased tooth while maintaining its function. Endodontic failure most likely remains hidden unless dental radiology is used. Follow-up radiographs at regular intervals throughout the patient's life are critical for ensuring the long-term success of any endodontic therapy.

The basic principles and concepts that govern the discipline of orthodontics are explored. The movement of teeth is mediated primarily through the periodontal ligament. When the periodontal ligament is stretched, bone apposition occurs. Conversely, in areas of compression, bone resorption occurs. The subject tooth moves in the direction of the force. The orthodontist must be cognizant of the prevailing ethical guidelines and the functional needs of the patient.

and of the factors contributing to the progression of resorptive lesions, reliable prevention cannot be offered.

Simple and Surgical Exodontia

Linda J. DeBowes

Preemptive and postoperative pain management is part of patient care when performing extractions. Simple extractions can become complicated when tooth roots are fractured. Adequate lighting, magnification, and surgical techniques are important when performing surgical (complicated) extractions. Radiographs should be taken before extractions and also during the procedure to assist with difficult extractions. Adequate flap design and bone removal are necessary when performing surgical extractions. Complications, including ocular trauma, jaw fracture, and soft tissue trauma, are avoided or minimized with proper patient selection and technique.

Maxillofacial Fracture Repairs

Loïc Legendre

Oral trauma remains a common presentation in a small animal practice. Most fractures are the result of vehicular accidents. Among other causes are falls, kicks, gunshots wounds, and encounters with various hard objects ranging from baseball bats and golf clubs to horse hooves and car doors. Next in popularity are dog fights, especially when a large dog and a small dog are involved, and fights with other animals. With cats, falls from various heights are responsible for a large percentage of presentations.

Mandibulectomy and Maxillectomy

Frank J.M. Verstraete

In an animal presented for evaluation of an oral tumor, the extent of the disease is based on the systematic evaluation of the tumor, including diagnostic imaging, and the assessment of regional lymph node involvement and distant metastases. The nature of the disease is determined by an incisional biopsy and histopathologic examination. The choice of treatment and expected outcome are based on the stage and expected biologic behavior, which is well known for many oral tumor types. The various mandibulectomy and maxillectomy techniques have been shown to give good functional and cosmetic results.

Regional Anesthesia and Analgesia for Oral and Dental Procedures

Judy Rochette

Regional anesthesia and analgesia benefit the client, the patient, and the practitioner, and their use is becoming the standard for care. Familiarity with the processes involved in the generation of pain aids in understanding the benefits of preemptive and multimodal analgesia. Local anesthetic blocks should be a key component of a treatment plan, along with opioids, nonsteroidal anti-inflammatory drugs, N-methyl-D-aspartate receptor antagonists, and other therapies. Nerve blocks commonly used for dentistry and oral surgery include the infraorbital, maxillary, mental, and mandibular blocks.

GOAL STATEMENT

The goal of the *Veterinary Clinics of North America: Small Animal Practice* is to keep practicing veterinarians up-to-date with current clinical practice in small animal medicine by providing timely articles reviewing the state of the art in small animal care.

ACCREDITATION

The *Veterinary Clinics of North America: Small Animal Practice* will be offering continuing education credits, to be awarded by a school of veterinary medicine, contract pending.

The aforementioned school of veterinary medicine is a designated provider of continuing veterinary education. Veterinarians participating in this learning activity may earn up to 6 credits per issue up to a maximum of 36 credits per year. Credits awarded may not apply toward license renewal in all states. It is the responsibility of each participant to verify the requirements of their state licensing board.

Credit can be earned by reading the text material, taking the examination online at *http://www.theclinics.com/home/cme*, and completing the program evaluation. Each test question must be answered correctly; you will have the opportunity to retake any questions answered incorrectly. Following successful completion of the test and the program evaluation, you may print your certificate.

TO ENROLL

To enroll in the *Veterinary Clinics of North America: Small Animal Practice* Continuing Education program, call customer service at 1-800-654-2452 or sign up online at http://www.theclinics.com/home/cme. The CE program is available to subscribers for an additional annual fee of $99.95.

FORTHCOMING ISSUES

RECENT ISSUES

VETERINARY
CLINICS
Small Animal Practice

ELSEVIER
SAUNDERS

Vet Clin Small Anim
35 (2005) xiii–xiv

Preface

Dentistry

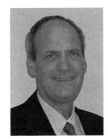

Steven E. Holmstrom, DVM
Guest Editor

"I did a dental" is a common statement by veterinarians and technicians. This issue of *Veterinary Clinics of North America Small Animal Practice* illustrates that there is no such thing as "a dental." Veterinary dentistry has continued to evolve, with many new concepts and techniques; as time goes by, there will continue to be advancements in veterinary dentistry. As interest grows, more practitioners become involved and all benefit.

The purpose of this issue is to provide the reader with information that facilitates a better understanding of veterinary dentistry. The text begins with the basics of anatomy and proceeds to articles on standards in veterinary dentistry, fundamentals of juvenile dentistry, diseases of the gums, diseases of the root canal system, and occlusion. Through the years, practitioners have been frustrated by two conditions in the cat, gingivostomatitis and tooth resorption; three articles have been devoted to these conditions. Oral surgery is an important area in veterinary dentistry. The fundamentals of surgery through extractions, maxillofacial fracture repair, and mandibulectomy procedures are covered in succeeding articles. Finally, the importance of pain control locally and systemically should not be overlooked.

I would like to thank the authors for their contributions to this edition. Also, I would like to thank all those who have participated in forwarding the profession through membership in the American Veterinary Dental

doi:10.1016/j.cvsm.2005.04.001

College, Academy of Veterinary Dentistry, and American Veterinary Dental Society.

Steven E. Holmstrom, DVM
Animal Dental Clinic
987 Laurel Street
San Carlos, CA 94070, USA

E-mail address: Steve@Toothvet.info

ELSEVIER
SAUNDERS

Vet Clin Small Anim
35 (2005) 763–780

VETERINARY
CLINICS
Small Animal Practice

Oral Anatomy of the Dog and Cat in Veterinary Dentistry Practice

Marco A. Gioso, DVM, DDS, PhD[a,b,*],
Vanessa G.G. Carvalho, DVM, MS[a,b]

[a]Department of Surgery, Comparative Dental Laboratory of the School of Veterinary
Medicine, University of São Paulo, Av. Prof. Dr. Orlando Marques de Paiva,
87, Cidade Universitária, São Paulo, SP, Brazil 05508-900
[b]Brazilian Veterinary Dentistry Association

Bones of the cranium

The head is the most important and specialized part of the body because it contains the brain and important sensory organs for hearing, seeing, eating, and smelling [1–4]. It is divided into the neurocranium (cranium) and viscerocranium (face) [2,5,6]. The cranium is a group of plain and irregular bones that are perfectly connected by sutures [7] to form a hollow box [5]. The sutures are open in a newborn, but they become ossified after growth [8]. The margins of each bone of the cranium can be identified in adult animals [7].

The bones of the cranium are the occipital, parietal, frontal, temporal (paired), interparietal, basisphenoid, presphenoid, ethmoid, pterygoid, and vomer (unpaired) bones (Figs. 1 and 2) [9].

The cranium cavity is separated from the nasal cavity of the face by a perforated plate called the cribriform plate [1]. The face is the most important part of the head for veterinary dentistry and needs to be fully understood by the practitioner [10]. It can be divided into orbital, nasal, and oral regions [1,3,11].

The orbital region is formed by portions of the frontal bone and lacrimal and zygomatic bones. The nasal airway is limited dorsally by the nasal bones, laterally by the maxillary and incisive bones, and ventrally by the palatine process of the maxillary bone as well as by the incisive and palatine bones. Fixed on the nasal cavity are the nasal turbinates (delicate curved

* Corresponding author.
E-mail address: maggioso@usp.br (M.A. Gioso).

0195-5616/05/$ - see front matter © 2005 Elsevier Inc. All rights reserved.
doi:10.1016/j.cvsm.2004.10.003
vetsmall.theclinics.com

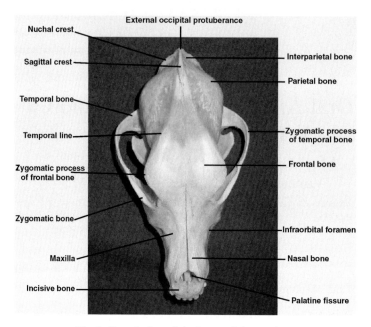

Fig. 1. Dorsal view of the bones of the cranium.

osseous laminas), which support the organs of smell, and the blood vessels [1,3,11]. The oral region has a long surface to support all the teeth [1].

The viscerocranium is composed of the following: incisive, nasal, maxilla, dorsal nasal concha, ventral nasal concha, zygomatic, palatine, and lacrimal bones and the mandible (see Figs. 1 and 2) [9].

The incisive bone divides the nasal cavity entrance and the palatine roof at the rostral end of the skull [6]. Some authors refer to the incisive bone as the premaxilla, but this is not a term used in veterinary anatomy [9]. This bone contains six incisive teeth that increase in size from the medial aspect to the lateral aspect. Laterally, the body of the incisive bone completes the medial wall of the canine alveolus [1]. The palatine process of the incisive bone forms a large groove to support the septal cartilage [11]. At this process, there are two large openings called palatine fissures that can be palpated in vivo and have a surface with a soft consistency. The palatine process contains the nasopalatine duct, which communicates between the nasal and oral cavity [12].

The nasal bone is long and thin, located at the dorsal surface of the face, and can be long or short depending on the breed of dog or cat. The ventral surface is covered by a mucous membrane, forming the dorsal nasal meatus [1]. The dorsal nasal concha (nasal turbinate), a simple and curved bone lamina inserted at the ethmoidal crest of the nasal bone [11], and the ventral nasal concha (maxillary turbinate), which is attached to the maxilla by a conchal crest [13], are located in the nasal cavity. The vomer bone forms

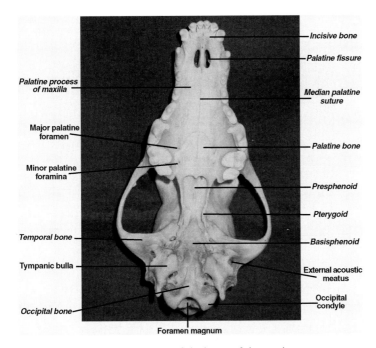

Fig. 2. Ventral view of the bones of the cranium.

the caudoventral portion of the nasal septum. The sagittal portion is formed by two thin lateral osseous laminas that are ventrally adhered to receive the cartilaginous nasal septum rostrally and the perpendicular plate of the ethmoid bone (osseous nasal septum) caudally [1].

The maxilla contains the canine, premolar, and molar teeth, and their roots are inserted into the bone, forming prominences that are called juga alveolaris or juga (Fig. 3). The most prominent jugals alveolaris are formed by the canine and fourth premolar teeth [1,12], because the maxilla has a thin lateral wall. This characteristic serves as a reference, helping the veterinarian to localize the roots during endodontic and exodontic procedures [10,14,15].

The infraorbital canal in dogs is present on the lateral face of the maxilla between the first molar roots and the fourth premolar roots (see Fig. 3). This canal begins in the pterygopalatine fossa (Fig. 4), and its opening is located in the infraorbital foramen distal to the upper third premolar. This canal contains the infraorbital vessels and nerves, which are important vascular structures in this region [1,11,12] and need to be carefully dissected and ligated during maxillectomy [10]. In cats, the infraorbital canal is short, and some animals have a double canal divided by a thin osseous lamina [13]. This infraorbital nerve can be easily reached by a needle through its rostral opening to accomplish regional anesthesia [14].

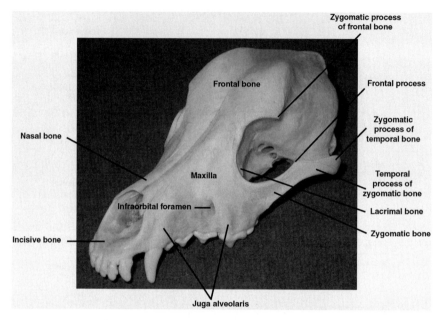

Fig. 3. Lateral view of the viscerocranium of the dog.

The lacrimal canal is also located in the maxilla. It is a tunnel that runs into the maxillary bone, beginning in the lacrimal fossa (at the lacrimal bone) and ending at the nasal cavity. The lacrimal canal drains lacrimal fluid from the conjunctival sac [2].

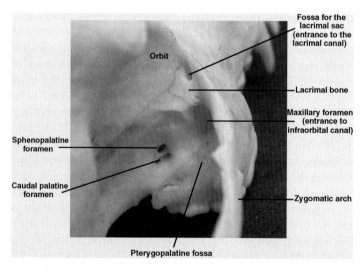

Fig. 4. Caudal view of the pterygopalatine fossa, lacrimal bone, and other important structures in the dog.

The palatine process of the maxilla comprises the hard palate, which separates the nasal and oral pathways. The ventral surface of the palatine process is in contact with the oral cavity. Its surface is demarcated with the palatine sulcus on both sides, beginning in the major palatine foramen and running rostrally to the palatine fissures. These fissures are large openings located at the rostral border of the palatine process (see Fig. 2) [1]. The major palatine foramen is located near or exactly at the transverse palatine suture between the median palatine suture and the alveolar border [11]. The major palatine artery that runs rostrally through the palatine sulcus emerges through this foramen. This artery is the most important vascular structure of the ventral palate mucosa and needs to be preserved during surgical procedures, such as cleft palate operations. Injuries to the major palatine artery can cause profuse hemorrhage and later dehiscence of the mucosa [10].

The palatine bone has no teeth. The horizontal plate forms the third caudal portion of the hard palate and has a variable number of minor palatine foramina with minor palatine arteries (see Fig. 2). These minor blood vessels form a secondary blood supply to the palate mucosa and do not cause significant hemorrhage if they are incised [10]. The lateral surface of this bone is free and forms the medial wall of the pterygopalatine fossa. The palatine canal begins in this fossa, opening at the sphenopalatine foramen (see Fig. 4), running into the palatine bone, and ending at the major palatine foramen. This canal contains the major palatine blood vessels and nerves [1]. The infraorbital canal also begins at the pterygopalatine fossa in the maxillary foramen (see Fig. 4), running into the maxillary bone and opening at the infraorbital foramen. This canal contains the infraorbital blood vessels and nerves [1,11] and is important during maxillectomies in this region [10,14].

The zygomatic arch is formed rostrally by the zygomatic bone and caudally by the zygomatic process of the temporal bone. The orbital ligament closes the orbit between the frontal process of the zygomatic bone and the zygomatic process of the frontal bone [1]. This ligament can be ossified in cats [6]. In cats, it is present in the postorbital process, making the orbit nearly closed [16] as well as causing some difficulty during positioning, with overlapping radiographs of the zygomatic arch into the teeth. The same problem occurs in brachycephalic dogs [14].

Two bilateral bones barely attached to each other by strong fibers at the intermandibular joint (Fig. 5) comprise the mandible [7] and are called the symphysis. The symphysis is easily disrupted during mandibulectomy because there are no bones on this region [10]. In old cats, this intermandibular joint can frequently be ossified [17], causing difficulties in separating the mandible during surgery [10].

The horizontal ramus (body of the mandible) has teeth (pars incisive and pars molaris) [7,15,18], and the vertical ramus (ramus of the mandible) contains the coronoid, condyloid, and angular processes (see Fig. 5) [7,15,19].

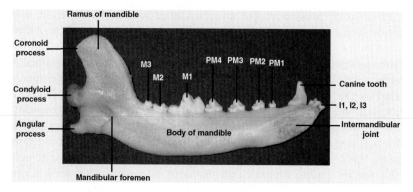

Fig. 5. Ventral view of the hemimandible of the dog.

The coronoid process is located between the zygomatic arch and the temporal bone. Most of the time, the zygomatic arch needs to be removed to obtain access to the coronoid process during surgery [10].

The body of mandible has an evident medullar cavity called the mandibular canal that begins at the mandibular foramen (see Fig. 5) in the ventral face near the angle of the mandible and opens at two or three mental foramina rostrally in the lateral face of the mandible [12]. The inferior alveolar nerve runs into the mandibular canal and is a part of the mandibular nerve, which separates into the mental nerves rostrally. The arteries and veins run together with the nerves [20] and need to be carefully located and ligated during mandibulectomies [10].

All the mental foramina are referred to by the same name, mental foramina [9], but they are different in size. There is a small one between the first and second lower incisive teeth, the largest one is ventral to the first lower premolar, and the third one is caudal to the largest foramen but can be absent [12]. These mental foramina need to be identified during rostral mandibulectomy as well, because there are blood vessels coming from these openings that can cause moderate hemorrhage when they are incised [10]. Regional block anesthesia can be performed at these large foramina if necessary [14].

Between the two horizontal rami, there is a space called the intermandibular space, where the tongue, pharynx, cranial portion of larynx, and hyoid apparatus are located [18].

The hyoid apparatus is dorsally attached to the skull and ventrally attached to the larynx and base of the tongue, suspending these structures in the caudal part of the mandibular space. It acts as a suspensory mechanism for the tongue and larynx [1,6,11]. The component parts, united by synchondroses, consist of the single basihyoid and the paired thyrohyoid, ceratohyoid, epihyoid, and stylohyoid bones as well as the tymphanohyoid cartilages [9]. The hyoid apparatus is an important reference point during pharyngostomy, because the incision is made between the hyoid apparatus and the angle of the mandible [10].

Temporomandibular joint

The articular (condylar) process of the mandible and the mandibular fossa of the temporal bone form the temporomandibular joint (Fig. 6). A cartilaginous disk divides the joint into two cavities: dorsal (or temporal) and ventral (or mandible) [12,15]. The joint is covered by a capsule that is attached around the joint surfaces, with synovial fluid inside [21]. Fibrous tissue is present around the capsule, forming a ligament laterally [12,15,22].

The movements of this joint are limited by all these structures [22]. The temporomandibular joint of dogs and cats can only move vertically. Characteristically, the cartilaginous disk is fibrous and thin but with evident rostral thickness to avoid anterior luxation during substantial vertical movements [23].

The perpendicular anatomic shape of the condylar process in dogs and cats is the most important characteristic permitting only vertical movement of this joint [24]. Especially in cats, the condylar process is transversally conic, and the mandibular fossa has a deep canal that intercepts any kind of lateral movement [25]. This conical shape in a lateromedial direction presents great difficulties when a condylectomy has to be performed [10].

Cranial types

As opposed to the case in human beings, the animal face is normally larger than the cranium [8], whereas the oral and nasal portions can be too

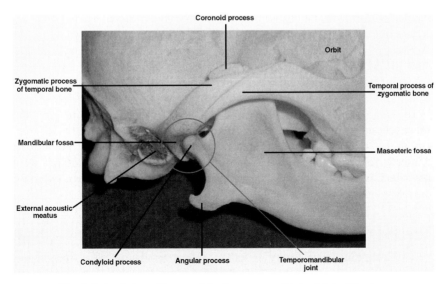

Fig. 6. Lateral view of bones of the temporomandibular joint of the dog.

long or too short, especially in dogs, because there is greater variation in breeds [3,18].

There are three kinds of cranium: brachycephalic, mesocephalic, and dolichocephalic. Brachycephalic means "short head," as in the Pekingese, Pug, Boxer, Bulldog, Shiatzu, and Lhasa Apso breeds. Mesocephalic means "medium head," as in the Labrador Retriever, Spaniel, Terrier, Beagle, Poodle, and Schnauzer breeds. Dolichocephalic means "long and straight head," as in the Collie, Dachshund, Doberman Pinscher, Greyhound, Saluki, Siberian Husky, and German Shepherd breeds (Fig. 7) [15,18,26–28].

Some characteristics are peculiar in dolichocephalic heads. This type of head has an extreme thin and long mandible, with distinct maxillary prognathism [27]. Normally, ample space is observed between the teeth [24]. Normal occlusion can occur if these animals have inherited abnormal maxilla and mandible length [27]. The dolichocephalic characteristics of the cranium are not yet observed in puppies; however, the long face appears when the puppies begin to grow [29].

A brachycephalic head always has maxillary brachygnathism and sometimes has mandibular brachygnathism also, and it is common to observe an anterior cross-bite in various degrees [27]. In fact, however, the real problem is the short maxilla; the impression of mandible prognathism is false [14] and can be referred to as relative prognathism [12].

Brachycephalic animals frequently have an airway obstructive syndrome because of the anatomic characteristics of the brachycephalic cranium, which results in a short and twisted pharynx, long soft palate, and straight nostril (in 50% of cases) [30].

Head shape and teeth positioning can each affect the other [26]. The wrong position of deciduous teeth can result in inappropriate occlusion of the permanent teeth and cause abnormal mandible or maxillary length. This is considered to be a genetic problem [24]. The most common kinds of skeleton malocclusion are brachygnathism (mandible or maxillary shortening), prognathism (mandible or maxillary lengthening) [14], or wry mouth (different length of each side of the mandible or maxilla) [14,31], which can be separated or organized by means of Angle classification [14].

In cats, head shapes are more uniform. Basically, there are the brachycephalic breeds (eg, Persian) and the dolichocephalic breeds (eg, Oriental) (see Fig. 7) [26,28]. Recently, another kind of classification of domestic feline head shapes was reported. Three different phenotypes were described, including triangular, cuneiform, and round head shapes, based on morphometric evaluation [32].

Teeth and support tissue development

The primitive oral cavity is called the stomodeum. The stomodeum comprises the primary epithelial band with a dental lamina (in which the tooth germs develop) and a vestibular lamina (in which the soft tissues develop) [33].

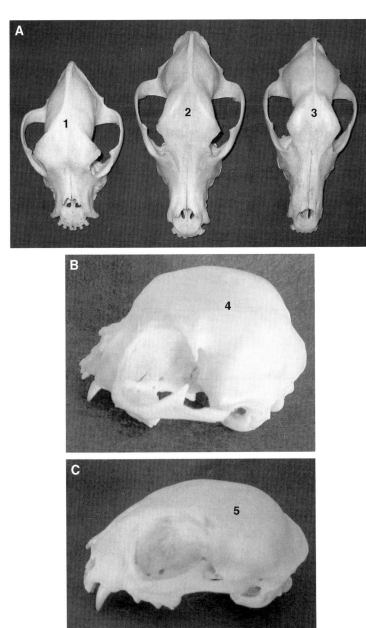

Fig. 7. Brachycephalic (1), mesocephalic (2), and dolichocephalic (3) craniums of the dog and brachycephalic (4) and mesocephalic (5) craniums of the cat.

Development of the tooth germ occurs in three stages: the bud, cap, and bell stages. It begins on approximately day 30 of gestation. The bud stage initiates tooth formation when the dental lamina forms a small bud. Afterward, in the cap stage, three different structures are observed: a dental organ (from which the enamel forms), a dental papilla (from which the dentin-pulp complex forms), and a dental follicle (from which the periodontal tissues form) [33].

Crown formation occurs during the bell stage. The end of crown calcification occurs approximately 20 days postpartum for the deciduous teeth and around the third month postpartum for the permanent teeth [27].

The formation of the roots is directed by Hertwig's epithelial root sheath, which is the epithelial extension comprising the junction at the cervical loop of the inner and outer enamel epithelium. As the roots end their development stage, the root sheath degenerates, leaving small clumps of epithelial cells (epithelial rests of Malassez) within the developing periodontal ligament [27]. With signs of inflammation, these epithelial rests of Malassez can proliferate, forming cysts on the apical region of the root [10].

Dental formulae

There are several kinds of tooth identification systems. In some systems, a specific number is given to each tooth, whereas other systems use symbols and numbers to designate individual teeth [34].

The deciduous dental formula for the dog is 3 incisors (I), 1 canine (C), and 3 premolars (PM) on each mandible and maxilla (total of 28 teeth). The permanent dental formula for the dog is 3 I, 1 C, 4 PM, and 2 molars (M) on the maxilla and 3 I, 1 C, 4 PM, and 3 M on mandible (total of 42 teeth) [10,14].

The deciduous dental formula for the cat is 3 I, 1 C, and 3 PM on the maxilla and 3 I, 1 C, and 2 PM on the mandible (total of 28 teeth). The permanent dental formula for the cat is 3 I, 1 C, 3 PM, and 1 M on the maxilla and 3 I, 1 C, 2 PM, and 1 M on the mandible (total of 32 teeth) [10,14].

The upper fourth premolar and the lower first molar are known as the carnassial teeth. In the maxilla of the dog, the last three upper teeth have three roots, the other premolars have two roots, and the canines and incisors have just one root. In the mandible, the incisors and canines have one root and the other teeth have two roots. In the cat, the only tooth with three roots is the upper fourth premolar. The upper and lower incisors and canines have one root, and the remaining teeth have two roots [12,14,24,28]. A study of 155 skulls of adult domestic cats showed anatomic variation in the teeth of cats, however. For example, the maxillary second premolar tooth can be absent, and this tooth can present a single root (27%), partly fused roots (55%), or two fully formed roots (9.2%). The maxillary first molar tooth can be absent (2.3%); when is present, it can have a single root

(35%), a partly fused root (34.7%), or two roots (28%). Supernumerary roots were found on the maxillary third premolar teeth (10.3%) [35].

The lumen (internal pulp space) of the pulp cavity of permanent teeth rapidly decreases in size until an animal is approximately 2 years of age. A thin or completely obliterated pulp can thus be expected in older pets. In younger animals, especially those less than 1 year of age, the pulp is much larger [24]. Radiographically, the apex of the mandibular first molar in dogs and cats is closed by 7 months of age, and the maxillary canine (the last to close) has a closed apex by 10 months of age in dogs and by 11 months of age in cats [36].

The alveolar process is the portion of bone that is located around the teeth and is composed of the cortical plate, trabecular bone, and cribriform plate. The cribriform plate is know as the lamina dura on radiographs, corresponding to a thin layer of bone in the interior of the alveolus [15], and has many perforations for the passage of vessels to the periodontal ligament [14]. The trabecular bone acts like a support between the cortical plate and the lamina dura. The alveolar crest (margin) is the occlusal portion of the alveolar process located next to the neck of the teeth [15].

The alveolar bone is a tooth-dependent structure. It is formed with the eruption of the teeth and is reabsorbed with extraction of the teeth. There are multiple tunnels in this bone called Volkmann canals, which are connected to the periodontal ligaments. Blood vessels, lymphatics, and nerves pass into these canals [20]. There are spaces between the teeth called interdental spaces, and the bone between the roots of the same tooth is called the interradicular septum [15]. When the interdental space is larger than usual, it is called a diastema, such as between the canine and first premolar. The space between the third incisor and the canine is called the occlusal space [24].

Muscles

The muscles of the head are composed of six groups: facial musculature (innervated by branches of the facial nerve), masticatory musculature (innervated by the mandibular branch of the trigeminal nerve), tongue musculature (supplied by the hypoglossal nerve), pharyngeal musculature (under the control of the glossopharyngeal and vagus nerves), laryngeal musculature (supplied by the vagus nerve), and eye musculature (innervated by the oculomotor, trochlear, and abducent nerves) [1]. The most important muscles manipulated by veterinarians during dental practice are discussed.

On the superficial muscles of the face, there are the muscles of the cheeks and lips and the muscles of the forehead and dorsum of the nose [1]. The muscles of the lips and cheeks are the orbicularis oris (closes the mouth and is a compressor of the labial glands), incisivus (raises the upper lip and pulls the lower lip), levator nasolabialis (increases the diameter of the external

GIOSO & CARVALHO

nose), levator labii superioris (lifts portions of the upper lip), caninus depressor labii superioris, depressor labii inferioris, mentalis, zygomaticus, and buccinator (returns food from the vestibule to the masticatory surface of the teeth) [1,6]. These muscles are situated on the superficial layer of the face and are known as the muscles of mimics. The platysma (draws the commissure of the lips caudally) is a cutaneous muscle located on the superficial muscle of the face (Fig. 8) [6].

The muscles of mastication are the masseter (see Fig. 8) (raises the mandible when closing the mouth), pterygoideus lateralis (raises the mandible), pterygoideus medialis (raises the mandible), and temporalis (same action as the masseter) [1,6]. These groups promote elevation of the mandible and permit the mouth to open, compression, and all mastication movements [6]. All are innervated by rami of the trigeminal nerve [28]. With this masticatory group can be included the superficial muscles of the mandibular space: the digastricus and mylohyoideus. They are referred to as superficial muscles of the larynx, with the function of supporting the masticatory muscles. The digastricus muscle is inserted in the lateral and medial portions of mandible at the ventral margins and promotes the opening of the mouth, moving the mandible in the back and down directions.

The mylohyoideus muscle is an auxiliary muscle of the tongue and mastication situated between the two medial faces of the mandible [6]. The muscles of the tongue are the styloglossus (draws the tongue backward), hyoglossus (retracts and depresses the tongue), genioglossus (depresses the tongue), and lingualis proprius (masticatory and deglutition functions).

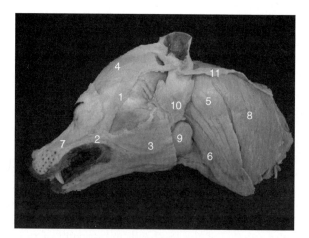

Fig. 8. Lateral view of the muscles of the dog: zygomatic (1), orbicularis oris (2), platysma (3), frontal (4), sternocephalicus pars occipital (5), sternocephalicus pars mastoidea (6), levator nasolabialis (7), cleidocephalicus (8), mandibular gland (9), parotid gland (10), rhomboideus (11), and masseter.

The muscles of the soft palate are the tensor veli palatini (stretches the palate between the pterygoid bones), levator veli palatini (raises the caudal part of the soft palate), and palatinus (shortens the palate and curls the posterior border downward).

Salivary glands

There are several salivary glands working in the oral cavity. The humidity of the mouth, its digestive proprieties, and its lubrication are dependent on the saliva secreted by these glands. There are minor salivary glands on the lips, cheek, tongue, soft palate, larynx, and esophagus. The largest volume of saliva production comes from the major and compact glands, which are not located in the mouth; however, the saliva is conducted to the oral cavity by long ducts [7].

The major salivary glands are the parotid, mandibular (see Fig. 8), sublingual, and zygomatic glands. The sublingual gland is divided into the polystomatic (diffuse) and monostomatic (compact) glands [7,28]. As opposed to the minor glands, the major glands produce a serous liquid with the enzyme ptyalin, which is important in the digestion of carbohydrates [7].

In cats, a membranous bulge is located lingual to the mandibular molar, extending from the middle aspect to the distal aspect of this tooth. The bulge is an irregular sphere approximately 7 mm in diameter containing a small mixed salivary gland. This gland is a tubuloacinar gland with multiple small openings through several short ducts to the surface of the lingual membrane, with a predominance of mucous acini. Studies have not demonstrated a specific function for this gland [37].

Nerves

The most important cranial nerve of the face is the trigeminal nerve (fifth cranial nerve). It is divided into the ophthalmic nerve, maxillary nerve, and mandibular nerve [28].

The maxillary nerve is the largest ramus of the trigeminal nerve. It is responsible for the sensory perception of the cheek, nose, soft and hard palate, upper teeth, and gingiva. In the pterygopalatine fossa, the maxillary nerve is divided into three pterygopalatine nerves: the minor palatine nerve that runs to the soft palate, together with the minor palatine artery; the major palatine nerve that runs to the palatine canal, together with the major palatine artery; and the accessory palatine nerve that runs to the caudal portion of the hard palate. Another maxillary nerve ramus is the nasal nerve, which passes to the nasal cavity by means of the sphenopalatine foramen in the pterygopalatine fossa [1].

The maxillary nerve then enters the infraorbital canal through the maxillary foramen, now called the infraorbital nerve, and has an alveolar connection to the upper teeth. After the infraorbital foramen, this nerve has multiple connections that run to the upper lips [1].

The mandibular nerve has a motor function in the mastication muscles, especially the masseter, temporal, and digastric muscles. It contains the pterygoid nerves (medial and lateral); the buccal nerve that runs to the masseter and temporal muscles; the temporal nerve that runs to the temporal muscle; the masseter nerve that runs to the masseter muscle; the auriculo-temporal nerve that runs to the ear, parotid gland, and temporomandibular joint; the mylohyoid nerve that runs to the digastric muscle and mylohyoid muscle; and the lower alveolar nerve that passes into the mandibular canal in the mandibular foramen with a connection to the lower teeth. This nerve forms the mental nerves, the nerves to the lower lips, and the lingual nerve to the tongue [7,28].

The ophthalmic nerve is the most important sensitive nerve of the orbit, dorsal skin of the nose, and nasal mucous and paranasal sinus, and it has three connections: the frontal, lacrimal, and nasociliary nerves [28].

The facial nerve (seventh cranial nerve) acts on the facial muscles and cranial portion of the digastric muscle, salivary glands of the tongue, sublingual gland, and muscles of the oral cavity [1,7].

Vascular system

The vascular system of the head depends on the external carotid artery, a bifurcation of the common carotid artery [7,11]. The branches that leave the external carotid artery are the occipital, cranial laryngeal (supplies most of the mucosa and intrinsic muscles of the larynx), ascending pharyngeal, lingual (principal artery of the tongue), facial (gives rise to a glandular branch and to muscular branches), caudal auricular, parotid, superficial temporal (constituting blood supply to masseter), and maxillary arteries [1].

The maxillary artery gives off many branches that supply the deep structures of the head lying outside the brain case. It may be divided into three important rami: the mandibular portion, the pterygoid portion, and the pterygopalatine portion [1].

In the mandibular portion, the mandibular branch carries the blood supply to the temporomandibular joint with the mandibular artery [1]. Some care needs to be taken during surgical manipulation of this region to avoid disruption of this artery [10]. The mandibular alveolar artery runs into the mandibular canal, exiting the bone as the mental artery [1]. During a mandibulectomy, much care needs to be taken to preserve the artery during osteotomy of the mandible. The two parts of the incised mandible contain the artery inside, and it needs to be ligated to avoid hemorrhage. If hemorrhage occurs, it can be controlled using bone wax [10]. The caudal mental artery, with its respective nerve and vein, exits the caudal mental foramen and runs to the lower lip. The middle mental artery is the largest of the three mental vessels and provides the principal blood supply to the

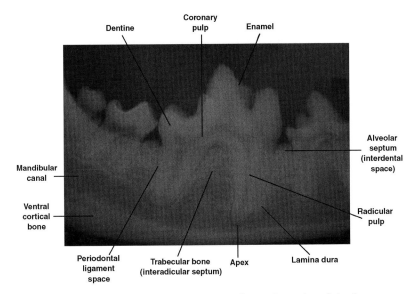

Fig. 9. Intraoral radiograph of the lower first molar region of the dog.

rostral part of the lower jaw. It is the main continuation of the alveolar artery of the mandible. The rostral mental artery is the smallest of the three mental arteries, running to the incisive-mandibular canal [1].

The pterygoid portion has no branches. The pterygopalatine portion has important rami, including the pterygoid (supplies part of the medial pterygoid), buccal (large wings are distributed to masseter, temporal, and buccinator muscles terminating in the region of the soft palate and the

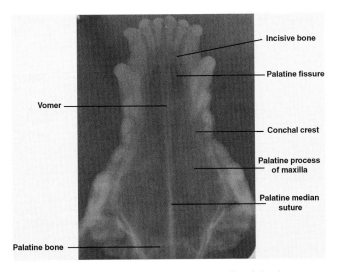

Fig. 10. Intraoral radiograph of the maxilla of the dog.

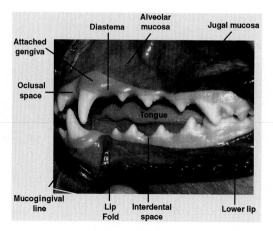

Fig. 11. Lateral view of the soft tissues of the dog.

pterygomandibular fold), minor and major palatine (supply the palatine glands, musculature, and mucosa of the hard palate), and infraorbital and sphenopalatine (supply the mucoperiosteum of the nose) arteries [1,7].

The branches of the sphenopalatine artery provide extensive vascularization of the dorsal and ventral nasal concha, which can cause extensive hemorrhage with trauma. When this happens, especially during nasal surgery, the region needs to be manipulated quickly and the hemorrhage controlled by compression [10].

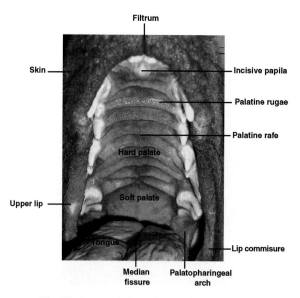

Fig. 12. Intraoral view of the mouth of the dog.

The palatine branches comprise a few small branches that leave the initial part of the ascending pharyngeal artery. They run ventrally in the lateral wall of the pharynx to the soft palate, where they supply the extensive palatine glands and the palatine mucosa and muscles [7].

The infraorbital artery is the continuation of the maxillary artery, exiting from the pterygopalatine fossa, entering the infraorbital canal, and exiting the maxilla by means of the infraorbital foramen [1,7]. This artery needs to be identified during maxillary surgery because it can cause extreme hemorrhage when it is accidentally incised [10]. It terminates by dividing into the lateral and dorsal nasal arteries [1].

Dental and oral anatomy on intraoral radiographs and oral anatomy of soft tissues

Normal radiographic aspects of the oral cavity need to be known by veterinarians who are practicing veterinary dentistry. Veterinarians need to be capable of recognizing normal structures and lesions so as to make a correct diagnosis [5]. Knowledge of the normal anatomy of soft tissues is also important in identifying oral lesions. Some examples of normal structures on radiographs and in soft tissues can be observed in Figs. 9 through 12.

References

[1] Evans HE. The skeleton. In: Miller's anatomy of the dog. 3rd edition. Philadelphia: WB Saunders; 1993. p. 128–68.
[2] Adams DR. La cabeza. In: Anatomía canina, estudio sistémico. Zaragoza: Acribia; 1988. p. 119–29.
[3] D'arce RD, Flechtmann CHW. Introdução à anatomia e fisiologia animal. São Paulo: Nobel; 1980. p. 37–9.
[4] Dubrul EL. Sicher and DuBrul's oral anatomy. 8th edition. Ishiyaku: Euro-America; 1991. p. 1–2.
[5] Madeira MC. Anatomia da face: bases anátomo-funcionais para a prática odontológica. 3rd edition. São Paulo: Sarvier; 2001. p. 3–113.
[6] Liebich H, König HE. Aparelho locomotor. In: Anatomia dos animais domésticos. Texto e atlas colorido. Rio Grande do Sul: Artmed; 2002. p. 1–66.
[7] Dyce KM, Sack WO, Wensing WO. Textbook of veterinary anatomy. 3rd edition. Philadelphia: WB Saunders; 2002. p. 113–20.
[8] Nusshag W. Compendio de anatomia y fisiologia de los animales domésticos. Zaragoza: Acribia; 1967. p. 67–72.
[9] Schaller O. International Committee on Veterinary Gross Anatomical Nomenclature. Nomina anatomica veterinaria. 4th edition. Zurich: Manole Ltda. 1994.
[10] Carvalho VGG. Ossos do sistema estomatognático e da articulação temporomandibular de cães e gatos: enfoque anátomo-cirúrgico [masters thesis]. São Paulo: Faculdade de Medicina Veterinária e Zootecnia of University of São Paulo; 2004. p. 22–74.
[11] Getty R. Sisson and Grossman's the anatomy of domestic animals. 5th edition. Philadelphia: WB Saunders; 1975. p. 1377–411.
[12] Harvey CE, Emily PP. Function, formation, and anatomy of oral structures in carnivores. In: Small animal dentistry. St. Louis: Mosby; 1993. p. 10–3.

[13] Gracis M. Radiographic study of the maxillary canine tooth of four mesaticephalic cats. J Vet Dent 1999;16(3):115–25.

[14] Gioso MA. Odontologia veterinária para o clínico de pequenos animais. 6th edition. São Paulo: I-editora; 2003.

[15] Wiggs RB, Lobprise HB. Oral anatomy and physiology. In: Veterinary dentistry. Principles and practice. Philadelphia: Lippincott-Raven; 1997. p. 77–9.

[16] Prince JH. The comparative anatomy of the eye. J Am Vet Med Assoc 1959;15:349–56.

[17] Chiasson RB. Laboratory anatomy of the cat. 7th edition. Dubuque: WC Brown Company; 1948. p. 6–12.

[18] Schwarze E, Schroder L. Compendio de anatomia veterinaria. Zaragoza: Acribia; 1970. p. 87–133.

[19] Boyd JS, Paterson C. A colour atlas of clinical anatomy of the dog and cat. 2nd edition. London: Wolfe Publishing Ltd; 1991. p. 15–27.

[20] Verstraete FJM. Self-assessment color review of veterinary dentistry. Ames: Iowa State University Press; 1999. p. 80–99.

[21] Bradley OC. Topographical anatomy of the dog. 5th edition. Edinburgh: Oliver and Boyd; 1948. p. 247–8.

[22] Umphlet RC, Johnson AL, Eurell JC, et al. The effect of partial rostral hemimandibulectomy on mandibular mobility and temporomandibular joint morphology in the dog. Vet Surg 1988;17(4):186–93.

[23] Gillbe GV. A comparison of the disc in the craniomandibular joint of three mammals. Acta Anat 1973;86:394–409.

[24] Shipp AD, Fahrenkrug P. Eruption and dentition. In: Practitioners's guide to veterinary dentistry. 1st edition. Glendale (California): Griffin Printing; 1992. p. 8–15.

[25] Autheville P, Barrairon E. Disposition anatomique. In: Odonto-stomatologie vétérinaire. Paris: Maloine SA; 1985. p. 13–6.

[26] Emily P, Penman S. Anatomy. In: Handbook of small animal dentistry. 2nd edition. Oxford: Pergamon Press; 1994. p. 1–4.

[27] Hennet P. Dental anatomy and physiology of small carnivores. In: Crossley DA, Penman S, editors. Manual of small animal dentistry. 2nd edition. Gloucestershire: British Small Animal Veterinary Association; 1995. p. 93–9.

[28] Whyte A, Sopena J, Whyte J, et al. Anatomia estrutural e nomenclatura dental. In: Román FS, editor. Atlas de odontologia de pequenos animais. 1st edition. São Paulo: Manole; 1999. p. 17–21.

[29] Onar V. A morphometric study on the skull of the German shepherd dog (Alsatian). Anat Histol Embryol 1999;28:253–6.

[30] Wykes PM. Brachycephalic airway obstructive syndrome. Probl Vet Med 1991;3(2):188–97.

[31] Weigel JP, Dorn AS. Diseases of the jaws and abnormal occlusion. In: Harvey CE, editor. Veterinary dentistry. Philadelphia: WB Saunders; 1985. p. 106–14.

[32] Kunzel W, Breit S, Oppel M. Morphometric investigations of breed-specific features in feline skulls and considerations on their functional implications. Anat Histol Embryol 2003; 32(4):218–23.

[33] Ten Cate AR. Oral histology: development, structure and function. 5th edition. St. Louis: Mosby-Year Book; 1998. p. 47–66.

[34] Holmstrom SE, Frost P, Gammon RL. Veterinary dental techniques for the small animal practitioner. Philadelphia: WB Saunders; 1992. p. 2–6.

[35] Verstraete FJM, Terpak CH. Anatomical variations in the dentition of the domestic cat. J Vet Dent 1997;14(4):137–40.

[36] Wilson G. Timing of apical closure of the maxillary canine and mandibular first molar teeth of cats. J Vet Dent 1999;16(1):19–21.

[37] Okuda A, Inouc E, Asari M. The membranous bulge lingual to the mandibular molar tooth of a cat contains a small salivary gland. J Vet Dent 1996;13(2):61–4.

ELSEVIER
SAUNDERS

Vet Clin Small Anim
35 (2005) 781–787

VETERINARY
CLINICS
Small Animal Practice

The Gold Standard of Veterinary Oral Health Care

Benjamin Colmery III, DVM

Vet Dentistry PLC, 5300 Plymouth Road, Ann Arbor, MI 48105, USA

Veterinary dentistry has evolved to the point that consumers now demand and expect the best oral health care possible for their pets. Through the efforts of the American Veterinary Dental Society, Academy of Veterinary Dentistry, and American Veterinary Dental College in conjunction with the American Veterinary Medical Association, Hill's Pet Nutrition, and other industry leaders, the public has been made aware of the significance of our pet's oral health problems. The industry has discovered the veterinary dental market, and a plethora of companies provide all sorts of products designed to "freshen breath" and "reduce gum disease." Pets are living longer because of better nutrition and health care. Most veterinarians recognize the need for examining the pet's mouth as well as the rest of the patient's body to determine areas of medical concern. Although the recognition of importance has improved, the delivery of care has not improved. It is time the veterinary health community elevates the care provided to satisfy consumer demand.

The "gold standard" of veterinary oral health care includes the following:

- Thorough physical examination and history
- Preoperative blood profiles, including blood gases
- Inhalation anesthesia with sevoflurane
- Regional and local nerve blocks
- Concurrent intravenous fluid therapy
- Blood pressure, electrocardiography (ECG), pulse oximetry, respiratory monitors, and body temperature monitors
- Intraoral dental radiology
- Air-driven high-speed dental equipment and complete hand instrumentation
- Trained dental operator
- Complete dental charting

E-mail address: Bhc3dvm@aol.com

0195-5616/05/$ - see front matter © 2005 Elsevier Inc. All rights reserved.
doi:10.1016/j.cvsm.2005.02.005   *vetsmall.theclinics.com*

- Home care
- Rechecks

The gold standard of veterinary oral health care encompasses clinical pathologic findings, anesthesiology, radiology, operative dentistry, oral medicine, and home care. The delivery system of oral health care must be as sophisticated as any other operative procedure in a small animal hospital. Dental prophylaxis is the cornerstone of operative dentistry and is technically more sophisticated than an ovariohysterectomy. Unfortunately, too many times, the oral procedure is delegated to an undertrained and ill-equipped veterinary technician whose sole responsibility is to perform as many "dentals" as possible in a day to increase practice revenues. This must stop.

Anesthesia and preoperative workup

Oral procedures require general anesthesia [1]. Hand scaling a patient's mouth while the patient is awake does not constitute professional dental prophylaxis but is instead much like tooth brushing. It does remove some supragingival plaque and calculus but is totally ineffective for subgingival pathologic findings and is limited in the number of teeth treatable. The reason why clients request and some veterinarians provide this inadequate procedure is the fear of anesthesia. This should no longer be an issue.

Pets requiring anesthesia should receive a thorough physical examination and workup. The minimum database for a patient of any age is a complete blood cell count (CBC) and blood gas study (eg, Heska's IStat 8, Heska Corporation, Denver, Colorado). Anesthesia alters physiology, and the best assessment is evaluation of parameters affected by metabolism. Blood pH and bicarbonate levels are the most critical tools for measuring the status of the patient (Fig. 1) [2–4]. Although the classic superchemistry profile provides some insight into the status of the patient, it does not relate to acid-base balance or to the hidden dangers of altering carbon dioxide and oxygen levels. The biggest trap veterinarians fall into is characterized by the patient with compensated metabolic acidosis or alkalosis. By adjusting the type of fluids given during anesthesia, these dangers can be avoided. In addition,

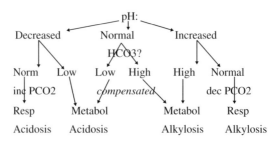

Fig. 1. Blood values.

blood gas analyzers, such as the IStat 8, provide insight into renal function, electrolyte levels, and hemoglobin levels. In addition to the minimum database, such tools as urinalysis, superchemistry profiles, and cardiac ultrasound (in patients with heart murmurs or arrhythmias) add to the confidence level of having a good outcome from the procedure.

All anesthetized patients receive intravenous fluids and are monitored for blood pressure, ECG, pulse oximetry, respirations, and body temperature. In addition, carbon dioxide monitors or other similar devices are used [3]. It makes little sense to reserve this equipment for patients in the operating room and to exclude patients undergoing dental procedures. In general, intravenous fluids are delivered at a minimum rate of 1.5 times maintenance (unless cardiac function is severely compromised). If blood pressure falls below a mean arteriole pressure of 50 mmHg the fluid rate is increased and anesthesia is reduced. Monitoring blood pressure is critical for renal function. Any patient emergency clinic can attest to the problem of acute renal failure in the postoperative dental patient that crashes several days after a procedure.

Preoperative agents include acepromazine for young and restless animals and butorphanol for all animals. Anesthesia induction can be accomplished with mask induction for most patients if sevoflurane is the agent. It is nonirritating to mucous membranes, and even cats rarely object to induction. In fact, cats do well wrapped in a towel with a face mask. If a dog is unruly, propofol works well to take the edge off and enable continuation of mask induction of any sized dog. Drugs like ketamine or xylazine are not used nor needed. The best features of sevoflurane are the rapid induction, rapid recovery, and stable blood pressure through a wide range of vapor settings.

In addition to general anesthesia, regional and local nerve blocks are used to minimize the need for general anesthesia and provide pain-free recovery [5]. These are easily accomplished using 25-gauge, 1.5-inch needles and bupivacaine or lidocaine. The mandibular nerve can be approached intraorally or extraorally. The palatine and infraorbital nerve can be reached dorsal to the distal edge of the hard palate. In addition, local blocks can be used if a single tooth is extracted and significant oral pain is anticipated. Regional and local nerve blocks can be performed by licensed veterinary technicians after induction of general anesthesia and are part of routine protocols.

Radiology

Radiology is critical to veterinary dentistry and oral surgery [6,7]. Veterinary surgeons would not consider operating on a fractured bone or open an abdomen without preoperative radiographs. The same is true for operating in the oral cavity. Failure to take radiographs of an area before extraction, oral biopsy, or another invasive procedure is malpractice. Intraoral dental radiology is essential and critical to practice (ie, the gold standard).

Radiology traditionally involves the use of conventional extraoral plates, placing the patient in lateral recumbency and radiographing the head. Superimposition is the biggest problem, along with minimal detail of the radiographed area. The trained veterinarian may be able to identify the lesion, but the casual observer is likely to miss it. The author affectionately refers to these films as "brain shots."

Dedicated intraoral dental radiography machines are affordable and versatile. They can be mounted on a wall or moved on a wheeled stand. They require simple 120-V current and are virtually indestructible. They are used each day and pay for themselves in a matter of months. Can the same be said of a "laser" surgery unit?

Intraoral dental films are high-detail films that offer great insight into any oral pathologic finding. The problems of superimposition are eliminated, and oral pathologic findings become easily identified with simple magnification. Apical granulomas, bone lysis, oral and nasal neoplastic lesions, dentigerous cysts, and feline resorptive lesions are a few of the lesions defined. Traumatic or pathologic fractures of the maxilla and mandible are correctly managed by determining the preexisting periodontic and endodontic status of the dentition. The nature of the fractures and complicating conditions, such as root and alveolar fractures, that may alter the healing process are identified and treated appropriately. Radiology is critical when endodontic therapy is performed. It is considered malpractice to fail to perform radiology when performing endodontics.

Intraoral radiology has now entered the digital age, making the procedure even easier to perform. Digital radiology is faster than conventional intraoral films and provides better quality images. Software programs allow for manipulation of the image, increasing diagnostic capabilities. In addition, the images are stored "on the hard drive," making retrieval much easier than fumbling through file cabinets. An additional feature is the ability to "e-mail" the image to a specialist for a consultation. In fact, digital systems are now available (eg, the Scan X Pro, All-Pro Imaging, Hicksville, New York) that take size 0 intraoral images up to 10 × 12 images. This eliminates processors, radiographic film, smell, and hassle. These images can be manipulated with software programs (eg, Tigerview, Tigerview Software, Morgan Hill, California) that make interpretation a much easier task. They can also be e-mailed to specialists for consultation.

If any oral cavity therapy is provided, even during the dental examination, failure to provide diagnostic radiography is unacceptable.

Periodontics

Terms

The term *dental* is now considered obsolete. Contemporary terms are as follows:

Conventional dental prophylaxis: to prevent periodontal disease and not alter tissue or structure in animals with minimal if any disease

Periodontal therapy: treatment of periodontal disease with closed curettage and scaling of areas of attachment loss

Surgical periodontal therapy: altering tissue, which includes extractions, open curettage, and surgical repositioning of tissue for the treatment of periodontal disease

Once the correct diagnosis has been made, the next step in the gold standard is to treat the condition correctly [8]. Most veterinary practices employ technicians to perform the dental prophylaxis (the dental). This should be limited to conventional dental prophylaxis. If the technician is properly, trained this is a good system. The technician should remove the gross calculus, radiograph the dentition, perform the nerve blocks if necessary, and step back for the veterinarian to perform periodontal therapy or surgical periodontal therapy as dictated by radiographic and probing findings. Periodontal therapy involves closed supragingival and subgingival cleaning. Probing, defining areas of attachment loss, and open and closed curettage are all part of the treatment. If these steps are not properly performed, the periodontal problems are likely to persist and, in reality, the disease is likely to last longer than if the teeth were ignored and allowed to be naturally exfoliated. If the teeth are to be treated, it needs to be done properly or not at all. If the pet does not require surgical intervention, the technician should finish the prophylaxis and waken the patient.

Critical in this arena is instrumentation. The minimum instrumentation in the gold standard includes the following [9,10]:

- Dedicated area for oral procedures, preferably a dental operatory
- Air-driven equipment with high-speed and low-speed handpieces
- Ultrasonic, piezoelectric, or subsonic scalers (avoid rotary instrument) [11]
- Hand instrumentation, including explorers, curettes, and scalers
- Periosteal elevators and dental elevators
- Surgical-length and standard-length burrs
- Prophy angles
- Dental mirrors
- Protective eyewear, masks, and gloves

Without this minimum equipment, it is impossible to perform thorough dental prophylaxis.

Dental charting is mandatory when performing dental therapy. Charting is a record of preexisting pathologic findings (ie, missing teeth) and therapies performed. Grading and staging diseases is a means to monitor success or failure of treatments. The author uses a grading system ranging from I to VI (Box 1). Regardless of the system used, it is imperative that the records be

---

Box 1. Dental charting: grading and staging diseases

Stage I: gingivitis
Stage II: chronic gingivitis not progressing to attachment loss
Stage III: attachment loss 1–3 mm
Stage IV: attachment loss 3–5 mm to furcation
Stage V: attachment loss 5–7 mm with complete furcation
    exposure, some tooth mobility
Stage VI: attachment loss to apical end, significant tooth
    mobility, apical disease present

---

consistent. Attachment levels, fractured teeth, extractions, and oral masses are all noted on the record. If a copy of the chart is given to the client with an explanation of the notes, the client is made aware of the efforts put forth in caring for the patient. If the client is not given this information, his or her understanding of the pet's problem is distorted and follow-up care is difficult to achieve. The more complete the dental chart is, the better clients are able to understand the care provided by the professional. Finally, intraoral digital photography is an excellent method of recording pathologic findings. Not only can these images be presented to the client, but they can be forwarded to a specialist for consultation if needed. The previous record-keeping entry of "dental, extractions, Rx amoxicillin 250 mg q12h × 7" is no longer acceptable.

Home care is important but must be realistic. Although tooth brushing is ideal, most clients are dismal failures. Products like T/D diet (Hill's Pet Nutrition, Inc., Topeka, Kansas), Science Diet Oral Care (Hill's Pet Nutrition, Inc., Topeka, Kansas), and Friskies Dental Diet (Friskies Corp., St. Louis, Missouri) for cats actually work for plaque, however. Iam's (Iam's Company, Ft. Wayne, Indiana) product with "DDS" (hexamethyl-phosphate) and IVD Dental Diet (IVD, St. Charles, Missouri) also help for calculus control. Together, these products do a pretty decent job of minimizing plaque and calculus reoccurrence. For those clients motivated and patients that tolerate tooth brushing, products with hydrogen peroxide as the active ingredient are helpful. Gly-Oxide (available over the counter) is a good choice because of its ease of application and tolerance by the patients. Products containing hydrogen peroxide as the active ingredient are generally regarded as safe. Products containing chlorhexidine are fine when used short term but should be used cautiously long term unless the patient learns to rinse and spit. Industry has provided a plethora of gadgets and devices that can be tried on an individual basis. The Veterinary Oral Health Council (VOHC) was established to certify efficacy of various dental diets and devices (www.vohc.org). Products with the VOHC seal actually perform as represented by the manufacturer.

The bottom line is that maintaining the oral cavity is the pet owner's responsibility. Any and all programs that encourage client participation are encouraged.

Rechecks

Rechecks are critical and an integral part of the gold standard. Unacceptable recommendations and observations to the client include: "the oral cavity doesn't seem bad today," "it doesn't appear to be causing the pet problems," or "let's watch it." Companion animals benefit from annual dental "prophys." This allows the veterinarian to provide a thorough oral examination on a regular basis. Recognition of endodontic disease, especially oral neoplasia, occurs earlier as a result of rechecks. If the practice is not equipped to handle these problems, referral to the appropriate specialist is suggested. The failure to diagnose and refer is a major reason for client dissatisfaction and loss.

In conclusion, the gold standard is an attainable goal for all veterinary practices that provide oral health care. If the practice chooses to improve its delivery system, the changes should be rewarding. Pets should be healthier, and clients should be happier. Everyone wins.

References

[1] Companion animal dental scaling without anesthesia. American Veterinary Dental College position statement adopted by the AVDC Board of Directors, April 10, 2004. Available at: www.avdc.org.
[2] Nelson RW, Couto CG. Essentials of small animal medicine. St. Louis: Mosby; 1992. p. 205–6.
[3] Birchard SJ, Sherding RG. Saunders manual of small animal practice. 2nd edition. Philadelphia: WB Saunders; 2000. p. 18–20, 78, 591, 918, 922.
[4] Merck veterinary manual. 7th edition. Rahway, NJ: Merck and Company. p. 1361–5.
[5] Lantz G. Regional anesthesia for dentistry and oral surgery. J Vet Dent 20(3):181–6.
[6] Mulligan T, Aller MS, Williams CA. Atlas of canine and feline dental radiography. Trenton, NJ: Veterinary Learning Systems; 1998.
[7] DeForge DH, Colmery BH. An atlas of veterinary dental radiology. Ames, IA: Iowa State University Press; 2000.
[8] Wiggs RB, Lobrise HB. Veterinary dentistry principles and practice. Philadelphia: Lippincott-Raven; 1997. p. 186–231.
[9] Holmstrom SE, Frost-Fitch P, Eisner ER. Veterinary dental techniques for the small animal practitioner. 3rd edition. Philadelphia: WB Saunders; 2004.
[10] Bellows J. Small animal dental equipment, materials and techniques. 1st edition. Ames, IA: Blackwell Publishing Professional; 2004.
[11] Brine EJ, Marretta SM, Pijanowski GJ, et al. Comparison of the effects of four different power scalers on enamel tooth surface in the dog. J Vet Dent 2000;17(1):17–21.

ELSEVIER
SAUNDERS

Vet Clin Small Anim
35 (2005) 789–817

VETERINARY
CLINICS
Small Animal Practice

Juvenile Veterinary Dentistry

Fraser A. Hale, DVM

Hale Veterinary Clinic, 159 Fife Road, Guelph, Ontario, Canada N1H 7N8

Certainly, the incidence and severity of periodontal disease and other oral problems increase with age, but young patients may also suffer from a number of dental and oral maladies. Often, early recognition and treatment of these problems can prevent more serious complications in later life. This article covers some of the more common dental concerns in dogs and cats during their first year of life. It is the intent of this article to teach the reader to recognize these conditions and their significance to the patient and to understand that treatment is indicated and available.

Normal primary dental formulas, dental morphology, and eruption times

The normal dental formulas for the primary teeth in dogs and cats are discussed in the article in this issue on anatomy. If the primary tooth fails to develop, the permanent tooth is also going to be absent. If the permanent bud fails to develop, the permanent tooth is going to be absent regardless of the normal development of the permanent tooth. For teeth with no primary precursor, the permanent bud forms at the same time as the primary buds but lies dormant until the time of permanent tooth eruption [1]. The eruption times for the primary and permanent teeth are listed in Table 1 [1,2].

The primary incisor and canine teeth are replaced by permanent (secondary) successors. These primary teeth are diminutive in form compared with their secondary successors but have the same basic morphology. There is no primary precursor for the first premolar tooth in the dog or for any of the molar teeth in the dog or cat. The primary fourth premolar tooth in each quadrant of the mouth of the dog and cat is anatomically and functionally similar to the first molar in each quadrant. Despite their appearance and function, the primary fourth premolars are named for the secondary tooth that they replace (Fig. 1).

E-mail address: toothvet@toothvet.ca

Table 1
Approximate eruption times (variations occur with breed and size of patient)

	Primary (weeks)		Permanent (months)	
	Puppy	Kitten	Dog	Cat
Incisors	3–4	2–3	3–4	3–4
Canines	3	3–4	4–6	4–5
Premolars	4–12	3–6	4–6	4–6
Molars			5–7	4–5

Juvenile dental problems recognized in the first weeks of life

Microglossia (bird tongue)

Microglossia is a lethal hereditary (autosomal recessive) abnormality that results in, among other things, an abnormally small tongue [3–5]. The puppies are usually presented for evaluation of difficulty in nursing because they are unable to latch on to the nipple properly. As well, these puppies seem mentally dull and disinterested in nursing and lack the swallowing reflex. It had been suggested that puppies dying of fading puppy syndrome are, in fact, afflicted with microglossia and fade because of an inability to nurse, with resultant malnutrition, dehydration, and aspiration pneumonia [3].

A litter of five affected Miniature Schnauzers was kept alive until 7 weeks of age through intensive nursing and medical care. Postmortem findings indicated that the condition is a complex multisystem birth defect with abnormalities noted in the tongue, pharynx, musculoskeletal system, and brain. The characteristic abnormality for which the condition is named was described as follows:

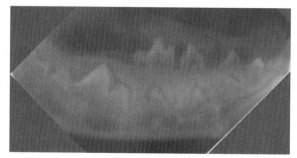

© Fraser A. Hale

Fig. 1. Radiograph of the right mandible of an 8-week-old pup shows the three primary premolars erupted and the developing permanent premolars and molars within the structure of the mandible.

"...the affected animals' tongues had grossly normal deep base muscular layers, but the lateral and rostral thin portions were missing or underdeveloped. Light fimbriation was present on the lateral surfaces. Their tongues initially moved only in a dorso-ventral direction action [sic], with the tongue commonly placed against the roof of the mouth."

The experience with this litter suggests that the prognosis is hopeless, even with heroic efforts; thus, immediate euthanasia seems to be the only reasonable recommendation [3,4]. Because this is a hereditary condition, the parents should be removed from the breeding pool [3].

Cleft palates

Clefts may be in the primary palate (rostral to the incisive foramen and including the lips) or the secondary palate (hard palate caudal to the incisive foramen and the soft palate) [5,6].

Defects of the primary palate (harelip) usually cause no problems with nursing or respiration and are largely of cosmetic significance only. In most cases, surgical treatment can be delayed until the patient is mature; at that time, the structures are larger and easier to work with and the anesthetic risks are lower. Primary palatal clefts may be unilateral or bilateral; when unilateral, they are almost always on the left side in dogs [6,7]. Standard surgical texts contain outlines of various surgical techniques for closing these defects.

Clefts of the secondary palate (hard palate caudal to the incisive foramen and the soft palate) pose a more immediate concern. Congenital hard palate clefts are almost always midline and usually associated with midline clefts in the soft palate. These clefts result in a direct communication between the oral and nasal cavities. During nursing, milk flows into the nasal passages, leading to sneezing, gagging, coughing, and nasal discharge. Affected animals are at great risk of developing aspiration pneumonia. Other signs include poor growth and weight gain and a general unthriftiness. The prognosis is guarded without surgical correction of the cleft to re-establish a functional separation between oral and nasal cavities. With successful closure of the defects, the prognosis is excellent [6–9].

The great challenge is keeping the patient healthy until anesthesia and surgery are acceptable risks. If the patient can be supported until 6 to 8 weeks of age, there is more tissue to work with and the anesthetic risk is more manageable than in a newborn. Delaying surgery longer is contra-indicated, because the defect often gets proportionally larger as the patient grows. Standard surgical and dental texts outline a variety of procedures for closure of midline hard and soft palate defects [6–10].

Clefts of the soft palate may be midline, unilateral, or bilateral with a thin strip of palatal tissue down the midline. If sufficient tissue exists, some of these clefts are amenable to surgical repair. Congenital bilateral absence of the soft palate has also been reported. In this case, the pharyngeal sphincter is incomplete; thus, the patient cannot swallow. It is not possible to create a soft palate with the necessary neuromuscular anatomy for a functional sphincter surgically; thus, the prognosis is hopeless [6].

The reader should be aware that repair of palatal defects can be frustrating. Complete healing does not often happen after the first operation. The constant motion of the tongue, changes in air pressure during respiration, and difficulty in obtaining a tension-free closure with connective tissue support under the suture line all conspire to cause dehiscence. Plan at the outset on more than one operation to effect complete closure of the defect.

Conversely, the reader should also be aware that the first operation has the best chance of success. If the first operation fails, subsequent procedures are compromised by the disruption of the vasculature, loss of tissue, and scarring from the first operation. Therefore, the first operation is planned as if it is the only chance at treating the condition, and everything possible is done to enhance its chances of success. Surviving patients affected by any form of cleft palate should not be allowed to breed because of the possibility of genetic involvement [5].

First visits: 8-week and 12-week checkups

Malocclusion

When a puppy or kitten is presented for a check-up at 8 weeks of age, it should undergo a thorough oral examination. By this age, the primary teeth should be well erupted and in place. The upper incisors of the puppy should just slightly overlap the lower incisors, and the lower canine tooth should be placed between the upper lateral incisor and the upper canine tooth. In kittens, the lower canine should be positioned as in the puppy, but the incisors may meet in a tip-to-tip fashion in a level bite.

Because the growth of the mandible and maxilla is under separate genetic control, the growth of one only influences the growth of the other in so far as they are "locked" together by the interdigitation of the teeth [11]. If the teeth are properly positioned, as the maxilla grows, its upper canine can push on the back of the lower canine and "drag" the mandible along. As the mandible grows forward, its incisors hit the back of the maxillary incisors and "push" the maxilla ahead. In this way, the proper mandible-maxilla relation should be maintained throughout the growth period and into adulthood [12,13].

An excellent review article by Hennet and Harvey [11] on craniofacial development of the dog details the complex interactions between genetics and function, soft tissues, and hard tissues in the development and growth of the maxilla and mandible. Among the salient points was the finding that up to day 50, the increase in the length of the mandible occurs as a result of growth in the rostral portion. After day 50, almost all the increase in mandibular length is a result of growth in the region of the ramus. A study in Labrador Retriever pups found that there was no change in the distance between the tips of the central incisors and the central cusp of the mandibular first molar between 3 and 6 months of age, indicating that all growth was caudal to the first molar during this period [11].

If the young puppy or kitten has a significant jaw length discrepancy such that there is an abnormal dental interlock (eg, lower canines digging holes in the hard palate or upper incisors trapped behind lower incisors), the potential for the short jaw to catch up is mechanically impeded.

In the example of an 8-week-old puppy with a short mandible (class II malocclusion), the lower canines often dig into the hard palate and the incisors are trapped behind the incisive papilla of the hard palate (Fig. 2) [13]. If the lower jaw attempts to go through a growth spurt to catch up to the maxilla, the interlock holds it back. The result can be that the mandible remains abnormally short or it may bend in the middle and bow ventrally.

A puppy or kitten with an obvious malocclusion is a candidate for interceptive orthodontics [12,13]. Interceptive orthodontics involves the selective extraction of any primary teeth that would impede the development of a proper bite. The general rule is to extract the teeth from the short jaw. Each case must be planned on its own merits, however. Extract those teeth that would impede desired growth, but retain those that would encourage desired growth or impede abnormal growth. For a class II malocclusion, extraction of the primary mandibular canines and incisors should alleviate the dental interlock. These procedures do not alter the patient's genetic makeup, nor do they make anything happen. Rather, they allow the patient to express its full genetic potential by removing any mechanical impediment

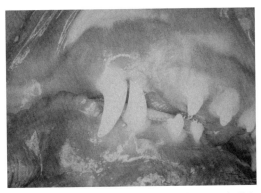

© Fraser A. Hale

Fig. 2. An 8-week old puppy with a class II malocclusion. The mandibular primary canine tooth is traumatizing the maxillary gingiva and causing pain. The abnormal dental interlock with the mandibular canine trapped in the palatal soft tissues and the mandibular incisors trapped distal to the incisive papilla imposes a mechanical impediment to the growth of the mandible.

to growth. Clients and breeders should be cautioned that even if the patient turns out normal, it required intervention and thus should be bred carefully if at all. A safer recommendation would be to neuter these animals at an appropriate age.

To maximize the benefit of interceptive orthodontics, it should be performed at the youngest age possible. The hope is that the jaw length relation normalizes before the permanent teeth erupt and recreate dental interlock. The more time between primary tooth extraction and permanent tooth eruption, the better are the chances of success. The owners should be made aware that most animals with jaw length discrepancies at 8 weeks of age do not "go normal" regardless of treatment and there are likely to be orthodontic problems when the permanent teeth erupt.

A second benefit of interceptive orthodontics is that it immediately relieves the oral trauma and pain associated with abnormal tooth-to-tooth or tooth-to–soft tissue contacts. On its own, this is sufficient cause to recommend surgery. The owners are often unaware of the pain their pet is experiencing because they have never known the patient without the problem. Once the traumatic occlusion is eliminated, clients typically report a noticeable improvement in their pet's quality of life.

Another common malocclusion is base-narrow or lingually displaced mandibular canine teeth. In these cases, the jaw length relations are normal but the mandibular primary canine tooth crowns are parallel to each other. Because the maxilla is wider than the mandible, if the mandibular canines are not tipped laterally (buccally), they contact and traumatize the maxillary gingiva or palatal mucosa. This causes pain and can lead to penetration or perforation into the nasal passage (Fig. 3). It also creates an abnormal dental interlock that can impede the lateral growth of the mandible. Finally,

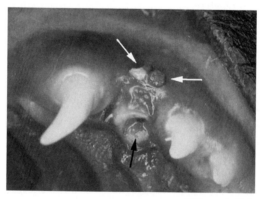

© Fraser A. Hale

Fig. 3. Although the jaw length relation was normal in this pup, the mandibular primary canine teeth were base-narrow and thus were traumatizing the palatal mucosa. The dark arrow indicates the deep traumatic pit caused by the malocclusion. The white arrows are pointing at some of the foreign matter removed from the palatal pit.

the permanent mandibular canine teeth erupt on the lingual side of the corresponding primary tooth (Fig. 4). Therefore, if the primary tooth is lingually displaced, there is a strong likelihood that the permanent canine tooth is also going to be lingually displaced.

The recommended treatment for lingually displaced primary mandibular canines is extraction of the primary mandibular canine teeth. Benefits of this operation include immediate relief of the traumatic occlusion and removal of the abnormal dental interlock, allowing unimpeded lateral mandibular growth. It also clears a pathway by which the permanent tooth can erupt in a more labial direction, tipped away from contact with the maxilla.

Fractured primary teeth

Primary canine teeth are long, thin, and are found in the mouths of puppies. These three factors make them subject to wear and fractures that expose the pulp of the tooth. The pulp is the soft tissue that is found inside a tooth and consists of blood vessels, nerves, lymphatics, and connective

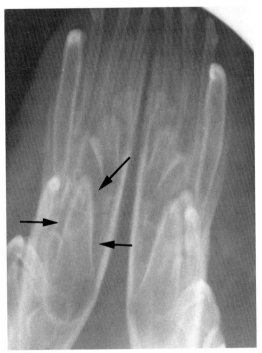

© Fraser A. Hale

Fig. 4. Radiograph of the rostral mandible of an 8-week-old pup. The length of the primary tooth roots is evident as is how thin the walls of these teeth are. The developing permanent canine tooth on the left side of the radiograph is indicated by the black arrows. Note its close proximity to the root of the primary canine tooth.

tissue. Once exposed to oral bacteria, the pulp quickly becomes infected and dies. During this time, there is significant pain, but once the pulp is dead, the pain subsides. Next, infection extends out through the root tip into the periodontal space around the root. This can cause a draining fistula, osteomyelitis, and damage to the developing permanent teeth (Fig. 5). The treatment for all primary teeth with exposed pulp is immediate and careful extraction of the entire crown and root. If the fracture is fresh (less than 24 hours), vital pulpotomy and direct pulp capping is also an option [1].

It is beyond the scope of this article to outline the procedure for primary tooth extraction in detail, but some general comments are appropriate:

- Always take a preoperative intraoral dental radiograph to document the presence and location of developing permanent teeth.
- Elevate carefully and avoid the area of the developing permanent tooth to prevent damage to it. Permanent teeth can be seriously damaged by careless extraction of primary teeth (Fig. 6).
- Use appropriately sized (small and delicate) elevators and forceps.

Delayed eruption of primary teeth

By 8 weeks of age, most of the primary teeth should all have erupted, and by 12 weeks, all should be evident in the mouth [1,2]. Occasionally, the primary teeth fail to erupt. In most cases, they are impacted below dense fibrous gingival tissue (Fig. 7). Small-breed dogs seem particularly prone to this condition. If the primary teeth fail to erupt, there may be insufficient room within the mandible and maxilla for normal development of the

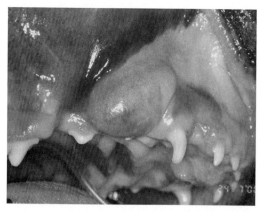

© Fraser A. Hale

Fig. 5. The right primary maxillary canine tooth has a small crown fracture that exposed the pulp to oral bacteria. The oral swelling is a result of infection passing through the canine tooth root, through the apex of the root, and into the maxillary bone. Osteomyelitis, bone fenestration, and cellulitis followed.

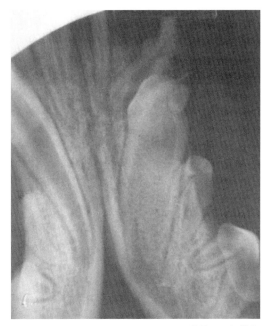

© Fraser A. Hale

Fig. 6. Radiograph of the rostral mandible of a 6-month-old dog shows seriously deformed incisors and canines on the right side of the film secondary to inelegant extraction of primary canine and incisor teeth.

permanent teeth. Also, impaction of the primary teeth may lead to impaction of the permanent teeth [14].

Treatment is preceded by dental radiographs (as are virtually all dental treatments) to document the shape, size, and location of the primary and

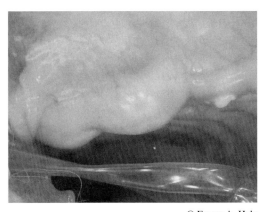

© Fraser A. Hale

Fig. 7. Soft tissue impaction of the primary third and fourth premolars in the right maxilla of a pup.

permanent dentition. Windows of gingiva are then resected (operculectomy) from around the crowns of the impacted primary teeth to reduce the resistance to eruption (Fig. 8). If this is done between 8 and 12 weeks of age, the primary teeth usually erupt and lead the way for the eruption of their permanent counterparts.

Bear in mind that the molars and first premolars have no primary precursors. Therefore, patients that have had soft tissue impaction of primary teeth should be monitored carefully because they may also suffer from soft tissue impaction of the permanent molars.

Third visit: 4-month checkup

Persistent primary teeth

By the time a pet is presented for rabies vaccine around 4 months of age, some of the permanent incisors should be erupting. The permanent canines and some of the premolars may also be erupting by this time. It is at this stage that you should start looking for persistent primary teeth. This is a problem commonly associated with small-breed dogs, but it can happen in cats and large-breed dogs as well. The rule is that if the permanent tooth crown is visible above the gum line, the primary tooth should be gone. If the primary tooth is still in place, it should be removed as soon as possible. Leaving a persistent primary tooth in place until 6 months (spaying or neutering time) is inappropriate because it forces the permanent tooth to erupt into an abnormal location. The interactions are complex; however, if the primary tooth is in place while the permanent tooth is erupting, you have two teeth occupying the space meant for one and this causes problems (Fig. 9).

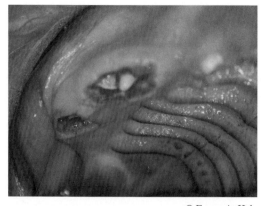

© Fraser A. Hale

Fig. 8. Postoperative view of the pup from Fig. 7. Operculectomies have been performed to remove the tough fibrous tissue that was impeding eruption of these primary teeth.

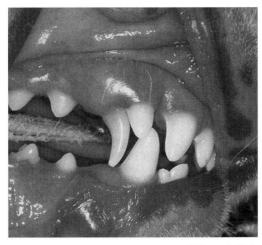

© Fraser A. Hale

Fig. 9. A persistent primary right maxillary canine tooth has resulted in mesial (forward) displacement of the erupting permanent canine tooth. The displacement of the maxillary permanent tooth is interfering with the eruption and occlusion of the mandibular permanent canine tooth.

When extracting persistent primary teeth, the operator must be careful to avoid causing damage to the root of the adjacent permanent tooth. In Fig. 10, it is clear that the solid wall of the permanent canine tooth is extremely thin and the pulp chamber is quite large. Using the permanent tooth as a fulcrum to elevate the primary tooth could result in a longitudinal crack in the permanent tooth extending directly into the pulp chamber, with disastrous results.

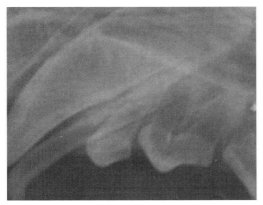

© Fraser A. Hale

Fig. 10. Radiograph of the left rostral maxilla of a 5-month-old pup shows an intact primary canine tooth root (no root resorption evident) and the thin-walled developing permanent canine tooth directly adjacent.

The mechanisms by which primary tooth roots resorb, allowing exfoliation, and permanent teeth erupt remain unclear [15]. There are complex interactions, and many things must go right for the primary teeth to vacate the mouth and the permanent teeth to erupt properly. Exactly which factors trigger the cascade of events is unknown; thus, the cause of abnormal exfoliation and eruption remains a matter of speculation. The general opinion is that when things go wrong, it is likely because of some genetic fault and the affected individuals should be removed from the gene pool.

Typically, the patient has been presented monthly for checkups and immunization. After this visit, it is often 2 months before the patient is presented for spaying or neutering. A lot happens in the mouth during those 2 months. It would be prudent to spend some time with clients to explain what should happen and what problems they should be watching for. It would also be worth making a 5-month checkup part of your puppy or kitten protocol so that developmental abnormalities (eg, persistent primary teeth, malocclusions of erupting permanent teeth) can be diagnosed early and dealt with in a timely fashion.

Six-month spaying or neutering visit

A patient presented for spaying or neutering at approximately 6 months of age represents a golden opportunity. The patient is going to be under general anesthesia, and you can do an unhurried thorough oral examination. In most breeds, all secondary teeth should be partially or fully erupted by this age. During your examination, you should note any missing or extra teeth, deformed or malpositioned teeth, or any other situations that might predispose to problems.

Dentigerous cysts

"Missing" teeth should always be documented with an intraoral radiograph. If the radiograph shows that the tooth is missing, it can be recorded as such on the patient's permanent dental record for future reference. Although this may be of no functional significance to the patient (depending on which tooth is missing), some breed standards have specific requirements for the number of teeth; thus, the breeder should be informed of this developmental abnormality.

Failure to detect and extract an unerupted tooth often leads to the development of a dentigerous cyst [16,17]. These cysts, although benign, are destructive of bone as they expand, which can lead to loss of adjacent teeth (Figs. 11 and 12). They have also been reported to undergo malignant transformation [18,19]. Treatment involves not only removal of the unerupted tooth but removal of the secretory lining of the cyst before closure of the incision [20]. In cases of large cysts that have created

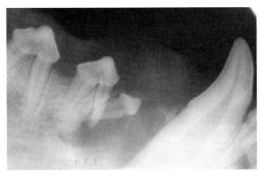

© Fraser A. Hale

Fig. 11. Radiograph of the right rostral mandible of a 3-year-old Golden Retriever with a dentigerous cyst formed around an unerupted first premolar tooth. Note the degree of bone loss affecting the periodontal support for the adjacent canine tooth and second premolar.

significant defects in the bone, removal of adjacent teeth that have lost their bone support and placement of bone grafting material before closure are indicated (see Fig. 12). Potentially large and destructive cysts are completely preventable by the timely identification and removal of unerupted teeth.

Soft tissue impaction

As is the case with the primary teeth, the permanent teeth may become impacted below a layer of dense fibrous gingival tissue. Typically, if there has been a primary tooth to lead the way, the permanent tooth does not have trouble breaking through the gingiva. There are no primary first premolars or molars, however; thus, these are the permanent teeth most likely to have soft tissue impaction. After intraoral radiography, treatment

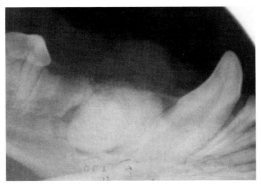

© Fraser A. Hale

Fig. 12. Postoperative radiograph of the dog in Fig. 11. The unerupted first premolar and the second premolar have been removed, the cyst lining has been curetted away, and a synthetic bone grafting material has been placed in the defect before closure of the wound.

involves an operculectomy to remove enough gingiva over the crown of the tooth to alleviate the physical barrier to eruption while leaving enough gingiva for proper periodontal health (Figs. 13 and 14).

Supernumerary teeth

Extra teeth also call for an intraoral radiograph to determine if there are two completely separate teeth or two crowns sharing a common root and pulp system. If you find that there are two completely separate teeth and the extra tooth is causing a crowding situation, the supernumerary tooth should be extracted in the near future. Failure to recognize the situation and to alleviate the crowding can lead to early onset of periodontal disease with loss of more than just the extra tooth (Fig. 15).

As well as crowding, supernumerary teeth may lead to malocclusions with abnormal tooth-to-tooth or tooth-to–soft tissue contacts (Fig. 16). Again, early intervention to remove the offending tooth is indicated to alleviate trauma, prevent permanent damage to other oral structures, and improve the quality of life of the patient. Although incisors and first premolars are the most common teeth to have supernumerary copies, the condition can be found with any tooth.

Dental crowding

Many brachycephalic and small-breed dogs have severe crowding and rotation of teeth. It has been shown that the smaller the dog, the larger the teeth are in proportion to the mouth [11,21]. Also, the shortened maxilla of the brachycephalic breeds does not lend itself to the proper alignment of the full compliment of teeth.

Crowding and rotation can lead to food impaction between teeth and early onset of periodontal disease. The suggested treatment is selective

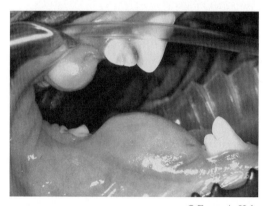

© Fraser A. Hale

Fig. 13. Soft tissue impaction of the permanent first maxillary and mandibular molars.

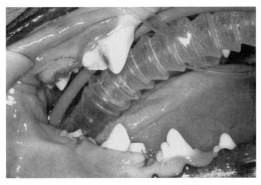

© Fraser A. Hale

Fig. 14. Postoperative view of the dog in Fig. 13 after operculectomies to remove the tough fibrous tissue interfering with the molar eruption.

extraction of less significant teeth to relieve the crowding and improve the periodontal prognosis for the remaining teeth. If there are three teeth crowded together, removal of the middle one may improve the outlook for the other two. Failure to extract crowded teeth can lead to tooth loss within a few years (Fig. 17).

Anteriorly, there may be crowding of the mandibular incisors and canines, putting the important canine teeth at risk. This risk can be reduced by selective extraction of the lateral incisors. Posteriorly, the distal shoulder

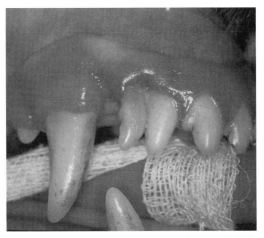

© Fraser A. Hale

Fig. 15. A supernumerary right maxillary lateral incisor was causing crowding in a 5-year-old dog. At this stage, the periodontal disease was such that the normal and supernumerary lateral incisors had to be extracted. Early removal of the supernumerary tooth (at 6 to 12 months of age) would have prevented the loss of the normal lateral incisor.

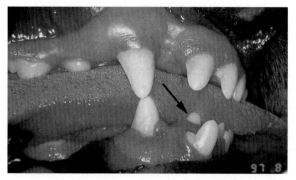

Fig. 16. A supernumerary right mandibular lateral incisor's (black arrow) root was interposed between the normal lateral incisor and the canine tooth. This extra tooth was displacing the permanent canine tooth distally, leading to malocclusion. Timely removal of the supernumerary tooth (at 6 months of age) allowed for resolution of the malocclusion with no further intervention.

of the maxillary third premolar may be impacted in the furcation between the mesiobuccal and mesiopalatal roots of the fourth premolar. Again, selective extraction of the partially impacted (and less important) third premolar can markedly improve the prognosis for the fourth premolar.

Malocclusions

Most orthodontic problems lead to abnormal tooth-to-tooth or tooth-to–soft tissue contacts. The resulting trauma can cause a variety of problems, including periodontal disease, root resorption, oronasal fistulas, and

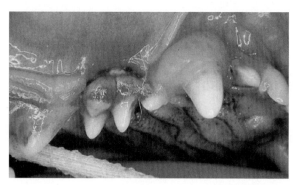

Fig. 17. Severe dental crowding in a brachycephalic dog has led to advanced periodontal disease affecting all permanent premolars in the right maxilla. Selective extraction of some premolars at an early age would have improved the prognosis for the remaining teeth. At this stage, all four premolars must be extracted.

endodontic (pulp) disease [22]. The treatment varies depending on the specifics of the condition but may involve selective extraction, crown reduction (with partial vital pulpotomy and direct pulp capping), or orthodontic movement of teeth to alleviate the abnormal contact [12,13, 23–26].

In all cases of malocclusion, there are ethical considerations to bear in mind [27]. Although it is difficult to produce absolute proof that a particular malocclusion in a particular patient is of genetic origin and heritable, the greatest likelihood is that most malocclusions are of genetic origin. Unless there is a specific history of some significant trauma (maxillofacial or mandibular fracture), it is best to assume that the condition is genetic [11]. Therefore, any plans to place the animal in the conformation show ring must be abandoned, and the patient must be permanently removed from the gene pool.

The practitioner should be careful about participating in someone else's fraudulent behavior. Patients that are genotypically abnormal should not be made to look phenotypically normal if there is any chance that the animal may then be used for showing or breeding. If there is a medically significant malocclusion, other options to allow the patient to have a comfortable and functional bite without masking its genetic faults are available.

One of the most common orthodontic problems is class II malocclusion as discussed earlier in this article. If the lower jaw remains short relative to the upper jaw into maturity, the permanent mandibular canine teeth are frequently trapped on the palatal side of the maxillary canine teeth and contact and traumatize the palatal mucosa. The trauma can result in oronasal fistulation, periodontal damage to the maxillary canine tooth, traumatic pulpitis in the mandibular canine tooth, and other problems.

One option for malocclusion is extraction of the mandibular canine teeth. In these cases, however, the lower jaw is already too short and removing the canines tends to cause further regression of the chin.

Another option might be to extract the upper canine teeth, remove the buccal cortical bone, and suture the defect so that the lower canines can slip into the groove where the upper canines used to be. The risk with this is that the lower canines contact the healing extraction site and may traumatize the flaps, leading to dehiscence.

Crown reduction

A less painful and less disfiguring option is crown height reduction, partial vital pulpotomy, direct pulp capping, and bonded composite restoration of the mandibular canine teeth. This is discussed in the article in this issue on endodontics.

Incline planes

In some cases of class II malocclusion and in cases of lingually displaced canines in dogs with normal jaw length relations, orthodontic movement of the mandibular canines might be considered. This treatment has the advantage of being the least invasive and giving a final result that is closest to normal.

There are several conditions that must be met before we can consider orthodontic procedures. There must be a vacant space to which the misplaced tooth can be moved. There must be a clear path for the tooth to take on its way to its new home. We must have a cooperative patient that allows daily examinations and cleaning of the appliance. We must have a compliant and motivated client who can be trusted to check and clean the appliance daily, keep regular recheck appointments, and keep the patient from chewing things that might damage the appliance. The client must understand that it takes one anesthetic procedure to install the appliance, one to remove the appliance, and possibly others for adjustments and repairs and that there can be no guarantees. Finally, it must be firmly established that the patient is not going to be used for showing or breeding, and the animal should be neutered before the start of orthodontic treatment. To orthodontically alter a show or breeding animal should be considered fraud. If all these conditions cannot be met, do not even consider orthodontic repositioning as an option.

An effective way to move mandibular canine teeth labially or forward and labially simultaneously is with the application of acrylic incline planes anchored to the maxillary canines and incisors. These passive force appliances act as wedges to direct the mandibular canine teeth to the desired location when the patient applies pressure by closing its mouth (Figs. 18–20) [23,25].

With the recent advent of early spaying and neutering protocols, more and more patients are being spayed or neutered before 6 months of age. For

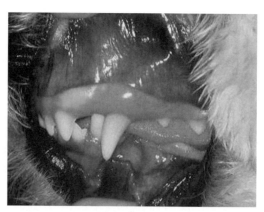

© Fraser A. Hale

Fig. 18. Preoperative view of a 6-month-old standard poodle. The mandibular canine tooth is displaced distolingually and is in traumatic occlusion with the palate. The situation was bilateral, although worse on the left side.

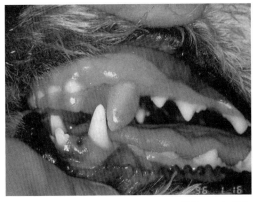

Fig. 19. The left lateral mandibular incisor has been sacrificed, and acrylic incline planes have been installed to act as wedges to direct the mandibular canine teeth to a desirable location.

these patients and for those that are not being neutered, plan on doing a thorough oral examination at 6 months of age with the patient awake. If there are any abnormalities or concerns, anesthetize the patient for a more detailed visual inspection and appropriate radiographs.

Class III malocclusion

In a class III malocclusion, the maxilla is short relative to the mandibles. In many breeds (eg, Boxer, Shih Tzu), this is actually a breed standard. Despite being selected for in some breeds, it is a significant skeletal deformity that frequently causes problems for the patient. Most obviously, there are often abnormal tooth-to-tooth contacts between the maxillary lateral incisors and the mandibular canines and abnormal tooth-to–soft

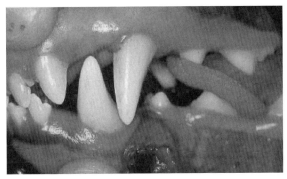

Fig. 20. One month after removal of the acrylic incline planes, the occlusion is comfortable and functional.

tissue contacts between the maxillary central and intermediate incisors and the floor of the mouth lingual to the mandibular incisors (Fig. 21). These contacts can cause pain, periodontal disease, and endodontic disease and can interfere with the eruption of teeth.

As is the case with all orthodontic cases, the treatment plan should be based on many factors, but options include selective extractions, crown height reductions (with treatments to protect the pulp), and orthodontic movement of teeth. Regardless of the treatment option selected, the goal should always be to allow the patient to close its mouth completely with no abnormal or traumatic contacts.

Deformed teeth

The various deformities possible in the permanent teeth of dogs and cats could easily fill this entire issue. This section mentions only a few of the deformities that the practitioner should be watching for.

The crown of each tooth should be carefully examined to ensure that there is a complete covering of enamel and that there are no apparent invaginations or abnormal fissures in the crown. Dens-in-dente is a condition in which the tooth has folded in on itself such that the endodontic chamber contains a "tooth within a tooth" [28]. Frequently, there is a communication from the surface of the tooth directly into the endodontic system, allowing bacteria to enter the tooth as soon as it erupts. Treatment usually involves extraction, although in some cases, the tooth might be salvaged with advanced endodontic and restorative procedures.

In small dogs of various breeds, it is possible to see a deformity on the mandibular molars characterized by a convergence of the roots. Typically,

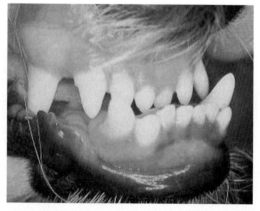

© Fraser A. Hale

Fig. 21. A class III malocclusion in which the maxillary central and intermediate incisors have caused trauma to the soft tissues on the lingual side of the lower incisors. Treatment is indicated to alleviate this traumatic occlusion.

a radiograph of the mandibular first molar reveals roots that diverge from the crown. In this condition (an example of dilaceration or bending of the tooth structure), the roots are parallel or actually converge toward the apices. Concomitant with this, there is often a groove evident in the enamel on the buccal side of the tooth leading into the furcation. The most significant deformity in this syndrome is an accessory canal into the endodontic chamber that communicates with the periodontal space in the furcation (where the roots separate from the crown of the tooth). Initially, this accessory canal is isolated from oral bacteria by the gingival attachment. The groove in the enamel of the crown traps plaque and conducts it into the furcation area below the gum line, however. Early on-set of periodontal disease in this location can allow bacteria direct access to the accessory canal and thence into the pulp chamber. Pulp necrosis and periapical infection follow. Affected teeth might have a reasonable prognosis if the deformity is found early in life and aggressive plaque control measures are put in place to prevent periodontal disease. In the author's experience, the problem is usually found after the damage has been done and extraction is the only option (Figs. 22–24).

Odontomas

Considered by some to be a benign tumor and by others to be a hamartoma (normal tissues in an abnormal location), odontomas are space-occupying masses composed of dental tissues [29–32].

Compound odontomas are characterized by the presence of a few to several dozen denticles. Each denticle has all the dental tissues (pulp, dentin, cementum, and enamel) in their normal relation, but there is a collection of them typically surrounding a deformed but identifiable permanent tooth.

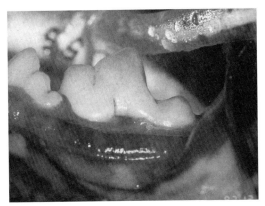

© Fraser A. Hale

Fig. 22. Clinical appearance of a dilacerated left mandibular molar in a 7-year-old Pomeranian. Note the groove in the enamel leading to the furcation and the periodontal disease evidenced by the gingival recession and furcation exposure.

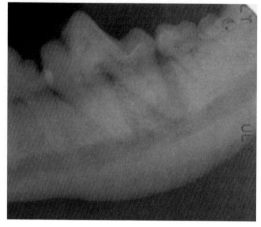

© Fraser A. Hale

Fig. 23. Radiograph of the molar in Fig. 22. Note how the roots are parallel rather than divergent. There is a dramatic radiolucency around the apex and along the entire distal aspect of the distal root as well as an apical lucency at the mesial root indicating chronic endodontic disease.

Often, the tooth on which the odontoma is based is impacted along with the denticles, and all these "teeth" are embedded in a fibrovascular stoma. Compound odontomas can be diagnosed radiographically by the presence of denticles surrounding a permanent tooth (Fig. 25) [32]. Complex

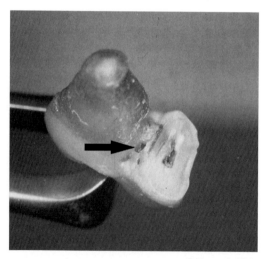

© Fraser A. Hale

Fig. 24. The molar in Fig. 22 was extracted. The tooth was sectioned and removed one root at a time. In this view of the mesial segment, the black arrow indicates the accessory canal that led from the furcation directly into the pulp chamber. This was the portal of entry for bacteria.

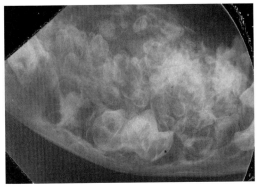

© Fraser A. Hale

Fig. 25. Radiograph of a compound odontoma in the right mandible of a 6-month-old Cocker Spaniel. A deformed but recognizable mandibular first molar tooth is seen below a mass of denticles.

odontomas differ in that all the dental tissues are present but with a deranged architecture such that the radiograph reveals an amorphous mass of dental density.

Treatment for odontomas involves surgical enucleation of all the denticles and associated teeth as well as the fibrovascular stroma from which they are growing. The prognosis is excellent if all the inductive dental tissue is removed.

Deep occlusal pits

Caries (bacterial dental decay) is not nearly as common in dogs as in human beings, and the author knows of no reported cases of true caries in cats (resorptive lesions were mistakenly referred to as feline caries years ago) [33,34]. Caries does occur in dogs on occasion, however, and when it does, it most commonly occurs in deep developmental pits in the center of the occlusal fossa of the maxillary first molar (Figs. 26 and 27). These anatomic features of the molars are prone to impaction of food, which oral bacteria ferment, producing acids that dissolve the hard tissues of the tooth. To prevent this, the permanent teeth, especially the molars, should be carefully inspected at spaying or neutering or any other time an anesthetic episode provides the opportunity. Prominent occlusal pits can then be filled with a pit and fissure sealant to exclude food impaction and prevent caries development. Large pits may require restoration with bonded composite materials.

Six months to 1 year

If the patient has developed a normal occlusal relation with the proper number of teeth all in their proper places, the rest of the first year should go smoothly from a dental standpoint.

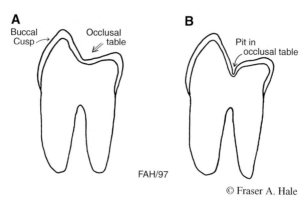

© Fraser A. Hale

Fig. 26. Cross-sectional illustrations of the maxillary first molar teeth of a dog. (*A*) The occlusal table is smooth, with no place for food impaction. (*B*) The occlusal table has a deep pit into which food would become impacted. Such a pit is prone to the development of dental caries.

Once all the permanent teeth have erupted and the pain of "teething" is over, it is time to start training the client and patient in the art of dental home care. Daily brushing of the teeth is the most effective means of controlling dental plaque and maintaining gingival health.

It is often suggested that clients should start introducing home care at a young age, when puppies and kittens are most easily trained. There is merit to this approach, but clients should suspend these efforts during the time of primary tooth exfoliation and permanent tooth eruption. Brushing during this mixed dentition period is likely to cause pain, thereby teaching the patient that home care is unpleasant. By waiting until the primary teeth

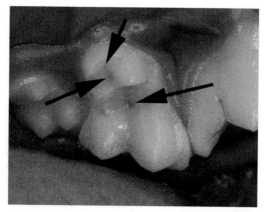

© Fraser A. Hale

Fig. 27. Photograph of the left maxillary first molar in a young dog. Three prominent occlusal pits are indicated by the arrows. A pit and fissure sealant is indicated to fill these pits so as to exclude impaction of food and to prevent caries.

are all gone and the permanent teeth have all erupted, the client can avoid this confounding factor. Home care programs should be introduced gradually and with plenty of positive reinforcement, as with any behavior modification program. Trying to proceed too quickly can result in a noncompliant pet and eventual failure of the program. Once a client has decided that he or she does not want to bother brushing a pet's teeth (because he or she tried and it did not go well), it is difficult to convince that person otherwise.

Fracture of immature permanent teeth

Young patients may suffer fractures of permanent teeth as a result of inappropriate chewing habits or accidental trauma. As is the case with mature patients, crown fractures that cause pulp exposure or near exposure (thin layer of dentin remaining over the pulp) require treatment. Treatment options are limited to extraction of the fractured tooth or endodontic treatment to save it. In a mature patient, endodontic treatment usually means full root canal treatment (removal of all the pulp and filling of the pulp chamber with dental materials). In a young dog or cat, full root canal treatment is often not an option.

When a permanent tooth erupts, the outside dimensions of the crown are established, but the wall of the crown, and especially of the root, is thin and the pulp chamber is large (Fig. 28). Until the tooth has fully erupted, the

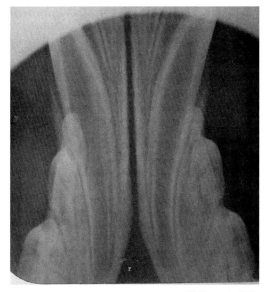

© Fraser A. Hale

Fig. 28. Radiograph of the mandibular canine teeth in a 6-month-old dog. Note the thin root and crown walls, the massive pulp chambers, and the wide open apices.

apex of the root is wide open. Once the tooth has erupted to its full length, the pulp produces dentin inside the tooth to create an apical delta and thicker root and crown walls (this posteruptive dentin production continues as long as the pulp remains alive and healthy).

If an immature tooth is fractured, it is desirable to keep the pulp alive so that the tooth can continue its normal internal development. This is accomplished by partial vital pulpotomy and direct pulp capping as is done after crown reduction. The procedure removes only a small amount of pulp from the crown of the tooth and then seals the tooth to protect the remaining pulp and keep it vital. The prognosis for this procedure is greatly affected by the amount of time between the injury and treatment. It is best if the tooth can be treated immediately before the pulp becomes contaminated and inflamed. The younger the patient, the larger the pulp is and the more forgiving it is; thus, in patients less than 1 year of age, a delay of 48 or even 72 hours is often acceptable. Beyond that, the prognosis decays exponentially with the passage of time. Therefore, crown fractures in dogs and cats less than 1 year of age (even up to 18 months) should be considered serious emergencies, and treatment should be sought without delay.

Conditions that can occur at any time

Maxillofacial fractures

Facial trauma with bone fractures can occur at any time. In the mature patient with a full set of permanent teeth, intraoral acrylic splints anchored to the teeth usually are the best option for stabilizing the fracture while allowing a rapid return to alimentation.

In young patients with primary or mixed dentition (some primary and some permanent teeth), there many be insufficient stable dental structures to act as anchors. Pins and plates are usually inappropriate, because the bone is too soft and too full of thin-walled teeth and roots (see Fig. 4). One concern is that placing pins and screws may cause serious iatrogenic damage to the dental structures. Another is that the appliances may become loose and ineffective quickly because the bone is so thin and soft. A third concern with rigid stabilization of any sort is that it may restrict facial growth and the eruption of the permanent teeth.

With these challenges imposed, facial fractures in young dogs and cats call for some creative approaches. One option is the use of a tape muzzle to hold the mouth closed enough that the interdigitation of the canine teeth holds the fracture in proper anatomic alignment during healing [6].

Another option is to use 2-0 polydioxanone suture material instead of wire for interosseous suturing, cerclage, and hemicerclage. This material can be tied tightly to appose the fracture and hold it relatively stable, but it then stretches and is less likely to restrict growth. It is also absorbed and thus

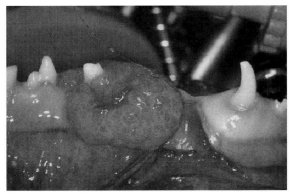

© Fraser A. Hale

Fig. 29. Clinical photograph of a papillary squamous cell carcinoma in a 4-month-old retriever cross. Surgical removal with wide margins was curative.

does not require removal. The only things that are then allowed to pass the patient's lips for the next 6 weeks are air, water, and extremely soft food.

Oral tumors

Although oral tumors are far more common in mature patients, papillary squamous cell carcinoma has a predilection for the juvenile patient (Fig. 29) [35]. These proliferative gingival tumors may be an expression of the papilloma virus [35]. Although considered malignant, they tend to be locally invasive rather than metastatic; thus, complete surgical excision offers a reasonable prognosis for cure.

Other juvenile oral tumors include those based on the tissues involved in the development of the teeth (inductive oral tumors, such as ameloblastomas). As is the case with all oral masses or swellings in a patient of any age, the diagnostic workup should include intraoral dental radiographs followed by an appropriate incisional or excisional biopsy.

Summary

The good news is that most dogs and cats live through their first year of life with no dental or oral problems requiring attention. For the others, being aware of the potential problems, recognizing them early, and instituting appropriate care in a timely manner can improve the quality of life immediately and avoid more serious problems in the long term.

References

[1] Harvey CE, Emily PP. Function, formation, and anatomy of oral structures in carnivores. In: Small animal dentistry. St. Louis: Mosby–Year Book; 1993. p. 3–18.

[2] Wiggs RB, Lobprise HL. Pedodontics. In: Veterinary dentistry, principles and practice. Philadelphia: Raven-Lippincott; 1997. p. 167–85.

[3] Wiggs RB, Lobprise HL, de Lahunta A. Microglossia in three littermate puppies. J Vet Dent 1994;11(4):129–33.

[4] Harvey CE, Emily PP. Oral lesions of soft tissue and bone: differential diagnosis. In: Small Animal Dentistry. St. Louis: Mosby–Year Book; 1993. p. 42–87.

[5] Barker IK, Van Dreumel AA, Palmer N. The alimentary system. In: Jubb KVF, Kennedy PC, Palmer N, editors. Pathology of domestic animals, vol. 2. Orlando: Academic Press; 1993. p. 1–257.

[6] Harvey CE, Emily PP. Oral surgery. In: Small animal dentistry. St. Louis: Mosby–Year Book; 1993. p. 312–77.

[7] GunnLips C. Oral cavity and salivary glands. In: Gourley IM, Vasseur PB, editors. General small animal surgery. Philadelphia: Lippincott; 1985. p. 193–231.

[8] Nelson AW. Upper respiratory system. In: Slatter D, editor. Textbook of small animal surgery. Philadelphia: WB Saunders; 1993. p. 733–76.

[9] Waldron DR, Martin RA. Cleft palate repair. Probl Vet Med 1991;3(2):142–52.

[10] Manfra Marretta S, Grove TK, Grillo JF. Split palatal U-flap: a new technique for repair of caudal hard palatal defects. J Vet Dent 1991;8(1):5–8.

[11] Hennet PR, Harvey CE. Craniofacial development and growth in the dog. J Vet Dent 1992; 9(2):11–8.

[12] Harvey CE, Emily PP. Occlusion, occlusive abnormalities and orthodontic treatment. In: Small animal dentistry. St. Louis: Mosby–Year Book; 1993. p. 266–96.

[13] Wiggs RB, Lobprise HL. Basics of orthodontics. In: Veterinary dentistry, principles and practice. Philadelphia: Raven-Lippincott; 1997. p. 435–81.

[14] Mendoza KA, Manfra Marretta S, Behr MJ, et al. Facial swelling associated with impaction of the primary and permanent maxillary fourth premolars in a dog with patent ductus arteriosus. J Vet Dent 2001;18(2):69–74.

[15] Stapleton BL, Clarke LL. Mandibular canine tooth impaction in a young dog. J Vet Dent 1999;16(3):105–8.

[16] Lobprise HL, Wiggs RB. Dentigerous cyst in a dog. J Vet Dent 1992;9(1):13–5.

[17] Gioso MA, Carvalhov GC. Maxillary dentigerous cyst in a cat. J Vet Dent 2003;20(1):28–30.

[18] Eisner ER. Surgical tooth extraction in two cases of impacted abnormally developed teeth. J Vet Dent 1989;6(1):17–9.

[19] Kramek BA, O'Brien TD, Smith FO. Diagnosis and removal of a dentigerous cyst complicated by ameloblastic fibro-odontoma in a dog. J Vet Dent 1996;13(1):9–11.

[20] Anderson JG, Harvey CE. Odontogenic cysts. J Vet Dent 1993;10(4):5–9.

[21] Gioso MA, Shofer F, Barros PSM, et al. Mandible and mandibular first molar tooth measurements in dogs: relationship of radiographic height to body size. J Vet Dent 2001; 18(2):65–8.

[22] Brine EJ. Endodontic disease of the mandibular first molar tooth secondary to caudal cross bite in a young Shetland Sheepdog. J Vet Dent 1999;16(1):15–8.

[23] Hale FA. Orthodontic correction of lingually displaced canine teeth in a young dog using light-cured acrylic resin. J Vet Dent 1996;13(2):69–73.

[24] Legendre LFJ. Anterior cross bite correction in a dog using a lingual bar, a labial bow, lingual buttons and elastic threads. J Vet Dent 1991;8(3):21–5.

[25] Pavlica Z, Cestnik V. Management of lingually displaced mandibular canine teeth in five Bull Terrier dogs. J Vet Dent 1995;12(4):127–9.

[26] Surgeon TW. Surgical exposure and orthodontic extrusion of an impacted canine tooth in a cat: a case report. J Vet Dent 2000;17(2):81–5.

[27] Hale FA. Orthodontic correction for breeding and show dogs: an ethical dilemma. J Vet Dent 1991;8(3):14.

[28] DeForge DH. Dens-in-dente in a six-year-old Doberman Pinscher. J Vet Dent 1992;9(3): 9–12.

[29] Hale FA, Wilcock BP. Compound odontoma in a dog. J Vet Dent 1996;13(3):93–5.
[30] Felizzola CR, Martins MT, et al. Compound odontoma in three dogs. J Vet Dent 2003; 20(2):79–83.
[31] Eickhoff M, Seeliger F, Simon D, et al. Erupted bilateral compound odontomas in a dog. J Vet Dent 2002;19(3):137–43.
[32] Regezi JA, Sciubba J. Odontogenic tumors. In: Regezi JA, Sciubba J, editors. Oral pathology. 2nd edition. Philadelphia: WB Saunders; 1993. p. 362–97.
[33] Hale FA. Dental caries in the dog. J Vet Dent 1998;15(2):79–83.
[34] Hale FA. Dental caries. In: Tilley LP, Smith FWK, editors. The 5-minute veterinary consultant. 3rd edition. Philadelphia: Lippincott Williams & Wilkins; 2004. p. 324–5.
[35] Stapleton BL, Barrus JM. Papillary squamous cell carcinoma in a young dog. J Vet Dent 1996;13(2):65–8.

ELSEVIER
SAUNDERS

Vet Clin Small Anim
31 (2005) 819–836

VETERINARY
CLINICS
Small Animal Practice

Management of Periodontal Disease: Understanding the Options

Colin E. Harvey, BVSc, FRCVS

School of Veterinary Medicine, University of Pennsylvania,
VHUP 3113, 3900 Delancey Street, Philadelphia, PA 19104, USA

We have all been told that "periodontal disease" is the most common disease occurring in domestic dogs and cats and that local severity and the impact on the rest of the body are reasons why all companion animal patients should receive an oral examination every time they are seen—"lift the lip." This article provides the background information on which an effective periodontal management program can be tailored for each patient.

The periodontal tissues ("periodontium") are the tissues that hold the tooth in the mouth: the alveolar bone, periodontal ligament, and gingiva, with the supporting connective tissue and blood vessels (Fig. 1A). Periodontal disease is defined as plaque-induced disease of any part of the periodontium. It is often separated into two conditions: gingivitis and periodontitis.

Gingivitis is inflammation of the gingiva. Inflammation is reversible: remove the cause, and the effect (the inflammatory response) disappears. Gingivitis is seen clinically as reddening and edema of the gingiva (initially the marginal gingiva, which is the gingival tissue that is touching the crown) and may progress in severity to visible ulceration and spontaneous bleeding. Gingivitis can be thought of as the "canary in the cage" in a mine—it is an indicator that conditions are right for permanent periodontal damage (periodontitis) to occur.

Periodontitis is inflammation of the nongingival periodontal tissues (ie, the periodontal ligament and alveolar bone). Periodontitis is in fact "alveolar bone osteomyelitis." It is impossible to recognize periodontitis separately from gingivitis, however. Periodontitis causes "loss of attachment" (ie, the connective tissue attachment between the root and the alveolar bone no longer starts at the level of the cementoenamel junction [CEJ] of the tooth; see Fig. 1).

Periodontitis is diagnosed when loss of attachment is recognized:

- Because "gingival recession" exposes part of the root (see Fig. 1B)

E-mail address: ceh@vet.upenn.edu

doi:10.1016/j.cvsm.2005.03.002 *vetsmall.theclinics.com*

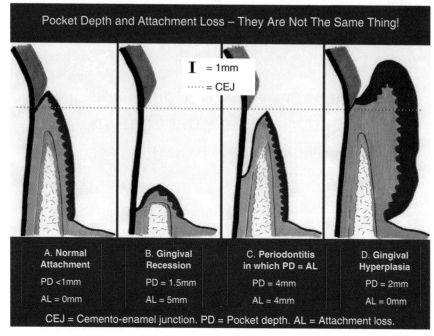

Fig. 1. Pocket depth and attachment loss—they are not the same. (*A*) Normal tooth and periodontal tissues. (*B*) Gingival recession reduces "pocket depth" relative to "loss of attachment." (*C*) Loss of attachment and pocket depth may be the same in the absence of gingival recession or hyperplasia. (*D*) Gingival hyperplasia increases pocket depth relative to loss of attachment. AL, attachment loss; CEJ, cementoenamel junction; PD, pocket depth.

- When a gently applied blunt-tipped probe can be passed apical to (ie, in the direction of the root tip) the CEJ (see Fig. 1C)
- Radiographically as loss of part of the "lamina dura" (the white line of alveolar cortical bone normally seen surrounding the root)

Note that loss of attachment does not indicate active periodontitis. If there is no evidence of gingivitis at the time of examination, any loss of attachment is presumed to be caused by past (sometimes referred to as "passive") periodontitis.

To understand periodontitis, it is helpful to know how the teeth and periodontal tissues function and how form relates to function.

Periodontal tissues

Teeth

Teeth are used to prehend and perform mechanical work on food material. Not surprisingly, they vary greatly depending on the natural diet of the particular species (herbivore, omnivore, or carnivore).

Whether the teeth tear, cut, shred, or crush the food material, a hard surface is required. The enamel covering the crown is the hardest tissue in the body. The crowns of teeth are the head of the hammer, the face of the rasp, or the blade of a knife or pair of scissors. No matter how hard they are, teeth cannot be effective without a platform or handle from which force can be directed. The jaws are the handles that permit application of this force. When one hard structure is struck against another hard structure with sufficient force, one of the two is damaged—it cleaves; this would be true of occluding teeth if they were rigidly fixed to jaws. Fortunately, the periodontal ligament is sandwiched between them.

Periodontal ligament

The periodontal ligament has three primary functions:

1. Hold the tooth in the jaw. The horizontally and obliquely oriented collagen fibers are the laces knitting the tooth to the bone and are locked into the cementum and alveolar bone.
2. Provide a shock-absorbing effect to prevent fracture of teeth during forceful occlusal action. It spreads the mechanical force around the full surface area of the root.
3. Maintain and repair the periodontal ligament tissues. Here is Wolff's law in action: occlusal force not only maintains the quality of alveolar bone but maintains the functional strength of periodontal collagen. If there is no or extremely reduced ongoing occlusal work, the quality of periodontal collagen is degraded.

Alveolar bone

The alveolar bone has the most rapid turnover of any bone in the body [1], followed by the cortices of the mandible and maxilla. This is why we observe "rubber jaw" as a clinical sign of hyperparathyroidism instead of "rubber leg." It is a reflection of the rich blood supply and multidimensional force to which the jaws are subject. Although a calcium-poor diet may enhance the progression of periodontitis, it is not the causative factor—plaque is [2]. The crestal bone (the tip of the alveolar bone closest to the crown) is the critical area in development of periodontitis. Think of the periodontal ligament as the zipper locking the bone and root together; the crestal attachment is the "open" end of the zipper. If it is not fully closed and locked by the zipper tab, the entire zipper closure is at risk.

Gingiva

The gingiva is the locking tab at the open end of the periodontal ligament zipper, and it provides a thick protective cap to the crestal bone. The marginal gingiva (the part abutting the crown and not attached to bone) moves with the tooth to keep the bony attachment protected.

Marginal gingiva is held in place by the hemidesmosomal attachment of the sulcular epithelium to the enamel surface—a chemical glue. The glue layer is itself protected by the external shape of the crown (dental or coronal bulge).

This finely engineered periodontal system works well under "normal" conditions. Of course, normal conditions include the daily janitorial effects of occlusion in wild carnivores. The mouths and teeth of many companion animals do not have the benefit of normal occlusal function. When the lack of normal occlusion is combined with the nonvascularized nature of the adjacent surfaces of the teeth, conditions are ripe for development of periodontal disease.

Oral environment

The teeth live in an open environment. Any inert surface exposed to the environment is covered with microorganisms. Think of the tongue as a dish rag used to mop up everything of emotional or gustatory interest to a dog, and one realizes why there is such a rich microflora in the oral cavity.

A moist surface supports more microorganisms than a dry surface. A warm environment encourages many organisms to grow faster. A fluid loaded with microbial nutrients encourages growth. The mouth is constantly moist, warm, and often loaded with nutrients. The teeth are constantly covered by oral fluid spread by the movements of the tongue and lips. Evaporation causes the oral fluid to become deposited as a glycoprotein layer (the "pellicle") on the crowns of the teeth. Think of it as flypaper snaring passing bacteria. Perfect conditions for development of a biofilm are thus present. When a biofilm forms on the inert surfaces of the teeth, it is called dental plaque. The microbes in the biofilm do not have completely free rein; the salivary fluid in which the teeth are bathed has antibacterial properties (eg, lysozyme, lactoferrins, IgA with specific antibodies), and the combination of this antibacterial activity and daily occlusal scrubbing works well to keep the enamel-based biofilm from getting out of hand under normal conditions.

Excellent long-term oral health is easy to achieve in dogs if daily oral care is impeccable [3]. When oral care is less than optimal and the biofilm is allowed to accumulate, it becomes thicker and more complex, and the protective oral fluids have less effect on the microbial inhabitants in the deeper layers.

The rigid nonvascularized enamel tooth surface is the ideal platform for development of a biofilm (dental plaque) and its cousin, dental calculus. Calculus forms when calcium carbonate and calcium phosphate salts in salivary fluid crystallize on the surface of the teeth, mineralizing soft plaque [4]. It takes 2 to 3 days for plaque to become sufficiently mineralized to form calculus that is resistant to being readily wiped off. This is the window that we work with in oral home care (whether for ourselves or our patients).

Calcium salts are more likely to be deposited on plaque in an alkaline environment. Unfortunately, the mouths of dogs and cats are slightly alkaline (oral fluid in human beings is usually slightly acidic). Thus, dogs and cats are more prone to deposition of calculus than people. The chemical composition of the diet influences oral deposits [5].

The bacteria found in dental plaque are not required for deposition of calculus. Germ-free dogs develop calculus deposits but do not develop the gingival inflammation and bone loss that occur in many pet dogs. Although the bacteria in plaque are the real cause of gingivitis and periodontitis, there are two clinically important attributes of calculus: (1) it provides a protected physical location for development of plaque, including deep crevices that promote growth of anaerobic bacteria, and (2) once formed, calculus cannot be removed except by mechanical action on the surface of the tooth.

When occlusal scrubbing is insufficient or infrequent, the biofilm on the enamel thickens and matures. Think of a biofilm as a microbial village constantly undergoing changes; the longer it is allowed to grow, the thicker and more complex it becomes. A tooth with thick calculus deposits and deep periodontal pockets has expanded beyond a village; it is a thriving microbial city with skyscrapers, tunnels, freeways, congested areas, dark alleys, and neighborhoods each unique unto itself. In the deeper part of the biofilm, equivalent to the back alleys of the older dilapidated parts of the city, the oxygen is strangled out of the fluid as a result of active growth of aerobic organisms and an anaerobic environment is established. Note that this is unique to the biofilm on the teeth because of the lack of vascularity of the enamel surface on which it forms—there is no replenishment of oxygen except by diffusion from the external surface.

Periodontal infection

Gingivitis and periodontitis are referred to as "bacterial infections"; however, Koch's postulate, the usual proof that a specific disease has an infectious cause, cannot be applied to periodontal disease because of the following:

- Any sample from an example of spontaneous clinical periodontal disease sent to a microbiology laboratory familiar with oral flora yields a wide variety of microorganisms. Which one(s) should be selected as the "pathogen"?
- Any healthy (non–germ-free) individual already has a rich oral microflora; thus, introducing a putative periodontal pathogen and finding that disease develops at the site of inoculation does not prove that the disease resulted from the inoculation of the organism.
- The putative pathogenic organism may not be found on culture of a sample from the area of induced disease if the sample is grossly contaminated with supragingival and commensal organisms.

- In a germ-free dog, although calculus accumulates on the surface of the teeth in the absence of oral hygiene, introduction of a putative pathogen in an attempt to prove Koch's postulate may be unrewarding, because the complexity of the biofilm that supports the growth of the pathogen in a dog with normal flora does not exist.

Plaque, the dental biofilm, is a complex mixture of organisms. Around 500 bacterial species have been identified to date in these microbial cities in normal and diseased mouths of dogs and cats [6].

Plaque development over the first few days on a clean tooth surface (ie, after dental scaling) follows a predictable pattern:

1. Colonization of the pellicle by aerobic cocci. Because they are small and round, they are not readily displaced by movements of the tongue, lips, or food material and grow well on the surface of the thin pellicle.
2. Adhesion of aerobic rods on the sticky and irregular surface provided by the growing coccal layer. The thickening biofilm allows aerobic and facultative rods to attach, aggregate, and grow.
3. The aerobic cocci and rods multiply, and as they do so, the oxygen gradient in the thickening biofilm changes so that at its deepest point, oxygen is no longer available. The occasional obligate anaerobes caught deep in the biofilm can now grow. The maturation of plaque to the point where it supports anaerobic organisms takes about 24 hours in the dog.
4. The biochemical environment changes as the biofilm continues to mature and is enriched by products of gingival inflammation. The mixture of microbial detritus and products of inflammation forms a physical and chemical environment that allows spirochetes to thrive; they are packed in dense palisades in mature subgingival plaque [7].
5. In biofilm parlance, a "climax community" results—a semistable state in balance with available nutrients and oxygen. This is made more complex in the case of dental plaque by the presence of calculus, which provides irregular chasms.

What are periodontopathogens?

"Periodontopathogens" are bacteria that are the putative cause of gingivitis and periodontitis. In the absence of being able to prove Koch's postulate, factors important in demonstrating periodontopathogenic significance are as follows:

1. The species is cultured more commonly from diseased individuals than from nondiseased individuals and from diseased areas of the mouth than from healthy areas in the same individual.
2. The bacterium produces products known to be toxins or tissue-destructive enzymes, such as metalloproteinases.

3. Cytotoxic effects are seen on tissue culture.
4. Other "virulence factors" are identified.

Because of the anaerobic ecologic niche, periodontal microbiology is a unique sphere of microbiology. Challenges to achieving expertise in veterinary periodontal microbiology include the following:

- Anaerobic culture techniques are absolutely essential. Many of the organisms of interest are obligate anaerobes and can only be grown on selective culture media.
- Spirochetes are common and are notoriously difficult to culture. DNA probe technology has allowed recognition of a group referred to as pathogen-related oral spirochetes (PROS) [8].
- Carnivore and human oral floras have many similarities but also some important differences. The gram-negative anaerobic rod *Porphyromonas gingivalis* is considered to be the key human periodontopathogen. A catalase-positive form of *P gingivalis* is found more commonly in canine and feline periodontal specimens, which is now a distinct species named *Porphyromonas gulae* [9].
- Other recently recognized canine and feline *Porphyromonas* organisms include *P cangingivalis*, *P canoris*, *P cansulci*, *P crevioricanis*, and *P gingivicanis* [10].

It seems likely that periodontopathogens act collectively in causing a destructive effect [11] by enhancing aggregation in the biofilm or promoting gingival cell attachment of other organisms as well as by specific cytopathic effects. The adherence-promoting fimbrial protein in human *P gingivalis* is also found in *P gulae* isolated from dogs [12].

Clinical and pathologic effects

As with bacterial infections in any other tissue, the initial effect is inflammation of the gingival tissues. What happens then depends on whether or not the local tissues are overwhelmed by the bacterial burden. In either case, neutrophils are attracted to the site; move onto the epithelial surface through the large intercellular spaces of the sulcular epithelium; and engulf, ingest, and digest the plaque bacteria. When a pathogenic plaque load is present, many of these neutrophils become overly full and burst, and some retire into the adjacent tissue before they burst; these bursting neutrophils release bacterial toxins and destructive enzymes, including metalloproteinases (eg, collagenase) within tissue, causing breakdown of the integrity of the connective tissue. The bursting neutrophils also release cytokines that propagate the inflammatory response.

When oral hygiene is poor, the bacterial load is constantly enlarging. This ratchets up the inflammatory response, and the mixture of bacterial and cell degradation products becomes destructive in its effect on the periodontal tissues. The sulcular epithelial layer ulcerates, exposing the more vulnerable connective tissue more fully to bacterial invasion. As the destructive inflammatory-infective mixture descends deeper into the tissue, inflammation-induced resorption nibbles away the alveolar bone to produce periodontitis (alveolar bone osteomyelitis).

Gingivitis does not predictably lead to periodontitis if left untreated. The ability of animals (including human beings) to resist a given gingival bacterial load varies greatly among individuals, depending on age, stress, nutritional status, immunologic competence, individual differences in protective constituents of saliva, concurrent infections (eg, feline immunodeficiency virus [FIV]), nonoral health status, and probably several other factors that are incompletely understood or not yet identified [13].

Continuing bone loss causes instability of the attachment of the tooth. The result is mobility, which causes the tooth to be pushed against the remaining bone during chewing. This further enhances alveolar bone resorption by squeezing the blood vessels adjacent to the tooth (an effect similar to that occurring during orthodontic tooth movement). In an aging toy-breed dog with severe periodontitis, there may be only a matchstick of mandibular bone present adjacent to the roots of the first mandibular tooth, and pathologic fracture of the mandible is possible.

If the process continues for long enough (which varies greatly from patient to patient), the eventual result is loss of the tooth. This is actually a defense mechanism; the remaining tissues can finally recover because there is no longer the constant presence of the overwhelming bacterial burden.

In the usually long period between the initial gingivitis and the final exfoliation of the tooth, bacteria that find themselves adjacent to capillaries may end up causing bacteremia. Bacteremia is frequent in patients with gingivitis and active periodontitis, and it is rapidly cleared by the reticuloendothelial system in otherwise healthy patients [14]. What are the long-term consequences of frequent bacteremic showering? It has been known for several years that there is an association between the severity of periodontal disease and distant organ abnormalities in human beings and dogs [15]. Studies are underway to determine whether the suspected cause (gingivitis and/or periodontitis) and effect (distant organ damage) hypothesis is correct.

Bacteremia is not the only likely cause of distant organ effects. Chronic body-wide release of inflammatory mediators and bacterial and cellular degradation byproducts may produce direct or immune-mediated distant organ pathologic changes.

Periodontitis is not a simple "infection" story. As veterinarians, we should emphasize the clinical importance of recognizing not just the extent of plaque and calculus deposition but the reaction of the periodontal tissues. In one patient, a tooth with extensive plaque and/or calculus buildup may be amenable to conservative treatment (scaling and polishing with follow-up home care), whereas another patient with the same extent of plaque and/or calculus buildup may have such a severe tissue response that extraction of the teeth in the involved area is the only practical option.

How can we recognize the extent of periodontitis? Even in a cooperative dog, we cannot reliably probe the pockets of an awake patient. "Pocket depth" is an unreliable measure; it may under- or overestimate the extent of periodontitis as a result of gingival recession or gingival hyperplasia, respectively (see Fig. 1). We can recognize gingivitis and gingival recession; however, particularly in dogs, there is often poor correlation between the severity of visible gingivitis and the extent of active or prior periodontitis. In a nonmobile tooth, the periodontal probe or a radiograph is the only accurate means of determining the severity of periodontitis, which creates a particular challenge for veterinarians compared with human dentists. The pathophysiology of gingivitis and periodontitis is summarized in Fig. 2.

Prevention

Prevention is primarily directed at prevention of accumulation of plaque and calculus or at suppressing the tissue-destructive effects of the inflammatory response. Frequent brushing (optimally daily) remains the "gold standard," although there are also some new approaches based on our

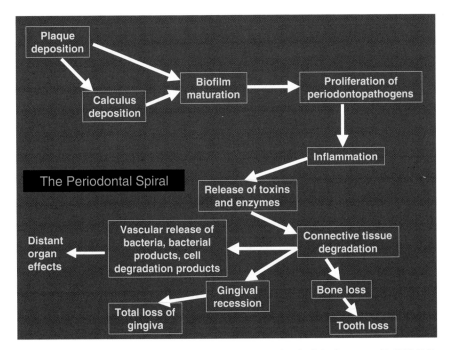

Fig. 2. The periodontal spiral: summary of periodontal pathophysiologic events. (© 2004 C.E. Harvey, BVSc, University of Pennsylvania, Philadelphia, PA.)

increased understanding of the formation of plaque and calculus and of the pathophysiology of periodontal disease.

Fig. 3 diagrams where a particular preventive approach works in the periodontal disease process. Combining strategies is likely to be more effective than relying on a single strategy. What is the owner willing and able to do, and what is the patient willing to accept?

1. Prevent accumulation of plaque. Daily cleansing is best, but cleansing every other day is also helpful in slowing down the progression of disease. Anything less frequent than this is of doubtful long-term value because of calculus deposition. Although oral home care is easy to describe to owners, it is difficult for many owners to practice over the long term:

    • Mechanical cleansing. In the wild and in controlled laboratory studies in dogs [16], mechanical cleansing resulting from natural chewing activity achieves moderate control of periodontitis in carnivores. In most pet dogs and cats, similar effectiveness can be achieved with consistent use of chew products and diets that are effective in removing plaque and calculus when combined with periodic professional examination [17,18]. The Veterinary Oral Health Council (VOHC)

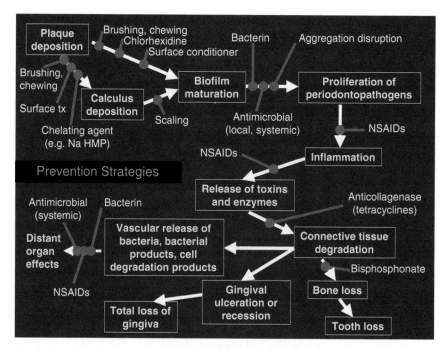

Fig. 3. Interrupting the periodontal spiral: summary of periodontal prevention strategies. (© 2004 C.E. Harvey, BVSc, University of Pennsylvania, Philadelphia, PA.)

recognizes products that achieve preset standards of effectiveness for plaque or calculus control in dogs and cats; check the VOHC web site (www.VOHC.org) for the up-to-date list of products that have been awarded the VOHC Accepted Seal.

- Chemical antiplaque effect. The long-term effectiveness of chlorhexidine in dogs has been well documented [19,20]. Many other "antiplaque" products are also marketed; however, there is little or no documentation of effectiveness available on which a recommendation for use can be made. Note that the use of antiplaque chemical agents alone does not prevent the gradual accumulation of calculus unless it is accompanied by mechanical action, and there is some evidence that chlorhexidine enhances the rate of deposition of calculus [21].

- Surface treatments extend the benefit of professional scaling. Polishing the tooth surface immediately after scaling is the standard. Newer surface treatments include application of a surface conditioner, such as silicone or wax, to the surface of the tooth. A veterinary product in two formats (one for professional use immediately after scaling and/or polishing and one for periodic reapplication by owners) was recently released (Ora-Vet; Merial, Duluth, GA).

2. Prevent accumulation of calculus.

- Mechanical scaling. This must be done professionally under anesthesia if it is to remove subgingival calculus effectively.
- Chemical effect. Some polyphosphates, such as sodium hexametaphosphate, have been shown to have a Ca^{++} chelating effect that reduces the rate of deposition of salivary or dietary calcium salts as mineralized calculus on teeth [22] and can be applied to dietary products and treats.

3. Correct host factors that may be exacerbating periodontitis (eg, diabetes or other systemic disease, poor nutrition, stress).

4. Prevent accumulation or reduce severity of the effects of pathogenic bacteria.

- Disrupt aggregation or adhesion. Clindamycin (Antirobe; Pfizer Animal Health), an antibiotic approved for management of oral infection in dogs and cats, retards the formation of the glycocalyx on the surface of bacteria, which reduces their ability to aggregate into larger clumps; this is in addition to the direct antibacterial effect of clindamycin.
- Suppress growth of or kill the bacteria.
- Systemic antibacterial treatment does have a short-term effect [20,23,24], and two antibacterial drugs (Antirobe and Clavamox; Pfizer Animal Health) have US Food and Drug Administration (FDA) approval for use in treating oral infections in dogs. Frequent or

intermittent use of systemic antibacterial drugs to control gingivitis and periodontitis is not recommended, however, because the effect is short term and there is a risk of bacterial resistance in the individual patient and others (people and companion animals). Use of an antibiotic drug is indicated as an ancillary part of periodontal treatment in some patients.

- Placement of an antibiotic drug at a high concentration in a carrier in a periodontal pocket does have a minor but measurable beneficial effect on attachment height, and a doxycycline product in an absorbable vehicle (Doxirobe; Pfizer Animal Health) is now available for clinical use in dogs.
- Replace pathogenic bacteria with nonpathogenic bacteria in the specific ecologic niche. "Good bug displacing bad bug" in the oral environment is now a topic of serious study in human dentistry, particularly in caries research. More research is required before this approach can be adopted in periodontal patients.
- Induce antibody reaction to specific pathogenic bacteria in oral fluids and serum using a bacterin made from periodontopathogens as a vaccine. Now that the specific effects of putative periodontopathogens are becoming clearer, attention is being paid to knocking out or suppressing growth of specific bacteria in the immediate periodontal neighborhood. Recent work with *P gulae* in experimental models suggests that this vaccine approach may be applicable to dogs [25] and that cross-reactivity may increase the effectiveness of this approach; however, clinical effectiveness has yet to be established.

5. Suppress the periodontal inflammatory reaction and related events.

- Although it has been shown that long-term use of nonsteroidal anti-inflammatory drugs (NSAIDs) reduces periodontitis in dogs [26], this strategy is not yet recommended as a clinically applicable approach to managing periodontal disease because the clinical effects of long-term use of NSAIDs have not yet been documented in dogs.
- Destruction of periodontal tissue results from the action of metalloproteinases and similar enzymes and toxic products. Compounds that counter these specific tissue-destructive effects locally are protective. The best-known example is the anticollagenase effect of sub-antibacterial doses of drugs in the tetracycline group; this is the basis for the approval for human clinical use of Periostat (20-mg doxycycline tablets).
- Suppress osteoclastic resorption of bone. The bisphosphonate class of drugs, such as alendronate and zoledronic acid, reduces the bone loss that results from the action of osteoclastic cells and thus has a protective effect on alveolar bone undergoing periodontitis in dogs [27]. There is no approved veterinary product or recommended dosage available at this time.

Approaches 3 through 5 should be regarded as auxiliary preventive strategies, and some are still in the experimental stage. If they deflect attention away from retarding plaque and calculus accumulation as the primary preventive approach, they may have a detrimental effect.

Treatment

In some patients, several different types of procedures may be indicated in an anesthetized patient. It is useful to differentiate between "preventive" procedures and "treatment" procedures (Fig. 4), both of which fit under the term *periodontal management*.

Dental scaling and/or polishing is a preventive procedure—it removes the cause of the disease and allows the tissues to restore themselves to health. The term *periodontal treatment* is often misused, and the terms *prophy* and *dental* (eg, "The dog is scheduled for a dental") should not be used in veterinary practice because they create the impression that a simple single procedure is all that is indicated.

Periodontal management is not like neutering a healthy young animal; every patient is unique in the extent of plaque and/or calculus deposition

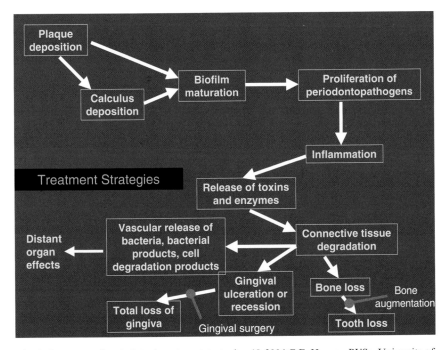

Fig. 4. Summary of periodontal treatment strategies. (© 2004 C.E. Harvey, BVSc, University of Pennsylvania, Philadelphia, PA.)

and in the tissue response and effects. "Examination" is the missing piece when the terms *periodontal treatment, dental,* and *prophy* are used.

Periodontal management under anesthesia without a prior awake oral examination (which provides initial appreciation of the severity of the disease) or without discussion of the potential procedures required with the owner is a common cause of consumer complaints about veterinary care and is likely to result in gross undercare in many patients, because the time slot available for that patient is not long enough for the indicated procedures. Veterinary technicians are often effective members of the veterinary dental team; however, keep in mind that gingivitis and periodontitis are "diseases" and that diagnosis and determination of the treatment of diseases are functions limited by state practice acts to a licensed veterinarian.

In a human patient with severe periodontitis, scaling and/or polishing is a pretreatment procedure; a decision on the actual treatment of the existing loss of attachment is often delayed for a couple of weeks until the effect of the scaling and/or polishing procedure is clear. Postscaling examination allows accurate assessment of the healthy attachment that is available, which indicates what specific surgical treatment, if any, is required. The need for sedation or anesthesia for complete oral and/or dental examination in veterinary patients limits what we know about our patients before anesthesia is administered. In many patients, two or more anesthetic episodes, allowing time for the periodontal tissues to heal in between, are impractical or unacceptable to the owner. Thus, even in some cooperative patients, veterinary dentists are often required to diagnose and complete treatment at one session, and the examination to determine need for surgical treatment is made on unhealthy tissues.

One partially successful way to manage this challenge is to pretreat patients with extensive periodontitis with an antibiotic drug for 7 to 10 days before anesthesia so that the tissues are less inflamed when they are examined. This is particularly useful when the owner wishes to retain as many teeth as possible, and it has the additional advantage that it provides a time window during which the owner can explore the practicality of a recommended active home care regimen.

Prioritizing treatment

Before anesthesia, two factors need to be determined: (1) is the patient healthy enough for the duration of anesthesia that may be required for dental scaling and/or polishing and specific treatment of severely affected teeth and (2) is the owner likely to be willing and able to apply home care consistently and long term?

Once the patient is under anesthesia, examination is critical. In some cases, scaling may be necessary before a tooth can be examined. In a mouth with complete dentition, there are 42 separate decisions to be made—one for each tooth, based on the worst affected root of that tooth. Triage each tooth as follows:

- No moderate or severe periodontitis: scaling and/or polishing is the only professional procedure required.
- The tooth can be retained but requires specific periodontal treatment in addition to scaling and/or polishing.
- The tooth is too diseased to retain: extraction is the only option.

Treatment is either (1) correction of existing loss of attachment so that remaining attachment is stabilized and further tissue loss is prevented or (2) extraction of the tooth.

There are many treatment options that permit retention of teeth that have severe loss of attachment. Which specific treatment procedure to use depends on several factors, including extent and health of gingiva surrounding the tooth, extent of loss of attachment, mobility of the tooth, and furcation exposure (loss of alveolar bone between the roots of multirooted teeth). If the owner wishes to retain the teeth to the extent practical and there is a good likelihood that home care is going to be provided long term, Fig. 5 summarizes the decision-making process to follow. Note that the health of the gingiva and the health of the bony attachment need to be considered separately.

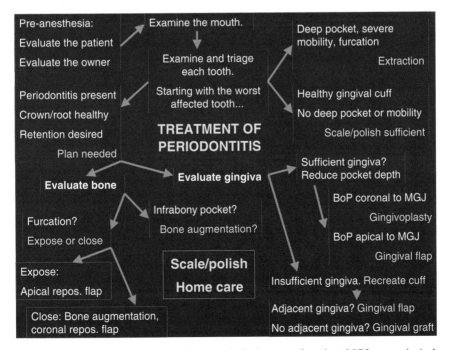

Fig. 5. Periodontitis treatment decision tree. BoP, bottom of pocket; MGJ, mucogingival junction.

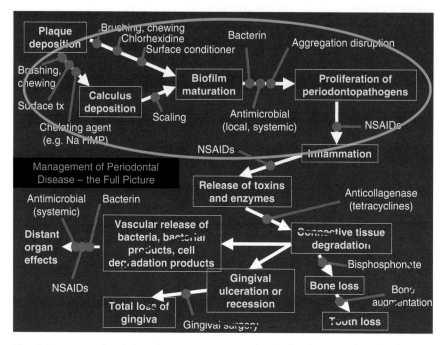

Fig. 6. Summary of periodontal management strategies. Performing procedures in the "red oval" without effective long-term "green-oval" effort does not produce good long-term results. (© 2004 C.E. Harvey, BVSc, University of Pennsylvania, Philadelphia, PA.)

Details of the specific procedures can be found in veterinary dental textbooks [28]. Be aware that many of these procedures have little documented information on long-term results in controlled studies of dogs or cats with spontaneous disease.

Prevention is a much more efficient option for the patient, and treating periodontitis does not make clinical sense if it is not accompanied by a prevention strategy that is likely to be followed long term (Fig. 6).

Whether periodontal disease should be ignored, prevented, or treated in our patients is no longer a question. The question is how to be optimally effective in each patient.

References

[1] Henriksen PA. Periodontal disease and calcium deficiency—an experimental study in the dog. Acta Odontol Scand 1968;26(Suppl 50):1–132.

[2] Svanberg G, Lindhe J, Hogoson A, et al. Effect of nutritional hyper-parathyroidism on experimental periodontitis in the dog. Scand J Dent Res 1973;81:155–62.

[3] Lindhe J, Hamp S, Löe H. Plaque induced periodontal disease in beagle dogs. A 4-year clinical, roentgenographical and histometrical study. J Periodontal Res 1975;10:243–55.

[4] Legeros RZ, Shannin IL. The crystalline components of dental calculi: human vs. dog. J Dent Res 1979;58:2371–7.

[5] Loux JJ, Alioto R, Yankell SL. Effects of glucose and urea on dental deposit pH in dogs. J Dent Res 1972;51:1610–3.

[6] Harvey CE, Thornsberry C, Miller BR. Subgingival bacteria—comparison of culture results in dogs and cats with gingivitis. J Vet Dent 1995;12:147–50.

[7] Soames JV, Davis RM. The structure of sub-gingival plaque in a beagle dog. J Periodontal Res 1974;9:333–41.

[8] Riviere GR, Thompson AJ, Brannan RD, et al. Detection of pathogen-related oral spirochetes, *Treponema denticola*, and *Treponema socranskii* in dental plaque from dogs. J Vet Dent 1996;13:135–8.

[9] Fournier D, Mouton C, Lapierre P, et al. *Porphyromonas gulae* sp. nov., an anaerobic, gram-negative coccobacillus from the gingival sulcus of various animal hosts. Int J Syst Evol Microbiol 2001;51:1179–89.

[10] Collins MD, Love DN, Karjalainen J, et al. Phylogenetic analysis of members of the genus *Porphyromonas* and description of *Porphyromonas cangingivalis* sp. nov. and *Porphyromonas cansulci* sp. nov. Int J Syst Bacteriol 1994;44:674–9.

[11] Ito R, Ishihara K, Nakayama K, et al. The mechanism of coaggregation between *Porphyromonas gingivalis* and *Treponema denticola* [abstract 3638]. In: Proceedings of the International Association of Dental Research. Honolulu, HI, March 2004.

[12] Hamada N, Kumada H, Hiyama T, et al. Purification and characterization of fimbriae from *Porphyromonas gulae* ATCC 51700 [abstract 3636]. In: Proceedings of the International Association of Dental Research. Honolulu, HI, March 2004.

[13] Schroeder HE, Attstrom R. Effect of mechanical plaque control on development of subgingival plaque and initial gingivitis in neutropenic dogs. Scand J Dent Res 1979;87: 279–87.

[14] Silver JG, Martin L, McBride BC. Recovery and clearance of oral micro-organisms following experimental bacteremia in dogs. Arch Oral Biol 1975;20:675–9.

[15] DeBowes LJ, Mosier D, Logan E, et al. Association of periodontal disease and histologic lesions in multiple organs from 45 dogs. J Vet Dent 1996;13:57–60.

[16] Egelberg J. Local effect of diet on plaque formation and development of gingivitis in dogs. Odontol Rev 1965;16:31–41.

[17] Lage A, Lausen N, Tracy R, et al. Effect of chewing rawhide and cereal biscuit on removal of dental calculus in dogs. J Am Vet Med Assoc 1990;197:213–9.

[18] Zetner K. Der Einfluss von Kollagen-sticks auf die Plaqueakkumulation bein hund. Kleinterprax 1983;28:315–9.

[19] Hamp SE, Lindhe J, Loe H. Long-term effect of chlorhexidine on developing gingivitis in the beagle dog. J Periodontal Res 1973;8:63–70.

[20] Yankell SL, Moreno OM, Saffir AJ, et al. Effects of chlorhexidine and four antimicrobial compounds on plaque, gingivitis and staining in beagle dogs. J Dent Res 1982;61:1089–93.

[21] Hull PS, Davies RM. The effect of chlorhexidine gel on tooth deposits in beagle dogs. J Small Anim Pract 1972;13:207–12.

[22] Warrick JM, Stookey GK. Overview of clinical trials using sodium hexametaphosphate for prevention of dental calculus. Proc Vet Dent Forum 2004;18:272–6.

[23] Listgarten MA, Lindhe J, Parodi R. The effect of systemic antimicrobial therapy on plaque and gingivitis in dogs. J Periodontal Res 1979;14:65–75.

[24] Sarkiala E, Harvey C. Systemic antimicrobials in the treatment of periodontitis in dogs. Semin Vet Med Surg 1993;8:197–203.

[25] Hardham JM, Dreier K, Wong J, et al. Efficacy of companion animal *Porphyromonas* spp. vaccines in the mouse model of periodontal disease. Proc Vet Dent Forum 2004;18:267–8.

[26] Jeffcoat MK, Willams RC, Wechter WJ, et al. Flurbiprofen treatment of periodontal disease in beagles. J Periodontal Res 1986;21:624–33.

[27] Ouchi N, Nishikawa H, Yoshino T, et al. Inhibitory effects of YM175, a bisphosphonate, on the progression of experimental periodontitis in beagle dogs. J Periodontal Res 1998;33: 196–204.

[28] Holmstrom SE, Frost-Fitch P, Eisner ER. Veterinary dental techniques. 3rd edition. Philadelphia: WB Saunders; 2004.

ELSEVIER
SAUNDERS

Vet Clin Small Anim
35 (2005) 837–868

VETERINARY
CLINICS
Small Animal Practice

Fundamentals of Endodontics

Brook A. Niemiec, DVM

*Southern California Veterinary Dental Specialties, 5610 Kearny Mesa Road,
Suite B1, San Diego, CA 92111, USA*

Etiologies and pathophysiology of endodontic disease

The endodontic system is the pulp tissue (blood and lymph vessels, nerves, odontoblasts, and connective tissue) that is in the root canals and pulp chambers in animals [1,2]. This living system supplies the vital tooth with the components it needs to live and mature. Endodontic disease refers to inflammation (pulpitis) [3] or necrosis (partial or complete) of the pulp tissues. Depending on the severity of the insult, the pulpitis may be reversible or irreversible. Reversible pulpitis is usually caused by a lesser insult that the tooth may survive. Irreversible pulpitis is secondary to significant pulpal inflammation and results in tooth death.

There are many possible etiologies of pulpitis. These include trauma (with or without pulp exposure), an ischemic event (avulsion or thromboembolism), or other pulpal exposures (caries, feline odontoclastic resorptive [FORL], class II perioendodontic lesion). In animal patients, however, traumatic pulp exposure is by far the most common cause. In general, this causes the tooth to fracture, exposing the endodontic system (or nerve) to the oral environment (Fig. 1). A recent study reported that 27% of domestic dogs have a fractured tooth. More concerning is that 10% of domestic dogs have one or more teeth with pulp exposure [4]. This means that of every 10 dogs entering the veterinary practice, one or more is likely to be suffering from endodontic disease. This does not include the approximately 20% of dogs with noncomplicated crown fractures, some of which are also nonvital. Teeth can break as a result of trauma (hit by a car, ball, or rock) or from chewing on hard objects. Any tooth can fracture, but certain teeth are more prone than others. The most commonly fractured teeth are the canine (cuspid) teeth of dogs and cats and the upper fourth premolar in dogs. In feline cuspids, the root canal system is close to the tip of the tooth. Therefore, almost any feline cuspid fracture overtly exposes the root canal [5].

E-mail address: dogbeachdr@aol.com

doi:10.1016/j.cvsm.2005.03.001   *vetsmall.theclinics.com*

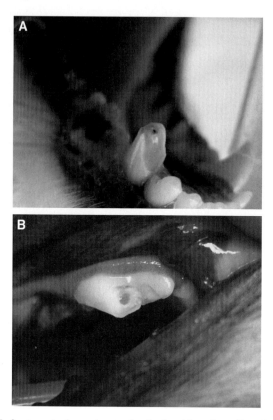

Fig. 1. Traumatic fractures to the canine tooth of a dog (*A*) and maxillary fourth premolar of a dog (*B*). Note points of pulp exposure to each tooth. The black pulp in (*A*) is indicative of nonvitality. The pink pulp in (*B*) shows that the tooth is still vital.

On occasion, a single tooth develops intrinsic staining (discoloration) (Fig. 2). The discoloration is caused by intrapulpal hemorrhage resulting from inflammation within the endodontic system of the dying tooth [6]. Intrinsic staining signals endodontic compromise as readily as a fractured tooth. Intrinsic staining occurs most commonly in cuspid and incisor teeth. In some (particularly young) patients, this staining may resolve, indicating reversible pulpitis [7]. Persistent staining likely indicates irreversible pulpitis. A recent veterinary study reported that 92.2% of discolored teeth in dogs are nonvital and in need of therapy despite apparently normal radiographic findings [7]. The etiology of the pulp necrosis is usually unknown, although trauma is a common cause in human dentistry. The intrinsically stained tooth may become infected via infiltration through the apex, a process known as anachoresis. This infected tooth acts as a bacterial reservoir just like a broken tooth.

Regardless of the etiology, acute pulpitis is an excruciatingly painful experience (as people who have had a fractured tooth or a deep carious

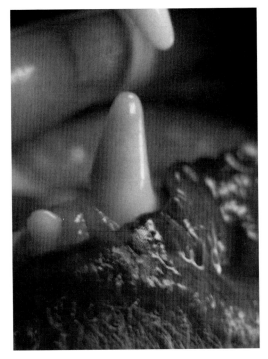

Fig. 2. Discolored maxillary canine in a dog. In all likelihood, this tooth is nonvital.

lesion can attest to) [8]. Oral pain in patients with pulp-exposed teeth was substantiated in a recent veterinary study demonstrating that pain on chewing was significantly increased in domesticated dogs with pulp exposure versus those without [4]. Unfortunately, our animal patients almost never demonstrate overt signs of oral pain because they are quite stoic, they cannot verbalize symptoms, or the condition occurs as a consequence of natural selection [9]. In the wild, animals that seem to be weak or painful may be culled from the pack, perhaps resulting in death. A fear of culling by a client who is perceived as alpha may prevent our pets from exhibiting any or, if any, only subtle (hence, often missed) signs of oral pain [9]. When the nerve dies, much of the pain goes away; however, it is replaced by infection, resulting in a chronic disease state that affects the patient daily [10,11]. This apparent lack of pain allows clients and veterinarians to dismiss a fractured tooth, because "it doesn't seem to bother him." Many a veterinary dentist can testify to numerous clients who have insisted that their pet is not bothered by the fractured tooth; when it is discovered, however, clients report that the pet acts "5 years younger" just 2 weeks after the staged or definitive endodontic treatment. These animals are being affected locally as well as systemically (as is detailed shortly), and neglecting the dentin- or pulp-exposed fractured tooth is not a viable option.

With irreversible pulpitis, the tooth eventually becomes nonvital because of pulpal necrosis [12]. With chronicity, the lack of immune competence of the pulp tissues to resist bacterial colonization results in bacterial contamination by the oral environment (most common) or via the systemic circulation [13]. Infection via the systemic circulation is called anachoresis and is defined as the preferential collection or deposit of particles, such as bacteria or metals, that have localized out of the bloodstream in areas of inflammation [14]. At this point, the affected tooth's endodontic system becomes purulent (Fig. 3). The bacteria are now fortressed against host immune defenses and antimicrobials, and the affected tooth's endodontic system is also a "superhighway" for oral bacteria. This bacterial superhighway has its on-ramp at the fracture site and its off-ramp at the apical deltas of canine and feline root apices. The bacteria and their byproducts occasionally stream through these openings into the alveolar bone and its blood supply.

With chronic pulpitis, the bacteria and host white blood cells, mediators, cell enzymes, and byproducts (eg, bacterial gasses) build up and pressurize in the unyielding endodontic chamber. These inflammatory products eventually result in bone destruction around the root apex, creating an apical abscess or granuloma (Fig. 4) [15].

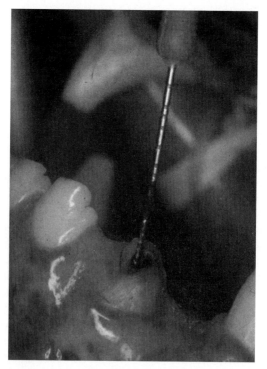

Fig. 3. Fractured maxillary incisor with pulp exposure and necrotic pulp is extirpated with an endodontic file.

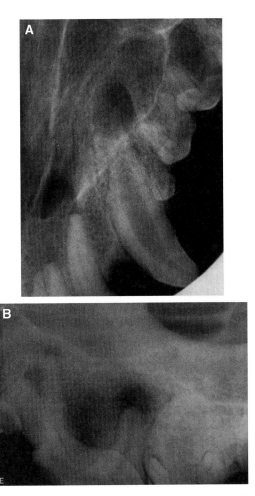

Fig. 4. Large periapical abscesses from a canine tooth (*A*) and maxillary fourth premolar (*B*).

This periapical bacterial abscess or granuloma results in the loss of the periodontal ligament and alveolar bone in the area of the tooth root apex, with potentially devastating consequences. The proximity of the tooth root apices of the maxillary molars and fourth premolars (carnassial teeth) in domestic dogs and of the maxillary cuspid teeth of cats risks compromise of the eyes and orbits during endodontic disease. "Apical blowout" (abscessation and/or granulation) can result in cellulitis of the orbit or globe, which may be vision threatening [16]. Because of the location of the root apexes of virtually all maxillary teeth, an endodontic infection can lead to a significant nasal infection. Finally, the proximity of the tooth roots of the permanent mandibular cuspids and first molars to the ventral cortex of the mandible can result in pathologic mandibular fracture [17].

Regardless of locale, the abscess at the root tips intermittently flares to the point of hard or soft tissue swelling or fistulates through the gingiva, mucosa (Fig. 5), or skin (Fig. 6). Such periapical flare-ups are termed a *phoenix abscess*. Phoenix abscessation is exceedingly painful [18]. In canine dentistry, this most commonly occurs secondary to endodontic disease of the maxillary fourth premolar (carnassial tooth); hence, the term *carnassial abscess*. Phoenix abscesses can occur in association with any tooth, especially the cuspids. In cats, the phoenix abscess is usually caused by a fractured canine. Because of the shortness of the feline nose, however, the infection from this tooth fistulates below the eye. Antibiotics control the acute infection, but the chronic infection remains; invariably, the problem reoccurs if the offending tooth is not treated effectively.

Painful local abscessation with or without fistulation is not the only problem that occurs with endodontic compromise. Systemic problems may also occur. The blood vessels in the area pick up the periapical bacteria and spread them to other areas of the body [19]. In human beings, oral bacteremias have been linked to valvular endocarditis, chronic obstructive pulmonary disease, diabetes mellitus, adverse pregnancy effects, strokes, and heart attacks [20]. It has been shown in animal studies that the liver and kidneys can be affected by oral bacteremias. This is a result of the formation of microabscesses on these organs, which, over time, decreases their efficiency [21].

Therapy

The goal of endodontic therapy is to maintain a vital pulp system. Failing in maintaining pulp vitality, the goal is to remove the infection from the endodontic system while leaving the tooth in place. Thus, endodontic therapy is composed of two main branches: vital pulp therapy (direct and

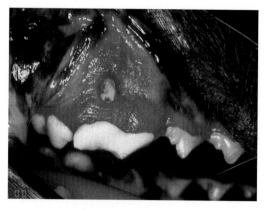

Fig. 5. Draining tract above a fractured maxillary fourth premolar in a dog.

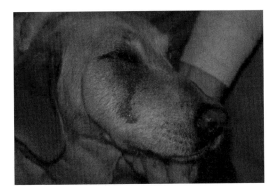

Fig. 6. Classic carnassial abscess in a dog.

indirect pulp capping) and nonvital pulp therapy (root canal, surgical root canal, and apexification).

Patient preparation

In many cases, fresh tooth fractures are the result of concussive trauma. It should be ensured that the patient is free of any neurologic or other systemic problems before the induction of general anesthesia by clinical examination and appropriate laboratory and radiographic evaluation. As important as prompt therapy is, the patient as a whole must be considered.

Endodontic therapy is an involved procedure; therefore, the patient must be in good health. Preoperative blood panels and three-view thoracic radiographs should be considered, especially in patients older than 7 years of age. If the tooth is a minor tooth and the patient is medically compromised, exodontics may be a better option.

Perioperative antibiotics (ampicillin or clindamycin administered intravenously over 15 minutes) should be administered in cases of abscessed nonvital teeth, especially in immune-compromised patients [14]. Pre- and postoperative antibiotic therapy is controversial for most endodontic therapies, and the decision is left up to the individual practitioner (vital pulp therapy by direct pulp capping is an exception).

A regional nerve block should be administered as well as some form of anti-inflammatory agent, and analgesic medication should be part of the anesthetic regimen, especially in the case of an infected tooth. A nonsteroidal anti-inflammatory agent given before the root canal therapy is an effective means of pain control [22].

Localized surgical site preparation

Perform a complete dental prophylaxis to prepare the oral cavity for as aseptic an oral procedure as possible. After the prophylaxis, the mouth should be rinsed with a 0.12% chlorhexidine gluconate solution. The surgeon should wear a cap, mask, and sterile gloves.

The tooth to be treated should be examined clinically and radiographically for periodontal pockets, potential neoplasms, significant periapical lucencies or incomplete apexes, and vertical or crown root fractures, because these findings can markedly affect the prognosis. The client should be informed of such findings as well as the effect of them on the prognosis before initiation of therapy.

Vital pulp therapy

Vital pulp therapy is the subdivision of endodontics that is concerned with maintaining the living tooth. Vital tooth maintenance is a common procedure in human dentistry but is less used in our veterinary animal patients for the following reasons:

1. Complicated crown fractures are not promptly discovered in veterinary patients.
2. Standard endodontic therapy (root canal therapy) has been shown to have a higher long-term success rate than vital pulp therapy in domestic dogs with prolonged pulp exposure.
3. Deep caries lesions (which are the most common reason for pulp capping in human beings) are less common in veterinary patients.
4. Veterinary patients are less likely to be presented for follow-up as a result of the need for anesthesia for dental radiology (partly because of our patients' failure to demonstrate pain and partly because of scheduling, fiscal constraints, or fear of anesthesia on the part of the client), which risks delayed or complete failure to recognize and treat the bacterial pulpitis [23].

Delayed diagnosis of complicated crown fractured teeth compromises the long-term success of vital pulp therapy. Studies have shown that the major prognostic indicator of vital pulp therapy is the duration of exposure [42]. A recent animal study showed that exposures between 48 hours and 1 week have a success rate of 41.4%, which drops to 23.2% with exposures longer than 1 week [2]. These statistics should be compared with the 100% success rate achieved with vital pulp therapy when it is performed after planned iatrogenic pulp exposure [23] and the 88.2% success rate if vital pulp therapy is performed less than 48 hours after pulp exposure because of a complicated fracture [2]. Thus, without prompt therapy, vital pulp therapy holds a poor long-term prognosis and should only be considered in cases of planned iatrogenic crown reduction procedures or near-complete or complete pulpal exposure during restorative procedures. An exception is made in the case of a fractured immature tooth of unknown duration in pets less than 2 years of age, with the aim of strengthening the tooth (by continued secondary dentin deposition) or achieving root end closure (apexogenesis) and hence a standard root canal therapy–ready tooth. Studies have shown that 75% (n = 4) immature (<18 months of age) teeth continued development and achieved apexogenesis sufficient to perform standard root canal therapy regardless of exposure duration [23]. Such use of vital pulp therapy requires committed and fiscally sound clients dedicated to radiographic monitoring of the therapy. Patients rarely show signs of oral pain. If therapy fails, the client generally does not know of the problem; therefore, the pet suffers until a phoenix abscess forms or radiographs are exposed. This may be a long time in coming. Subjective client assessment of tooth vitality in vital pulp therapy– treated teeth has been proven to be unreliable [9]. Inability of clients and veterinarians to monitor vitality of the teeth subjectively, combined with the much higher rate of success with standard root canal therapy, makes this a poor choice when the time of exposure is not known. Hence, complicated crown fractures of prolonged (>48 hours) or unknown duration in mature (>18 months of age) canine patients should immediately be treated with standard root canal therapy [23].

   Taking this into consideration, the indications for vital pulp therapy are
      as follows:
 1. Pulpal and near-pulpal exposures during restorative procedures
 2. Crown reduction procedures for orthodontic (Fig. 7) or disarming
    procedures
 3. Fractures of immature permanent teeth (those without a radiographic
    apex) of less than 2 weeks (Fig. 8) in which there is no radiographic
    (periapical lucency) or clinical (necrotic pulp or intrinsic staining) sign of
    pulpal nonvitality
 4. Complicated crown fractures of acutely fractured teeth (<48 hours) [9]

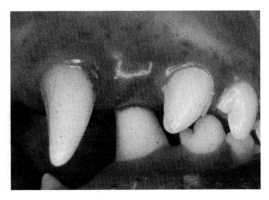

Fig. 7. Palatine trauma secondary to a base-narrow bite in a Standard Poodle, which could be corrected by coronal amputation and vital pulp therapy. This could also be seen in class II malocclusions as well as in wry occlusions. Another option for this case would be orthodontic therapy.

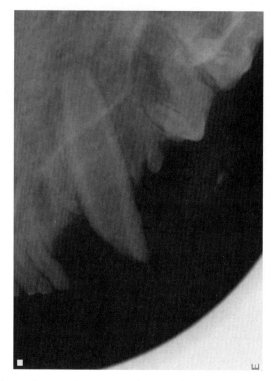

Fig. 8. Incomplete apex in a recently fractured feline maxillary canine tooth.

Indirect pulp capping

The indication for indirect pulp capping is near-pulpal exposure [9,24]. Near-pulpal exposure typically occurs in cases of significant tooth structure removal for restorative procedures, but it can also occur with mild fractures. This procedure is performed to protect the pulp from environmental contaminants (eg, bacteria) by sealing the dentinal tubules with two to three layers of restoratives.

Technique

Step 1: Ensure that there is no pulpal exposure by exploring the entire surface of the defect with a sterile explorer or sterile fine endodontic file (pathfinder).

Step 2: Expose a dental radiograph and evaluate for any signs of pulpal nonvitality. Any sign of nonvitality is a contraindication for vital pulp therapy, and nonvital therapy should be performed.

Step 3: Remove any carious or diseased dentin and enamel with a carbide or diamond burr or spoon excavator. Perform the restorative preparation necessary for the selected final restorative.

Step 4: Medicant placement. There are currently three materials in use for the initial layer of this procedure: calcium hydroxide, zinc oxide eugenol (ZOE) and glass ionomer cements. Calcium hydroxide and ZOE have been shown to rid carious dentin of bacteria almost completely when used as the base layer. These materials should be placed in a thin layer according to the package directions. The purpose of this layer is to protect the pulp from the acid etching. In addition, if this is used for a deep carious lesion in which some carious dentin is intentionally left behind, it helps to decrease the bacterial contamination.

Step 5: Place the selected restoration (typically composite) by standard methods and finish smoothly.

Recheck dental radiographs in 6 months and, ideally, every 6 months for 3 years.

Direct pulp capping

Indications for direct pulp capping include accidental pulpal exposure during restoration preparation or after crown reduction, pulp exposure of any duration in a vital immature tooth as long as radiographic follow-up is ensured, and pulp exposure confirmed to be less than 48 hours in mature teeth (controversial) [9,21,24,42].

Direct pulp capping after coronal crown or pulpal exposure during restorative procedures carries a good prognosis [23]. This is likely attributable to aseptic technique, a short duration of exposure, and a decrease in the amount of inflammatory trauma. Direct pulp capping performed as a result of iatrogenic exposure during cavity preparation carries a good prognosis but less than iatrogenic crown height reduction likely because of contamination with bacteria from the carious dentin. Acute (<48 hours) fractures can do well when treated with vital pulp therapy. Prolonged pulp exposure is a poor prognostic indicator for a long-term successful outcome with vital pulp therapy regardless of the age of the animal. Thus, vital pulp therapy is generally not recommended in pulp exposure of longer than 48 hours in mature patients. Some veterinary dentists think that any exposure in a mature tooth should not be treated in this manner because of the relatively high failure rate of 11.8% in exposures less than 48 hours and increasing with longer exposures [2]. Vital pulp therapy is an effective procedure in immature teeth regardless of the duration of exposure. Although the procedure generally fails long term after prolonged exposure, almost all teeth treated in this manner survive long enough to achieve apexogenesis and to receive standard root canal therapy [23].

Technique

The reader should refer to the previous section regarding general guidelines for patient preparation for endodontic therapy; however, for vital pulp therapy, antibiotic therapy is initiated to decrease bacterial contamination [25]. Fast-acting corticosteroids (Solu-Delta-Cortef; Pharmacia and Upjohn, Kalamazoo, MI) may be administered parentally to decrease pulpal inflammation caused by the trauma or the procedure.

Step 1: If treating a fractured tooth, determine the vitality of the tooth as evidenced by a pink pulp that bleeds on gentle superficial probing.

Step 2: Expose a dental radiograph and look for signs of nonvitality (eg, periradicular osseous rarefaction, increased root canal diameter). If present, proceed to nonvital therapy.

Step 3: The oral cavity is prepared with an antiseptic solution (0.12% chlorhexidine gluconate [25]), and as sterile a technique as can be achieved in the oral cavity is followed throughout the procedure.

Step 4: Remove all the diseased pulp, and achieve a depth in the canal sufficient to allow deposition of the materials that are used to seal the tooth (generally, approximately 5–7 mm). Removal of the inflamed pulp with minimal disturbance of the underlying healthy pulp to be maintained is accomplished with a spoon excavator or sterile round carbide [25] or diamond [21] burr. This author's choice is a diamond burr because it is less inflammatory than the carbide burr and, in addition, seems to control hemorrhage effectively, thereby decreasing procedure time. Use copious amounts of water or sterile saline during a partial coronal pulpectomy to avoid heat necrosis of the remaining pulp.

Step 5: Hemorrhage is controlled with dampened sterile paper points or cotton pellets. Hemorrhage that is not controlled within 5 minutes is usually indicative of inflamed pulp. If this is the case, amputation of another 1 to 2 mm of pulp is indicated to ensure that only healthy pulp remains.

Step 6: Placement of pulp dressing. Classically, the first layer of pulp medicament is calcium hydroxide [42] in the form of a powder or a self- or light-cured paste (Ultrablend Plus; Ultradent Products, Jordon, UT). This is a basic substance (pH 13), such that it is not only antibacterial but irritates the remaining odontoblasts into apical retreat. These apically retreating odontoblasts deposit a dentinal bridge of tertiary and/or reparative dentin in their wake to protect the pulp, which is visible radiographically [9]. Given that calcium hydroxide is irritating to the dentinal pulp, the product should be carefully placed on the healthy coronal pulp stump (eg, placement with a retrograde filler) and gently tamped down (eg, with sterile paper points). Forceful apical thrusting of this or any medication is contraindicated because it forces the product into the pulp, creating significantly more inflammation and risking pulpal death [21]. A new product called mineral trioxide aggregate (MTA) (ProRoot; Densply, Tulsa, OK) has shown promise as a pulp dressing [24]. It is effective in stimulating new calcified material. In addition, the neutral pH does not increase the pulpal inflammation. The negative aspect of this decreased inflammatory effect is the loss of the antibacterial effect. An additional drawback has been the dark staining of the tooth that this product can cause. The recent development of a tooth-colored MTA makes this less of a concern, however. This author's choice is still calcium hydroxide; however, either product is acceptable. Other recommended pulpal dressings include direct application of glass ionomer or filled composites to the pulp. It has been reported in the human literature that placing composite directly onto the pulp is no less effective than other means of direct vital pulp therapy [24].

Step 7: An intermediate layer is then placed on top of the direct pulp dressing to act as an additional layer of protection versus bacterial contamination as well as a base for the final restorative. A glass ionomer is generally chosen for this purpose [9,26] because it forms a chemical bond with the dentin without the need for etching or adhesive application [27].

Step 8: A dentinal bonded composite resin is used to seal the access site. Dental adhesives applied according to the package directions are critical because they enhance the marginal seal and decrease microleakage [28].

Step 9: A postoperative radiograph is taken to evaluate the filling.

Step 10: The restoration is finished with the operator's choice of equipment (fine diamond burr or polishing disk). After this, it is recommended that an additional coating of unfilled resin be placed over the final restoration [29]. This fills in any microdefects created in the seal by means of polymerization shrinkage.

For step-by-step illustrations of this procedure, the reader is referred to an article by Niemiec [26].

Follow-up

Recheck radiographs 6 months after surgery and, ideally, every 6 months thereafter for at least 3 years to ensure continued pulpal vitality. This is recommended because of the common finding of vitality at 6- and 18-month radiographic follow-ups but nonvitality at the 3-year radiographic follow-up [2]. Therefore, client compliance must be gauged before the performance of vital pulp therapy. Signs of continued pulp vitality include a decrease in the width of the root canal system, lack of periapical lucency, and a root canal system that is the same width as the contralateral canal (Fig. 9) [30]. The canals are not a perfect cylinder, and a change in angle affects the apparent canal size; therefore, evaluate the size of the canal with knowledge of the angle [30]. Dentinal bridge formation alone is not a reliable marker of vitality.

Reasons for failure of vital pulp therapy (Fig. 10) are numerous [9]. In human dentistry, the most common reason for continued pulpal

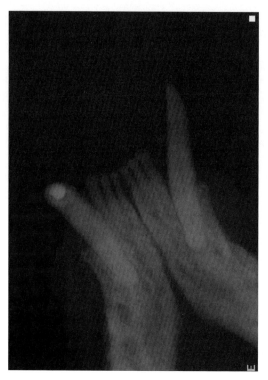

Fig. 9. Two-year vital pulp therapy recheck radiograph. The root canals appear to be of the same diameter, and there is no evidence of periapical lucency. This seems to be a successful procedure.

inflammation is microleakage of bacteria around the final restoration [31]. Studies have shown that the dentinal bridge is not an effective bacterial barrier [32]; therefore, the intermediate layer and coronal restoration are critical in ensuring a successful outcome. Meticulous patient and oral cavity preparation and attention to asepsis are also important, as is constant vigilance (during tooth brushing or radiographic follow-up) for any obvious loss of the coronal seal. Other causes of vital pulp therapy failure include infection before or during therapy and inadequate removal of inflamed or infected pulp tissue. Significant pulpal hemorrhage is also a reason for vital pulp therapy failure. Therefore, gentle tissue handling throughout the procedure, administration of copious coolant during the partial pulpectomy procedure, and nonforceful application of the pulp medicants onto the pulp tissue are crucial. Corticosteroids can be used to pretreat or ameliorate the inflammation.

Nonvital pulp therapy

Nonvital pulp therapy treats not only dead and infected pulp but significantly diseased pulp tissue that is suspected of becoming nonvital.

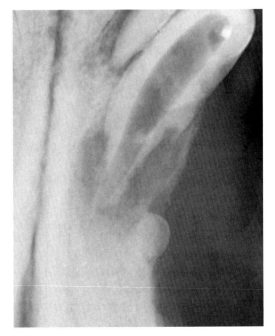

Fig. 10. Nine-year follow-up of vital pulp therapy (none performed previously). Note the severe periapical lucency and root resorption. This is a case of obvious failure.

Apparently vital teeth of unknown pulp exposure duration or pets belonging to noncompliant clients are correctly and definitively treated in this manner. Treatment modalities include standard root canal therapy, Weber root canal therapy, apexification, and surgical root canal therapy with retrograde filling. If these therapies fail or if the client is not interested in such therapies, extraction is an alternative.

Standard (nonsurgical) root canal therapy

Standard root canal therapy is a highly effective means of controlling the pain and infection of endodontic disease [43] while retaining the function of the tooth for the patient.

Any tooth can be treated endodontically. The decision for root canal therapy versus extraction should be influenced by the relative importance of the tooth to the animal (strategic teeth [cuspid and carnassials]) and the client (esthetic teeth [incisors]).

Extraction procedures should be considered only as a salvage procedure for the canines in dogs and cats and for the upper fourth premolar and lower first molar (carnassial teeth). There are several reasons why extraction should be avoided whenever possible. Extraction is a much more painful option because of the root sizes of our veterinary patients (eg, the root of the cuspid is wider and approximately twice as long as the crown). These are not simple extractions. They are complicated oral operations usually requiring a surgical approach via a gingival incision as well as bone removal and suturing; as such, carry an inherent risk of surgical complications. Finally, extraction causes the patient to lose the function of the tooth as well as that of its opposing counterpart in most instances.

When considering adding endodontic therapy to one's practice, the clinician must carefully consider several important points. First of all is the cost of the armamentarium. The cost to equip a dental operatory for basic endodontic therapy is greater than $20,000. This includes dental radiography and development equipment, a high-speed air-driven drill system, all sizes of files and gutta percha points in human and veterinary lengths, several endodontic cements, spreaders and pluggers, and restorative materials (including a light curing gun). An additional concern is the tremendous technique-related sensitivity of the procedure. If not performed absolutely perfectly, the endodontic therapy is likely to fail and the patient is no better off than if nothing was done. Perfection is paramount and necessitates that the practitioner spend hours in laboratories as well as practicing on cadavers or extracted teeth perfecting skills before treating an actual patient. Finally, the practitioner should determine how many root canals are likely to be performed. It is likely not worth the expense or in the patient's best interest to offer endodontic therapy unless the practitioner would be doing three standard root canal therapies per week on average. That being said, when 10% of dogs need a procedure, there are many potential candidates.

Root canal therapy has three ordered components: access, cleaning and shaping, and obturation [21]. They are separate steps, but each one builds on the prior step, such that if one is not performed correctly, the next step is more difficult if not impossible. Therefore, perform each step while anticipating the needs of the next component step, and you are more likely to stay on the right track.

Step 1: access

Access is the hole made in the tooth surface for the introduction of files and filling material [33]. As previously stated, the operator should take the needs of the next step into account during this step. The needs of the next step (cleaning and shaping) are straight-line access to the apex (or as straight as possible) and enough room at the access so that the master file and cone can move freely in the access opening. Therefore, the fracture site is generally not a good access point. For some incisor teeth and feline canines, however, the fracture site can be used against a tooth-weakening additional access site [9].

Outlining access sites for all teeth is beyond the scope of this article; however, there are some guidelines. First, using your knowledge of tooth anatomy as well as palpating the juga, you should be able to approximate the apex. The point that provides the straightest and shortest line is ideal. Do not make access holes over incisal edges, cusp tips, or developmental grooves if at all possible, however [21]. For canines in dogs, the access is on the mesial aspect 2 to 3 mm above the gingival margin directed at the apex (Fig. 11) [9]. The distal and mesial buccal roots of the maxillary carnassials are prepared by palpating the juga and making an access site above them approximately half of the way up the crown on the buccal surface (Fig. 12). The palatine root of this tooth can be accessed through the same hole as the mesiobuccal via the transcoronal approach, or a separate hole can be made directly over the root (Fig. 13) [9]. Molar teeth are generally accessed through a V- or Y-shaped hole in the occlusal surface [21]. The exception is the lower first molar, whose mesial root is accessed on the lingual side of the mesial developmental groove.

Access size is an art. The law of tooth conservation dictates as small a hole as possible so as to retain as much strength as possible in the tooth [35]. Accordingly, inexperienced operators create a small access hole, thus leading to insufficient access and making the procedure more difficult [21]. This results in three common problems. First, it makes finding the actual canals difficult, because access only enters the pulp chamber in most instances. The root canal is much smaller and often more difficult to find than the accessed pulp chamber or its horn. A small access site can make this difficult, increasing anesthetic time. Next, if the access is too small, the master file or cone binds in the access, giving the erroneous feeling that the canal is completely cleaned. This leads to short fills and the necessary refiling and refilling. Finally, a small access hole binds the file in the coronal third, which prevents the file from easily following the canal curves or irregularities. This results in errors of instrumentation, such as ledging, gouging, or zipping. Once errors of instrumentation have occurred, correction is difficult and may make successful endodontic therapy nearly impossible.

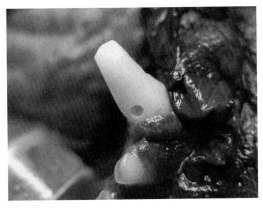

Fig. 11. Approximate access site for the canine tooth in a dog.

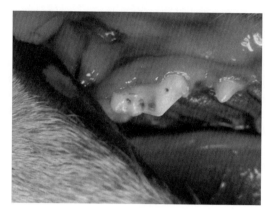

Fig. 12. Approximate access sites for the maxillary fourth premolar in a dog.

This author's recommendation is to approximate the master file size based on preoperative radiographs. By using a file and measuring a rough working length, you should be able to judge the approximate diameter of the master file at the access before making your approach. By looking at the master file, make the access slightly larger than the diameter of the file at that point. This avoids having to increase the access size after wasting time and possibly damaging the root canal. In large-breed young dog canines, expect the access hole to be large.

Step 2: Sterilization (cleaning and shaping the canals)

Sterilization is the longest and most tedious part of root canal therapy; however, when performed correctly, it facilitates the final step. The final step, obturation, requires a completely clean canal that is slightly tapered

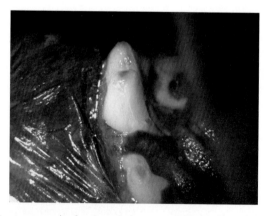

Fig. 13. Approximate access site for the palatine root of the maxillary fourth premolar if not using the transcoronal approach.

toward the apex. The taper avoids binding the filling cones in the coronal section of the canal.

The first step of sterilization is to determine the working length [9]. The working length is approximated by measuring the distance on the preoperative radiographs and gently introducing a small file to the apical constricture. With the file tip at the apex, a dental radiograph is exposed (Fig. 14). This should show the file at the apical constricture. If it is not, the file needs to be repositioned apically by means of a gentle watch-winding technique until radiographic confirmation of the working length is achieved. The working length is then recorded in the patient's file. In stenotic canals of old dogs, the canal is too constricted to fit even a number 15 file to the apex.

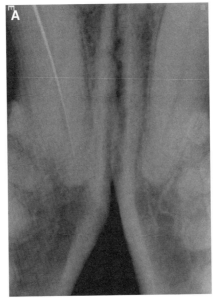

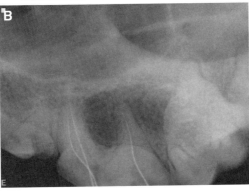

Fig. 14. Working length determination in a canine tooth (*A*) and maxillary fourth premolar (*B*) in a dog.

If this is the case, follow the crown-down procedure to achieve the working length. A file should never be forced.

There are two main methods for achieving the desired cornucopia shape of the sterilized canal: crown down and step back. The step-back technique [9] is performed as follows. The entire canal is filed until the master file size reaches the apex. After this, increase the file by one size and take this and each subsequent file 1 mm shorter than the previous file.

The crown-down technique [36] is initiated with files several sizes larger than the anticipated master file. The filing starts by opening the coronal third of the canal wide enough to accept the wider nonworking portion of the master file without binding. The middle third is then instrumented to approximately three file sizes larger than the master file. Once the coronal two thirds of the canal has been instrumented (before enlargement), a small file is gently introduced to the working length. After this, subsequent files are carefully worked at the apex as evidenced by measured endodontic stops until the master file moves freely in the canal.

The crown-down technique is preferred over the step-back technique for the following reasons. Both techniques place more pressure on the initial files than on the later ones. In the crown-down technique, these are the larger files, which are less prone to separation. In addition, this technique risks less damage (eg, transportation, gouging, zipping, perforation) of the fragile apex. This is because fewer files actually work the apex and the increased size of the coronal two thirds of the canal allows freer movement of the files in the apical third, which allows the file to follow the canal curvatures more readily. Finally, by opening up the coronal section, it allows for easier irrigation of the canal. Therefore, coronal debris is not carried to the apex or forced apically, allowing more complete irrigation as well as decreasing the chances of forcing the irrigation solution and bacteria periapically. This is especially important when using 5.25% sodium hypochlorite as the irrigant.

There are two major types of instrumentation: hand and rotary. Rotary files are generally made of nickel titanium (NiTi) and are designed to work with a special slow-speed handpiece. The handpiece should ideally have an automatic reverse system that "backs off" in the case of undue binding or pressure. These are excellent if somewhat expensive units for rapid preparations of canals (ProSystemGT, Tulsa Dental Products, Tulsa, OK; Lightspeed, Lightspeed Technology, San Antonio, TX). NiTi files can and do break and must be used carefully because they can easily damage the canal if used improperly. The reader is referred to the manufacturer's instructions for the particular instrument for directions on use.

Hand files are still the most common type in veterinary endodontics. There are three types of hand files: Hedstrom or H-files, K-files, and K-reamers.

Hedstrom files [21] are the sharpest and the most fragile of the endodontic files. These are metal blanks that are machined down to a spiral groove. This makes them more prone to fracture than a similar sized K-file. Therefore, they are only used in a push-pull fashion. They are best used in the coronal two thirds of the canal, because the push-pull motion does not tend to follow canal curvature well. These are the most efficient files and quickly achieve the crown-down technique.

K-files [21] are twisted triangular blanks. They may be used in a push-pull fashion or in an insert one-quarter turn and pull technique. K-files cannot be twisted (reamed) more than one-quarter turn without risk of fracture. These are of intermediate aggressiveness and can be used at the apex.

K-reamers [21] are similar to K-files but are less twisted, making them less aggressive but stronger than K-files. K-reamers can be used in a push-pull or one-quarter turn technique but are best used as a reamer with numerous clockwise turns. When used in a reamer fashion, they not only file the canal but carry the debris out of it. They are also useful at the apex, and because they can be highly rotated, they are good in curved canals. Because of the longer spiral cutting edge of the veterinary length (K-Reamers; Dr. Shipp's Laboratories, Tucson, AZ), which better matches the veterinary length gutta percha points, they are this author's choice when performing root canal therapy on large-breed canine cuspids.

Regardless of the method or file chosen, filing (especially at the apex) must be performed with a feather-light touch. If files are forced in any way, there are dire consequences. Ledging or gouging the canal is a common complication when too much apical force is applied. If the file is turned excessively, binding and file separation can occur.

Once the operator has begun filing at the apex, irrigation is critical. The canal should be irrigated between the use of at least every other (if not each) file size, with full (5.25%) or half-strength sodium hypochlorite [36] at a dose of at least 1 mL. This should be done with a side-exit endodontic needle without excessive pressure. The apex should be opened to at least an International Standards Organization (ISO) size 25 file before irrigation to avoid forcing the irrigant periapically.

Between the use of every other file size, a small file should be introduced to the apex and quickly worked (recapitulation) [9]. Recapitulation stirs up any diseased dentinal debris and avoids packing it at the apex, which makes further instrumentation more difficult.

The operator should have a rough idea of the master cone size based on the preoperative radiograph, but there are two additional indications that filing is complete: completely clean white filings are achieved and file binding at the apex. Most texts recommend filing until the third file after the first to bind at the apex [21]. Once the operator thinks that he or she has completely filed the canal, a gutta percha point is inserted to the apex. Ideally, the point should reach the apex and fit snugly so that when it is removed, "apical tug back" is felt. A radiograph should be exposed at this point to ensure that the point fills the apex and, ideally, the remainder of the canal (Fig. 15). Once the master cone has been documented, the canal is flushed liberally and

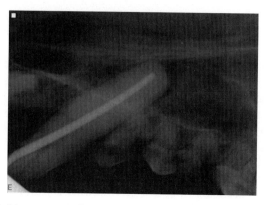

Fig. 15. Master cone radiograph to ensure proper fit of the master cone.

dried with sterile paper points. If the paper points are dirty or bloody, this is an indication of incomplete cleaning (underinstrumentation) or apical perforation (overinstrumentation). Determine the repeatable position of the debris or blood on the paper points to aid causal determination in addition to exposing a dental radiograph to ensure that apical perforation has not occurred. Once perforation is ruled out, reinitiate cleaning and shaping until the paper points are clean.

Step 3: Obturation

The goal of obturation is to eliminate all pathways of leakage into the endodontic system from the oral cavity or periradicular space as well as sealing within the endodontic system any infective agents that cannot be removed by cleaning and irrigation (dentinal tubule infection) [34]. There are two components of the endodontic fill: gutta percha and sealant cement. Gutta percha consists of an inert rubber with zinc oxide and silver additives. Gutta percha is soft and pliable in the beta stage and can be softened by heat or chemicals. There are numerous types of sealant cements that function to fill in any imperfections of the canals that the gutta percha may miss as well as to seal the dentinal tubules and any accessory or lateral canals. The sealer selected depends on the type of obturation as well as on different endodontic presentations or complications. There are different cements for different indications, and practitioners should have several types available and know how and when they are best used. When used correctly, the combination of gutta percha and sealer cement provides a bacteria-tight seal that resists the apical migration of bacteria. It should be noted that most of the fill should be with gutta percha.

The first step in obturation is application of the sealant [34]. There are several methods available: paste injection, spiral filler, file placement, and placing on master cone. When performing cold obturation techniques, a relatively large amount of sealer cement is used because some is placed on each accessory cone. This is because of the inferior three-dimensional fill with cold gutta percha techniques; the paste helps to fill and seal any irregularities or lateral and/or accessory canals [34]. As the first step in cold gutta percha application, this author fills the canal with sealant, using a spiral filler. In the case of large canals, paste injection is used before spiral filling. When performing softened gutta percha techniques, however, the walls should only be coated with a small amount of sealant cement, allowing the softened gutta percha to fill any irregularities [34].

Paste injection is accomplished by mixing a sealer cement and injecting it into the canal with a syringe attached to a needle (in large-breed canine cuspids, a spinal needle is used). The needle tip should be placed at the apex and the cement injected slowly until the canal is full. Once sealer cement is extruded from the access point, the needle is slowly withdrawn while injecting the paste to fill the canal and minimize air voids. Because this method can leave air voids, it is not recommended as a sole means of fill. Paste injection is not an acceptable means for softened gutta percha techniques.

Spiral filling is performed with lentulo paste filler on a 10:1 reduction gear low-speed handpiece. The filler is coated with paste and inserted to the apex. The file is started in a forward (clockwise) direction and pumped carefully to the apex. This is performed a couple of times to coat the walls or is repeated until the canal is full.

File filling is accomplished by coating a sterile small file with paste and inserting it to the apex. The file is turned counterclockwise while being slowly withdrawn. This process is repeated at least three times depending on the obturation method chosen.

Master point coating

Master point coating involves excessively coating the master point (and any accessory points) with sealant before placement into the canal to the apex. This technique is obviously not an option in softened gutta percha techniques and should not be used alone in cold gutta percha techniques, except in straight canals, because it can leave voids.

Gutta percha application

Gutta percha may be placed "cold" or softened. Cold gutta percha techniques refer to those in which the gutta percha is placed in its solid state. The major means of softening (plasticizing) the gutta percha is by heating (or partially melting). Softening by means of chemicals has become outdated since it was recognized that significant shrinkage occurs on setting. Thermo-mechanical (McSpadden) filling is currently experiencing a renascence with NiTi instruments (Microseal condensers; SybronEndo, Orange, CA).

Cold lateral condensation

Cold lateral condensation [9,34] is performed by placing a master cone in the canal that is the same size as the last file to reach the apex. A radiograph is exposed to ensure that the point reaches the working length. It is this author's experience that selecting a point that stops 1 to 2 mm short of the apex is ideal, because the point can be plugged to the apex, thus creating an even tighter seal (like a plug). Once the master cone has been selected, squeezing with cotton pliers at the access site should mark it. This allows the operator to know if it binds short of the apex during obturation. The addition of cement can be enough to make the master cone not fit.

The sealer cement is then placed into the canal by means of one of the aforementioned methods. After this, the master cone is placed into the canal. The previously placed mark should come to or within 1 mm of the access. Next, the gutta percha is excised flush to the access point with a red-hot beaver tail instrument or other heated device. The transected point is then compressed (plugged) toward the apex with an endodontic plugger. A radiograph should be exposed at this point to ensure a good apical seal as evidenced by lack of voids in the apical area. If the radiograph reveals a less than ideal apical fill, the cone should be removed and replaced. If the point stopped short, it should be replaced with one of a smaller size; if it does not fill the apex, a point one size larger should be selected. If obturation of the apex is not optimal after a few attempts, cleaning and sterilization should be repeated.

Once the apical seal is radiographically verified, the process of obturation can continue, with lateral condensation as necessary. An endodontic spreader is chosen based on canal size (the larger the canal diameter, the larger is the spreader). The spreader is inserted firmly toward the apex until it stops. The same or one ISO size smaller than the spreader-sized accessory cone is coated with sealer cement. The spreader is carefully removed from the canal by rotating the spreader 180° to avoid dislodging the master cone, and the accessory cone is immediately inserted into the canal, cut off, and plugged. This process is continued until the pulp canal is full.

Softened gutta percha techniques

Currently, the most common way to soften gutta percha is by heat. There are several methods of placement of heat-softened gutta percha [9,21,34].

Vertical condensation

In vertical condensation, the gutta percha is heated and injected via a cannula (Obtura II; Obtura Corporation, Fenton, MO) or placed with a file (SucessFil; Hygenic, Whaledent, Manwah, NJ) into the pulp canal, after which it is compacted (vertically condensed via endodontic pluggers) to the apex. Vertical condensation of heat-softened gutta percha is best done in approximately 5-mm increments. To accomplish this, coat the walls of the canal with sealant cement, select a cannula based on the master file, and place approximately 5 mm of gutta percha to the apex. Using a veterinary endodontic plugger, compress it to the apical constricture. Failing this, ensure an adequate apical seal radiographically. If the apex is filled correctly, proceed to back-filling with additional gutta percha to the access hole. If the apex is poorly filled, remove the gutta percha and reinitiate the obturation process.

Vertical and lateral condensation

Vertical and lateral condensation of heated gutta percha is performed by lightly coating the pulp canal walls as previously described. Select a gutta percha cone slightly larger than the master cone so that it stops just short of the apex, and insert until it binds in the canal. Using the hot tip of the electric spreader (System B; EIE Analytic Technology, San Diego, CA), the gutta percha is heat softened as well as condensed apically and laterally simultaneously. If this fills the apex well as evidenced radiographically, accessory cones are selected and the pulp canal is filled in a similar manner.

Core carrier

The core carrier method employs heated gutta percha using plastic or titanium blanks as carriers of softened gutta percha [34]. These blanks (Thermafil plus; Tulsa Dental Products, Tulsa, OK) (Soft-Core; Soft-Core Systems, North Richmond Hills, TX) are the same size as the rotary endodontic files and provide effective and fast obturation. Unfortunately, their taper is matched to rotary and not ISO hand instruments; therefore, they are not useful after hand instrumentation unless special files are obtained. A recent veterinary study has proved that coating sterile stainless-steel files in heated gutta percha and intentionally separating them at the coronal access site can be an effective means of obturation [37]. This is an especially valuable technique for use in the stenotic canals of older large-breed dogs.

Chemically softened gutta percha

Gutta percha can be softened using chemicals [9,34]. The most effective chemical for this is chloroform because it is fast and effective at softening gutta percha. Chloroform is carcinogenic, however. Eucalyptus oil and xylol are other chemicals that can affect gutta percha softening, although they are not nearly as effective. To perform chemical softening of gutta percha, soak the point in the solution until it is soft (occurs in seconds with chloroform) and then insert the chemically softened point into the canal and compress. Such fitting of the cone can be performed before sealer cement placement in that the custom cone is removed after a few minutes. The sealer cement is then placed, followed by replacement of the "custom cone," which is vertically condensed with a cold endodontic plugger to the apex. A less preferred method (by the author) involves placing the chemically softened gutta percha in the canal after it has been standardly coated with cement and the point has been plugged to the apex. Finally, cold lateral condensation is performed to back-fill the canal.

Thermolateral condensation [34] is a new spin on an old technique called the McSpadden technique. The theory behind thermolateral condensation is that a file-like instrument (compactor) on a low-speed handpiece simultaneously chops up and heats the gutta percha using friction. The softened gutta percha is then compressed and forced into irregularities by the instrument. A master cone one size larger than the master file is selected, and the canal is coated with cement. The master cone is inserted into the canal as far as it goes. The "compactor" is placed into the canal, turned on, and then advanced toward the apex. Verify adequacy of the apical fill radiographically. If it is deemed satisfactory, commence the back-fill with additional points.

Regardless of the obturation method chosen, a complete homogeneous fill of the entire canal without voids is critical to crucial to ensure nonsurgical endodontic success (Fig. 16) [34]. Complete obturation of the apex is critical. If the apex is incompletely obturated, failure is likely. In addition, recent studies have proven that complete obturation of the entire canal and a good coronal seal are important for a successful endodontic outcome [34].

After endodontic obturation, all access sites are cleaned and restored with the material of the operator's chosen restorative material(s). An intermediate layer (generally of glass ionomer) is recommended below the final restorative [21] to act as a base for the final restoration while adding an additional layer of protection from the oral environment. It is considered an absolutely critical step if using a eugenol-containing sealer cement and a composite restoration, because the eugenol has been reported to interfere with the setting of the composite [38,39]. There is a recent study indicating that eugenol-containing cements may not adversely affect the bonding of composite, however [40]. Composite restorations are typically used after endodontic therapy. This final step must also be performed correctly, because it has been shown that the coronal restoration is also critical to a successful endodontic outcome [41].

Reasons for failure

There are numerous causes of failure of standard root canal therapy. The various causes of standard endodontic failures can generally be traced to continued infection stemming from improper technique during any of the three stages of standard root canal therapy or when the coronal seal is lost

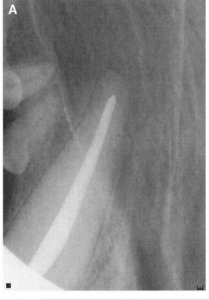

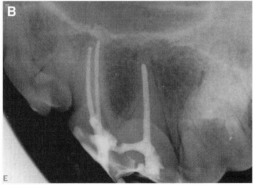

Fig. 16. Complete obturation of a canine tooth (*A*) and maxillary fourth premolar (*B*) ensures a good prognosis.

after root canal treatment. Regardless of the initial cause, the cause of all failure is leakage [43]. Problems can occur at any point during therapy from access, to cleaning and shaping and sterilization, to obturation, and, finally, to coronal sealing (Fig. 17). Therefore, the steps discussed previously must be followed to the letter to ensure successful therapy.

Signs of failure

Unfortunately, clinical signs of failure are often inconspicuous and rarely observed. The classic clinical sign of standard endodontic failure is phoenix abscessation (swelling or fistulous tract) from the treated tooth (see Figs. 4

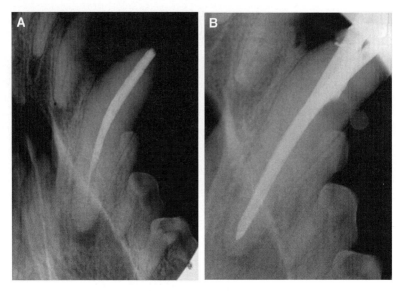

Fig. 17. This root canal was improperly obturated (by a human dentist) several years previously. (*A*) The fill is short by several millimeters, resulting in continued infection as evidenced by the periapical lucency. The tooth was retreated by a veterinary dentist and properly obturated. (*B*) Same tooth at a 6-month recheck.

and 5). Such phoenix abscessation of the standardly treated tooth is rarely observed. The only effective objective way to assess endodontic success is by means of dental radiology. The tooth should be evaluated 9 to 12 months after therapy by dental radiology and at regular intervals thereafter to monitor for any signs of endodontic failure [21]. Radiographic evidence of standard endodontic success is a lack of a novel or resolution of a previous periapical lucency. In the case of a previous periapical lucency, a decrease in the size of the defect is considered to be a positive indicator of success. An endodontically treated tooth that develops a novel periradicular lucency or one with a previously observed periapical lucency that has enlarged since treatment or the last follow-up is radiographic evidence of failed standard root canal therapy (Fig. 18). A lucency that stays the same or initially decreases but then stagnates is a questionable result. This could indicate a noninfected granuloma or cyst, or possibly a low-grade infection. Close monitoring of this tooth clinically and radiographically for signs of failure is recommended. Any negative change in the defect or any clinical signs would be grounds for diagnosing failed root canal therapy.

Treatment of failed standard endodontic therapy

There are several options for treatment of failed standard root canal therapy–treated teeth [9,43]. If the obturation from the standard root canal

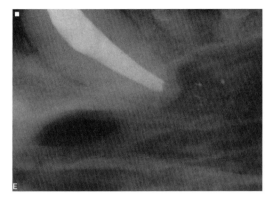

Fig. 18. This root canal failed despite adequate apical fill. This is an indication for surgical root canal therapy and retrograde filling.

therapy is radiographically inadequate, reinstrumentation, including attentive recapitulation and obturation, using a nonsurgical technique is the logical first step. If the obturation appears radiographically sufficient, similar reinstrumentation (including recapitulation) can be attempted, but success is much less likely. There are two basic options for radiographically apparent well-performed initial therapy that fails: surgical endodontic therapy and retrograde filling or extraction. Extraction techniques are covered elsewhere in this issue; surgical root canal therapy is beyond the scope of this article.

Follow-up

Our patients do not show signs of oral pain, and clinical abscesses (phoenix abscess) are rare in dogs and cats. The success or failure of any endodontic therapy cannot be determined without dental radiography. Veterinary patients must have recheck radiographs 6 to 9 months after standard root canal therapy and, ideally, every 6 to 12 months for the remainder of the patient's lifespan. This is easily integrated during the general anesthesia for routine complete dental prophylaxis. Recheck radiographs should at least be performed on a semiannual basis regardless of the need for a prophylaxis in a large-breed dog or a cat in which the clients perform meticulous home care.

Summary

Endodontic disease is a highly prevalent (>10% of all dogs) and insidiously painful process that can have significant local and systemic effects. The root canal system is a delicate organ and is prone to inflammation, infection, and partial and complete necrosis. Vital pulp therapy must be performed quickly, gently, and meticulously if it is to be effective. The relatively high rate of failure in direct pulp capping makes regular follow-up radiographs of critical importance to ensure patient health.

Once a tooth is dead, there are often no obvious clinical signs; therefore, clinicians must be educated in the diagnosis of the disease processes. Once properly educated, the practitioner must remain vigilant for subtle signs of the disease process. Standard root canal therapy is an effective method of removing the inflammation, infection, and associated discomfort of the endodontically diseased tooth while maintaining its function. Like vital pulp therapy, standard root canal therapy must be performed meticulously, because nonideal treatment, in all likelihood, results in failure. Endodontic failure most likely remains hidden unless dental radiology is used. Follow-up radiographs at regular intervals throughout the patient's life are critical for ensuring the long-term success of any endodontic therapy.

Acknowledgments

The author thanks Dr. Lee Jane Huffman for her tireless efforts in editing this article.

References

[1] Trowbridge H, Kim S, Suda H. Structure and functions of the dentin and pulp complex. In: Cohen S, Burns RC, editors. Pathways of the pulp. 8th edition. St. Louis: Mosby–Year Book; 2002. p. 423–34.

[2] Clarke DE. Vital pulp therapy for complicated crown fracture of permanent canine teeth in dogs: a three-year retrospective study. J Vet Dent 2001;18(3):117–21.

[3] Cohen S. Diagnostic procedures. In: Cohen S, Burns RC, editors. Pathways of the pulp. 7th edition. St. Louis: Mosby–Year Book; 1998. p. 17–8.

[4] Golden AL, Stoller NS, Harvey CE. A survey of oral and dental diseases in dogs anesthetized at a veterinary hospital. J Am Anim Hosp Assoc 1982;18:891–9.

[5] Holmstrom S, Frost P, Eisner E. Restorative dentistry. In: Veterinary dental techniques. 2nd edition. Philadelphia: WB Saunders; 1998. p. 319–94.

[6] Sheets CG, Paquette JM, Wright RS. Tooth-whitening modalities for pulpless and discolored teeth. In: Cohen S, Burns RC, editors. Pathways of the pulp. 8th edition. St. Louis: Mosby–Year Book; 2002. p. 751–2.

[7] Hale FA. Localized intrinsic staining of teeth due to pulpitis and pulp necrosis in dogs. J Vet Dent 2001;18(1):14–20.

[8] Gluskin AH, Cohen AS, Brown DC. Orofacial dental pain emergencies: endodontic diagnosis and management. In: Cohen S, Burn RC, editors. Pathways of the pulp. 7th edition. St. Louis: Mosby–Year Book; 1998. p. 20–5.

[9] Holmstrom S, Frost P, Eisner E. Endodontics. In: Veterinary Dental Techniques. 2nd edition. Philadelphia: WB Saunders; 1998. p. 255–318.

[10] Harvey C, Emily P. Periodontal disease. In: Small Animal Dentistry. St. Louis: Mosby–Year Book; 1993. p. 89–144.

[11] Holmstrom S, Frost P, Eisner E. Dental prophylaxis. In: Veterinary dental techniques. 2nd edition. Philadelphia: WB Saunders; 1998. p. 133–66.

[12] Trope M, Chivan N, Sigurdsson A. Traumatic injuries. In: Cohen S, Burns RC, editors. Pathways of the pulp. 7th edition. St. Louis: Mosby–Year Book; 1998. p. 552–99.

[13] Wiggs RB, Lobprise HB. Clinical oral pathology. In: Veterinary dentistry, principals and practice. Philadelphia: Lippincott-Raven; 1997. p. 104–39.

[14] Baumgartner JC, Hutter JW. Endodontic microbiology and treatment of infections. In: Cohen S, Burns RC, editors. Pathways of the pulp. 8th edition. St. Louis: Mosby–Year Book; 2002. p. 501–20.

[15] Simon JHS. Periapical pathology. In: Cohen S, Burns RC, editors. Pathways of the pulp. 7th edition. St. Louis: Mosby–Year Book; 1998. p. 425–61.

[16] Ramsey DT, Maretta SM, Hamor RE, et al. Ophthalmologic manifestations and complications of dental disease in dogs and cats. J Am Vet Med Assoc 1996;32(3):215–24.

[17] Mulligan TM, Aller S, Williams C. Atlas of canine and feline dental radiography. Trenton: Veterinary Learning Systems; 1998. p. 176–83.

[18] Cohen S, Liewehr F. Diagnostic procedures. In: Cohen S, Burns RC, editors. Pathways of the pulp. 8th edition. St. Louis: Mosby–Year Book; 2002. p. 28–9.

[19] Xiaojing L, Kolltveit KM, Tronstad L, et al. Systemic diseases caused by oral infection. Clin Microbiol Rev 2000;13(4):547–58.

[20] Garcia R, Grossi S, Lacopino A, et al. The Periodontal-Systemic Connection: A State-of-the-Science Symposium. April 18–20, 2001. Bethesda, MD.

[21] Wiggs RB, Lobprise HB. Basic endodontic therapy. In: Veterinary dentistry, principals and practice. Philadelphia: Lippincott-Raven; 1997. p. 280–324.

[22] Hargreaves KM, Hutter JW. Pediatric endodontic pharmacology. In: Cohen S, Burns RC, editors. Pathways of the pulp. 8th edition. St. Louis: Mosby–Year Book; 2002. p. 665–82.

[23] Niemiec BA, Mulligan TM. Assessment of vital pulp therapy for nine complicated crown fractures and fifty-four crown reductions in dogs and cats. J Vet Dent 2001;18(3):122–5.

[24] Camp JH, Barrett EJ, Pulver F. Pediatric endodontics. In: Cohen S, Burns RC, editors. Pathways of the pulp. 8th edition. St. Louis: Mosby–Year Book; 2002. p. 804–7.

[25] Harvey C, Emily P. Endodontics. In: Small animal dentistry. St. Louis: Mosby–Year Book; 1993. p. 189–90.

[26] Niemiec BA. Vital pulp therapy. J Vet Dent 2001;18(3):154–6.

[27] Wiggs RB, Lobprise HB. Basic materials and supplies. In: Veterinary dentistry, principals and practice. Philadelphia: Lippincott-Raven; 1997. p. 29–54.

[28] Roeber LB, Tate WH, Powers JM. Effect of finishing and polishing procedures on the surface roughness of packable composites. Oper Dent 2000;25(5):448–53.

[29] Donly KJ. Sealants: where we have been and where we are going. Gen Dent 2002;50(5): 438–40.

[30] Mulligan TM, Aller S, Williams C. Interpretation of endodontic disease. In: Atlas of canine and feline dental radiography. Trenton: Veterinary Learning Systems; 1998. p. 124–52.

[31] Murray PE, Hafez AA, Smith AJ, et al. Bacterial microleakage and pulp inflammation associated with various restorative materials. Dent Mater 2002;18(6):470–8.

[32] Cox CF, Subay RK, Ostro E, et al. Tunnel defects in dentin bridges: their formation following direct pulp capping. Oper Dent 1996;21(1):4–11.

[33] Burns RC, Herbranson EJ. Tooth morphology and cavity preparation. In: Cohen S, Burns RC, editors. Pathways of the pulp. 8th edition. St. Louis: Mosby–Year Book; 2002. p. 173–230.

[34] Gutmann JL, Witherspoon DE. Obturation of the cleaned and shaped root canal system. In: Cohen S, Burns RC, editors. Pathways of the pulp. 8th edition. St. Louis: Mosby–Year Book; 2002. p. 293–364.

[35] Wiggs RB, Lobprise HB. Operative dentistry. In: Veterinary dentistry, principals and practice. Philadelphia: Lippincott-Raven; 1997. p. 395–433.

[36] Ruddle CJ. Cleaning and shaping the root canal system. In: Cohen S, Burns RC, editors. Pathways of the pulp. 8th edition. St. Louis: Mosby–Year Book; 2002. p. 246–75.

[37] Niemiec BA. Success rate of utilizing a stainless steel carrier for heated gutta percha in stenotic canine canals. In: Programs of the 17th Veterinary Dental Forum: San Diego: Walker Management; 2003. p. 179.

[38] Woody TL, Davis RD. The effect of eugenol-containing and eugenol-free temporary cements on microleakage in resin bonded restorations. Oper Dent 1992;17(5):175–80.

[39] Yap AU, Shah KC, Loh ET, et al. Influence of ZOE temporary restorations on microleakage in composite restorations. Oper Dent 2002;27(2):142–6.

[40] Peters O, Gohring TN, Lutz F. Effect of eugenol-containing sealer on marginal adaption of dentine-bonded resin fillings. Endod J 2000;33(1):53–9.

[41] De Moor R, Coppens C, Hommez G. Coronal leakage reconsidered. Rev Belge Med Dent 2002;57(3):161–85.

[42] Trope M, et al. Traumatic injuries. In: Cohen S, Burns RC, editors. Pathways of the pulp. 8th edition. St. Louis: Mosby; 2002. p. 610.

[43] Ruddle CJ. Nonsurgical endodontic retreatment. In: Cohen S, Burns RC, editors. Pathways of the pulp. 8th edition. St. Louis: Mosby; 2002. p. 878.

ELSEVIER
SAUNDERS

Vet Clin Small Anim
35 (2005) 869–889

VETERINARY
CLINICS
Small Animal Practice

Fundamentals of Small Animal Orthodontics

Thoulton W. Surgeon, DVM

ANC Veterinary Center Dental and Surgical Services, 1 Cottage Place,
New Rochelle, NY 10801, USA

To understand the fundamental principles involved in veterinary orthodontics, it is necessary to become familiar not only with the normal anatomy [1] and the anatomic variations that exist but to acquire a firm grasp of the underlying biologic and biomechanical principles that govern orthodontic tooth movement. The anatomic variations and their classification have been adequately documented [1,2].

Most of the orthodontic procedures undertaken in veterinary dentistry relate to the mandibular and maxillary incisors and the canine teeth. The premolars and molars are rarely involved in orthodontic abnormalities that justify or warrant intervention (Fig. 1).

With due consideration of the guiding principles of veterinary medical ethics [3–7] and our vow to provide a pain-free and optimally functional existence to the animals in our care, we embark on the sometimes frustrating and occasionally gratifying specialty of veterinary orthodontics.

This article discusses orthodontic principles; specific case treatments are discussed in the article in this issue on juvenile dentistry.

Periodontitis and orthodontics

The self-cleaning mechanism of the oral cavity is predicated on the presence of a normal anatomic alignment of the dentition in an anisognathic configuration with a pinking shear premolar orientation and a scissor incisor occlusion. When this normal state is altered because of genetic or developmental abnormalities, the net result is the development of periodontal disease [2,8]. Gross dentition displacement as occurs in linguoverted mandibular canines can cause palatal trauma (Fig. 2), and

E-mail address: surgeon668@cs.com

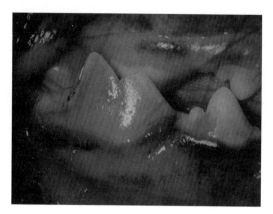

Fig 1. Posterior cross-bite in a Collie.

the resultant pain fosters the accumulation of plaque with subsequent gingivitis. If the orthodontic condition is left untreated, generalized periodontal disease develops. Similar calculus and plaque accumulations have been noticed in cases of anterior cross-bites, posterior cross-bites, individually rotated teeth, and moderate to severe dental crowding. In as much as tooth movement should not be initiated during episodes of active periodontal disease, it is known that orthodontic correction can facilitate resolution of orthodontically induced periodontitis.

Tooth movement stimulates resorption and deposition of bone. Osteoclasts, which originate in the bone marrow, where they are protected from the site of periodontal inflammation, tend to be unaffected by infection and continue to reabsorb bone. Osteoblasts are of vascular origin and are strongly suppressed by inflammatory disease [8–10].

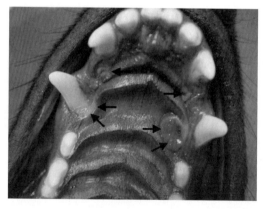

Fig 2. Palatal trauma from a linguoverted canine. Arrows indicate trauma sites caused by mandibular canines (caudal) and lateral incisors (rostral).

In periodontal disease situations, bone resorption is normal but bone formation is inhibited, and the resultant loss of alveolar supporting bone is exaggerated. Orthodontics, although a useful adjunct for enhancing periodontal health if undertaken in the presence of active periodontal disease, is invariably disastrous [8].

The cellular inflammation produced by orthodontic tooth movement should not be confused with the infection associated with periodontal disease, however. This condition quickly resolves after the end of orthodontic movement.

Periodontal ligament

The periodontal ligament (PDL) mediates the bony response to pressure applied to the dentition. Tooth movement is primarily a PDL phenomenon.

Forces applied to the teeth, whether extrinsic as from an appliance or intrinsic as a consequence of the normal dental interlock, can affect bone apposition or resorption at sites distant to the contact location. The ventral bowing of the mandible and changes on both sides of the temporomandibular joint are vivid examples of distant effect of the dental interlock in developing individuals with a propensity for excessive mandibular growth.

The supporting structure of each tooth is the network of collagenous fibers, which are inserted into the cementum of the root and the lamina dura of the alveolus. The cellular elements of the PDL are undifferentiated mesenchymal cells, fibroblasts, osteoblasts, cementoblasts, fibroclasts, and multinucleated giant cells. The PDL contains blood and lymph vessels, unmyelinated nerves for pain perception, and myelinated fibers for proprioception. The PDL space also contains tissue fluid, which acts an important ingredient of the hydraulic shock absorption system.

The composition of the PDL allows for its adaptation to heavy chewing forces that are applied for brief durations. Light forces applied over a prolonged period result in movement of the teeth within the alveolus, however [8–11].

Control of tooth movement

Presently, there are two theories: the biologic electricity theory and the pressure-tension theory. These two theories are neither incompatible nor mutually exclusive and may, in fact, be complementary. The pressure-tension theory is more easily explainable and is thus the basis of most orthodontic discussions [8,11].

The bioelectric theory involves the production of piezoelectricity by the deformation of bone, collagen, and fibrous proteins. Electricity is produced in the deformation process and the relaxation process, thereby providing a constant flow of bioelectric energy. There is also the "bioelectric potential" which is an integral component of biologically active tissue. The exact mechanism has not been elucidated, but the application of exogenous electrical signals has been known to affect cellular activity.

When force is applied to a tooth, the PDL is compressed in some areas and stretched in other areas. The areas of compression would correspond to the direction in which the movement is taking place, whereas the area of stretch would correspond to the direction from which movement is occurring. If the pressure does not exceed the capillary pressure, frontal resorption occurs and movement of the tooth begins. If, however, the pressure is excessive, sterile necrosis develops in the compressed area. The cells cut off from adequate blood supply die. The remodeling of bone occurs subjacent to the necrotic layer, delaying the process of tooth movement several days to weeks. Because the osteoclastic activity is separated from the moving tooth by this necrotic layer of PDL, the process is referred to as "undermining resorption."

After application of a continuous load, tooth movement can be classified into three distinct phases. The first phase is the initial strain, with displacement of approximately 0.4 to 0.9 mm, which occurs within the first week as a result of PDL compression, bone strain, and extrusion. A number of factors influence the initial response. The width of the PDL, root length, force magnitude, periodontal health, and anatomic configuration determine the initial response to force application. Initial tooth displacement occurs early after force application, but compression of the PDL requires 1 to 3 hours.

The second phase is the lag phase, which can vary from 1 to 3 weeks depending on the age of the patient, the degree of PDL necrosis (hyalinization), and the density of the alveolar bone. Undermining resorption subsequently removes the necrotic tissue, vitality is restored, and progressive tooth movement occurs. This constitutes the third phase of tooth movement.

Within 4 hours of sustained pressure, cyclic adenosine monophosphate (AMP), an important ingredient in cell differentiation, is elaborated. The levels of prostaglandin E increase rapidly. This results in the stimulation of osteoblast and osteoclast cells. Osteoclastic activity results in alveolar bone resorption at areas of increased PDL pressure, whereas osteoblasts lay down new bone in areas of PDL tension [8,11].

Biomechanical manipulation of bone is the physiologic basis of orthodontics. Orthodontics is bone manipulation therapy. In patient selection, it is thus imperative that the calcium homeostatic mechanism be fully operational and maintained at the optimal 10-mg/dL level. There is usually scant concern about this, because most veterinary orthodontic cases involve young actively growing animals in which calcium homeostasis is adequately maintained by active osteoblastic and osteoclastic activity. Within physiologic limits, it is possible to support calcium homeostasis without resorbing bone [8,11].

In clinical practice it is probably a combination of undermining and frontal resorption that occurs. The forces applied to the dentition are approximations, and the moments are, at best, rough estimates based on human studies, which are not necessarily applicable to the dog and cat.

There are a few fundamental principles that need to be understood to undertake the discipline of orthodontics successfully.

Anchorage

Anchorage is the resistance to unwanted tooth movement. Because each action results in an equal and opposite reaction, the functional definition of anchorage is the resistance to reaction provided by other teeth or structures. The desired result is to maximize the target tooth movement and minimize the undesirable side effects. The anchorage value of a tooth is a function of its root surface area.

A single tooth may be used as anchorage for moving a distant tooth by taking advantage of the greater force required for translation versus the lower force requirements of tipping. This type of anchorage is often referred to as simple anchorage.

Reinforced anchorage

Adding more units to the anchor segment or designing an anchorage appliance that takes advantage of the wedge configuration of the mandible to prevent forward movement of the anchorage unit can achieve reinforced anchorage. This is referred to as an anchor plane (Fig. 3).

Stationary anchorage can be obtained by pitting the translation movement of the anchorage unit against the tipping movement of the target tooth (Fig. 4). The forces used in all these instances should be kept at the lowest possible level to effect movement of the target tooth.

Reinforced anchorage can also be achieved by changes in appliance design to take advantage of the principle of recruitment. The application of the Mann incline plane with a telescoping bar in a young growing subject tends to end up with the appliance significantly removed from the palate coronally as the teeth erupt. The additional torque placed on each maxillary canine results in mesial tipping. A simple design change in the telescoping bar to prevent the independent rotation of the anchor canines recruits both canines as a single anchor unit, reducing the incidence of torque that would otherwise occur. Two square rods are clasped together so that the telescoping effect is maintained but planar rotation is eliminated. In instances in which just one mandibular canine is linguoverted, the antitorque effect of the appliance now prevents the reciprocal tipping of the maxillary canines (T.W. Surgeon, DVM, unpublished observation, 1995) (Fig. 5).

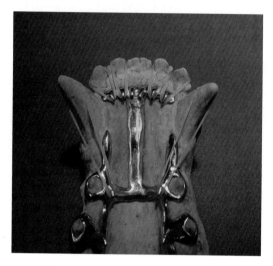

Fig 3. Mandibular plane on stone model.

Absolute anchorage

There is always some degree of reciprocal movement irrespective of how many units are included in the anchor. Absolute anchorage implies that there is no movement in the anchor unit. This can be achieved with the use of osteointegrated endosseous implants. Absolute anchorage occurs when an appliance is attached to a partly or fully ankylosed tooth. These endosseous implants behave in a similar fashion to ankylosed teeth and have the advantage of being able to be loaded immediately after placement. Only one surgical episode is needed, and because the unit is placed subgingivally, there are minimal problems with oral hygiene.

Friction and anchorage

When moving objects contact each other, frictional forces develop at the interface. There is resistance to the desired direction of movement. The frictional resistance occurs as a result of the surface irregularities of the contacting entities. These forces are concentrated at high points called asperites. Frictional resistance can be used advantageously to create a force couple, which can be beneficial in controlling unwanted tooth movement. Using this concept, an appliance that embodies the principles of reinforced anchorage with an attached glide rail of polished composite or metal and a metal cast band with a directional groove that fits over the glide rail is fabricated. The cast band is cemented to the target tooth (an upright mesolingually displaced mandibular canine requiring translation rather than tipping), and the directional groove and glide rails are aligned. When appropriate force is applied to the target tooth, it moves along the guide rail,

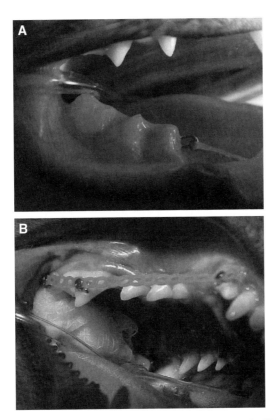

Fig 4. (*A*) Stationary anchorage in a cat. The unit includes the PM3, PM4, and M1. (*B*) Stationary anchorage in a dog. The unit includes the PM4 and M1.

with the frictional resistance creating a force couple that maintains the upright position with minimal tipping and almost pure translational movement (T.W. Surgeon, DVM, unpublished observation, 1994) (Fig. 6).

For significant differential tooth movement, the ratio of PDL area in the anchorage unit to the PDL area in the target (moving) unit should be at least 2:1 without friction. With the frictional component designed in the appliance, the PDL ratio should be a minimum of 4:1.

Similarly, the force magnitude required to overcome frictional resistance and translation is approximately double the anticipated levels. Bodily movement of a tooth requires a moment to force ratio of 8:1 to 10:1.

Force is defined as a load applied to an object that tends to move it to a different place. The unit of measure is the Newton or centiNewton (cN) but is usually expressed in weight units of ounces or grams. Force can be applied continuously or intermittently but should not exceed the normal capillary pressure of 20 to 26 g/cm^2. Many of the variables in orthodontic

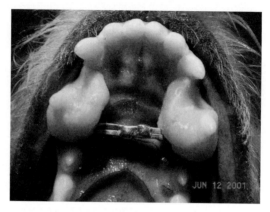

Fig 5. Telescoping bar for reinforced anchorage.

tooth movement cannot be controlled, such as growth and tissue response to appliances; however, the force placed on the tooth is a controllable variable. It is thus the duty of the clinician to understand the physics of these forces so that he or she can control this one variable that he or she is in a position to affect so strongly.

The center of resistance is the approximate geometric midpoint of the embedded portion of the tooth root or midway between the alveolar crest and the root apex. The center of rotation is the point around which rotation occurs when a tooth is being moved. In translation, the center of rotation is at infinity, whereas in tooth rotation, the center of rotation is near the center of resistance. The stress level is zero at the center of rotation during tooth movement. The center of rotation could be equated to the fulcrum if the tooth were to be regarded as a simple lever. To appreciate these centers, the tooth needs to be visualized in three dimensions.

When two forces equal in magnitude and opposite in direction are applied to an object, a pure moment is created; this results in rotation. Bodily movement can be achieved by the application of a coronal force with an opposing frictional resistance, creating a couple.

A moment is defined as the product of the force (F) applied to the target tooth times the perpendicular distance (d) from the point of force application to the center of resistance measured in units of grams per millimeter:

$$M = F \times d$$

The moment created by the application of a force away from the center of resistance results in rotation around the center of resistance. By varying the distance, a larger moment can be created without increasing the force magnitude. The moment arm is the distance between the point of force application and the center of resistance.

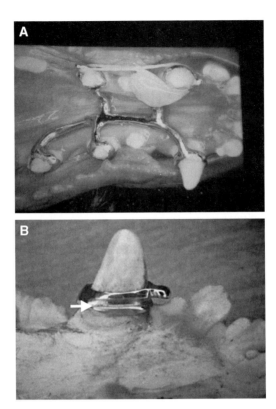

Fig 6. (*A*) Friction couple for translation of a canine tooth. (*B*) Stone model with a cast metal band with directional groove (arrow) for translation of a canine tooth.

Rate of tooth movement

The rate of tooth movement is inversely related to the bone density and volume of bone resorbed. The three principal variables that determine the rate of tooth movement are as follows:

1. Bone density
2. Type of tooth movement
3. Age of the patient

The ratio of cortical to cancellous bone is higher in the mandible than in the maxilla; correspondingly, tooth movement is faster in the maxilla than in the mandible. Tipping movement requires less bone resorption than translation and consequently occurs at a more rapid rate.

In young dogs with open apices, root formation results in extrusion of the crown. Orthodontic movement during this phase of development would be the equivalent of "guided eruption." The resorption and apposition of bone are only minimally affected, because this is an active part of the eruption process [2,12–14].

Types of tooth movement

Different types of tooth movement [2,5,6,12–16] are discussed in the following sections.

Tipping

In this type of tooth movement, the force is applied to the crown with the intent to move the tooth around its center of rotation. The apical portion of the tooth consequently moves in the opposite direction. The pressure side in the root is opposite to the direction of the applied force, and the coronal portion on the pressure side results in resorptive remodeling under the influence of osteoclasts, whereas additive remodeling occurs on the tension side as a result of osteoblastic action. Simultaneously, a similar set of events occurs at the apical portion of the tooth. Extrusion occurs coincidental to the tipping movement, partly because of the architecture of the alveolar socket and the stretching of the PDL fibers. Tipping of the tooth using light continuous force invariably results in a greater amount of movement within a shorter period of time than obtained by any other method. The optimal force range for tipping is 50 to 75 g. Tipping movement invariably results in some degree of hyalinization just below the alveolar crest. There may be an appreciable loss of alveolar crestal bone as a consequence of the tipping movement, which is particularly noted in older patients. Tipping movements can be achieved by using incline planes, rubber balls, springs, elastics, and screw-activated devices.

Bodily movement or translation

Bodily movement can be effected by creation of a force couple or by transposing the point of force attachment toward the center of resistance. The net effect is to achieve movement of the tooth with a minimum of tipping action. A tooth may be moved along an arch wire using springs or elastics to slide it along the wire while taking advantage of the frictional force to maintain the tooth in an upright position. Similarly, a tooth equipped with a cast band that is designed to slide along a glide rail uses the friction couple to maintain an upright position during movement. Because the entire tooth moves in a planar fashion, the force required for translation is higher than that needed to effect tipping. The usual force range for translation is 100 to 150 g (50–60 cN).

Rotation or torsion movement

In this movement, all the periodontal fibers are stretched in a spiral fashion. In the coronal region, rotation causes displacement of the fibrous structures. The supra-alveolar fibers and the periosteal structures are intimately attached, and this results in displacement of tissue some distance from the site of the rotated tooth. There may be areas of pressure in regions of the PDL adjacent to the subject tooth because of overlap of the fibers in rotation. Rotation requires light forces over an extended period. Because recoil is a major problem after rotation, an extended retainer period is necessary. The use of nickel titanium (NiTi) wires in an edgewise application is ideal for effecting rotation. The bracket placement needs to be precise to achieve the desired effect with minimal adjustments. Force requirements for rotation are in the range 50 to 75 g (25–30 cN).

Extrusion

This type of tooth movement may be regarded as controlled extraction. The tooth is moved out of the alveolus under light axial force to facilitate the coronal migration of the alveolar process. Here again, the use of an edgewise appliance or other specially designed devise greatly facilitates this procedure, the easiest of tooth movements. In situations in which impaction of the tooth is a complicating factor, surgical intervention in the form of an operculectomy and subgingival attached devices to bring the tooth into occlusion may be necessary [15]. The force requirements for extrusion are 50 to 75 g (25–30 cN).

Intrusion

The PDL is intrinsically designed to resist axial compression as occurs during mastication. To achieve intrusion, extremely light forces (15–25 g) need to be used. The area of force concentration is at the apex of the tooth, and the possibility of inadvertent root resorption is likely if loading is excessive. Relapse is a likely sequel, and an appropriate retention period is advisable.

Types of orthodontic appliances in current use

There are basically two types of orthodontic appliances: fixed appliances and removable appliances.

Fixed appliances consist of those designed to be firmly attached to the teeth and oral structures and can be made of composite, acrylic, metal, or a combination of these components. A fixed appliance may incorporate the use of elastics, springs, bone screws, or osteointegrated components to achieve the desired tooth movement.

Bite wing appliances are generally made of composite or acrylic and are generally used for minor cases involving base-narrow canines. These appliances can be made and installed chairside, requiring only a single visit. An impression and model should still be made, however, to document the presenting problem medicolegally. Typically, the attachment is to the maxillary canine with incorporation of the third incisor [17] or the first premolar for rotational stability. The latter attachment is preferred in young growing animals in which it is important not to hinder growth at the incisive suture. In older subjects, the first to third incisors and canines can be incorporated in the bite wing appliance (Fig. 7).

Incline planes can be made chairside using acrylic or composite or may be fabricated of metal or composite in a laboratory. Rubber play toys have been used with good results in some cases of lingually deviated canines [18]. The metal incline planes with telescoping bars allow for continued lateral maxillary growth. Orthodontic movement of base-narrow canines can also be effected with the use of W-wires, quad helix devices, spring-loaded devices, or screw-activated devices.

Edgewise appliances

These can be applied using steel or NiTi memory type or heat-activated wire. The most important component related to orthodontic wire use is bracket placement. It is important that the brackets be placed in proper vertical alignment so as to prevent inadvertent intrusion or extrusion events during therapy. For precision movement intrusion, rotation extrusion, and torquing, the slotted brackets are preferable. For tipping movements, ram cleats can be used to anchor the wires (Fig. 8). Because the forces generated by edgewise appliances are light, the duration of application has to be extended to achieve the target location. Probably because of the light forces generated, there is a minimum of discomfort associated with the use of heat-activated NiTi wire. The heat-activated wires require relatively low temperatures ($37°C$) for activation. The normal warmth of the oral cavity produces significant activation and efficient tooth movement. Because of its superelasticity and resistance to permanent deformation, NiTi wire has to be flame treated and quenched to place permanent bends in the wire [19,20].

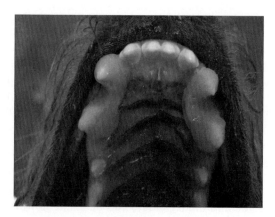

Fig 7. Bite wing "incline plane" appliance.

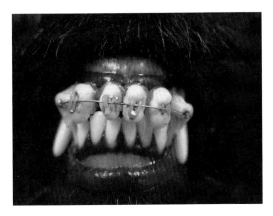

Fig 8. Nickel titanium edgewise appliance with ram cleat anchors.

The use of edgewise wires necessitates familiarization with the variations in the incisal arch form. There are three basic arch forms: the tapered arch form seen in most dolichocephalic head shapes, the square arch form seen in some brachycephalic head shapes, and the ovoid arch form of most mesocephalic heads. The arch form is determined by the underlying bone initially and is influenced by the dentition and masticatory musculature [21]. There is great variability in canine and feline arch form; even within head types, genetic and environmental differences produce great variations. There is therefore no ideal arch form. The selection of the appropriate arch form wire determines to a large extent how successful the outcome of the orthodontic movement is likely to be.

Arch bars

Arch bars can be applied to the maxilla and the mandible. In the maxilla, the usual location is on the buccal aspect so as to move the incisors facially to correct anterior cross-bites or level traumatic bites.

The mandibular location is usually the lingual aspect of the incisors so as to move them distally. These bars can be cast in a laboratory with small hook points for anchoring elastics used in moving the teeth (Fig. 9). The tooth attachments are metal, acrylic, or composite buttons bonded to the target teeth. The design should incorporate allowance for growth in younger patients.

In the orthodontic movement of the incisors, it is not unusual to have to strip the interproximal enamel to provide room for proper alignment. Small amounts of enamel should be taken from each tooth rather than excessively stripping a single tooth. Although caries secondary to enamel reduction is not a cause for concern, the reduced surfaces should be finished to a smooth final form [22].

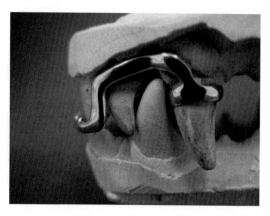

Fig 9. Maxillary arch bar.

Arch expansion devices

These devices use a screw apparatus embedded in acrylic or welded to a metal template (Fig. 10). The screw is activated every fourth day using the metal key to turn it one-quarter turn or 90°. The screws available result in 0.18 to 0.25 mm per one-quarter turn [7]. Because the force declines over time, this type of movement is referred to as intermittent movement. Arch expanders with springs or screw activation can be used in moving single or multiple teeth in either arch.

Incline capping

Incline capping is the process of bonding acrylic or composite to create tooth extensions or camouflage. By extending the contours of a tooth, the opposing teeth or the tooth with the extension can be made to move to a predetermined location within the arch (Fig. 11). These extensions can be

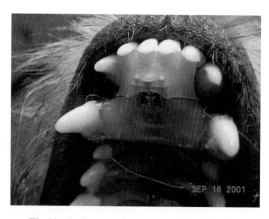

Fig 10. Arch expansion screw-activated device.

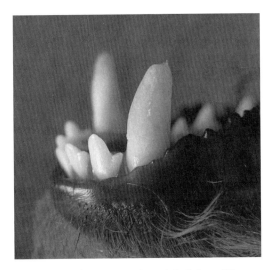

Fig 11. Acrylic tooth extensions to cause buccal deviation of linguoverted canines.

used for finishing mechanotherapy or as the primary mechanism for moving teeth. The tooth extensions are made of composite or acrylic bonded to the target tooth. Addition of composite or acrylic lingually results in labial movement of the capped tooth. With mesial and distal additions to the mandibular canines, the interdental space between the maxillary canine and lateral incisor can be widened to create room for the mandibular canine (Fig. 12). Tooth capping can be used in selected situations as the sole orthodontic device to guide the mandibular canines from a base-narrow occlusion to a normal occlusal orientation. In certain anterior cross-bite cases, a mandibular incisal bite cap is used as an incline plane to guide the

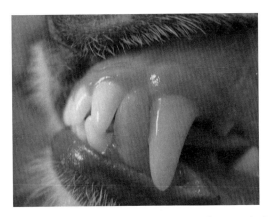

Fig 12. Acrylic tooth extension to widen the interdental space between the lateral incisor and the canine tooth.

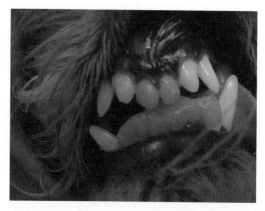

Fig 13. Mandibular incisal bite cap and maxillary central incisor tooth extensions for correcting an anterior cross-bite.

maxillary incisors into proper occlusion (Fig. 13) [2]. At the end of the orthodontic movement, the extensions are removed using a six-sided flame burr or diamond in a high-speed handpiece with copious water irrigation.

Gingival contouring

In some mild cases of base-narrow conditions, the gingiva can be contoured to eliminate the entrapment of the mandibular canine cusp. This can be done using a carbon dioxide laser, diamond burrs, electrocautery, or a scalpel blade. The obvious advantage of the laser is that in addition to no bleeding, there is minimum pain sensation associated with the procedure (Fig. 14).

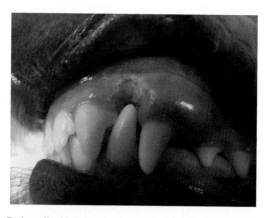

Fig 14. Carbon dioxide laser gingival contouring for base-narrow canines.

Force delivery in orthodontics

The incline planes, bite wing appliances, and incline caps all make use of the animal's own bite forces to effect tooth movement. The design and mechanics take advantage of the powerful axial forces generated to cause the tipping action needed to position the teeth in the desired location. These devices have a proven track record and are probably the most frequently used devices in veterinary orthodontics.

Elastics for orthodontic use are available as chains, rings, ligatures, and tubes. There are numerous instances in which elastic is the preferred force delivery medium. Not only is there a fairly long interval between changes, but the force delivery is gentle and the force decay rate is slow. With appropriate button placement, elastics can be used for intrusion, extrusion, tipping, and rotation movements. With careful control of the placement, a longer moment arm can be created, which results in more efficient tipping movement. Elastics are helpful in correcting buccally inclined canine teeth.

NiTi and steel wires have been used less frequently. The springiness, memory capability, and versatility in applications of the NiTi wires are advantages that allow for light force application and reduction in patient discomfort. The limiting factors in this force delivery modality are client compliance and the patient's attitude. With the advent of staged mechanotherapy, the application of arch wires in veterinary orthodontics is likely to see increasing use. NiTi wires can be used in the correction of anterior cross-bite malocclusions as edgewise appliances.

Surgical intervention in orthodontics

In a young growing animal in which asynchronous arch growth has resulted in primary dentition entrapment, selective extraction [23,24] can be helpful in reversing the asynchrony at a subsequent growth spurt. If the patient is genetically programmed to have a class II or class III malocclusion, this attempt at interception is not likely to succeed. Alternative strategies include crown amputation and vital pulp-capping and jaw-lengthening procedures using the stair-step osteotomy technique [25] or the distraction osteogenesis technique [26,27]. Similarly, jaw shortening can be accomplished by ostectomy and miniplate fixation. These latter techniques are best undertaken by individuals trained in orthopedic surgery.

In extraction therapy in which there is mixed dentition or supernumerary teeth and occurrence of minor tooth displacement, a partial tooth extraction can be done without disruption of the apical region, and a wedge of tooth root from an extracted primary tooth can be inserted into the space between the alveolus and the tooth to maintain the tooth in proper occlusion (Fig. 15). If the tooth wedge is securely placed beneath the gingiva, it may become resorbed. It could, however, be extruded or need to be removed once the tooth has stabilized.

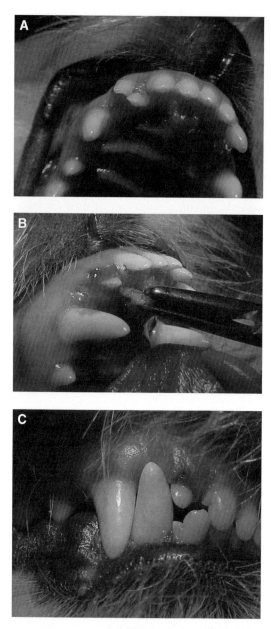

Fig 15. Surgical repositioning of a supernumerary tooth (*A*) using the root of the extracted tooth as a wedge (*B*) to maintain stability in the arch (*C*).

Exodontia is frequently needed to create space so that the target tooth has room to move and also to prevent embrication [2]. The surgical removal of soft and hard tissues is often needed to facilitate eruption of impacted teeth. This is achieved by an operculectomy when soft tissue is the cause of entrapment and alveoloplasty when bone is the offending tissue.

Retainers

If the scissor bite is achieved after incisor tooth movement and if the canines are in their proper interdental configuration, there may be no need to apply retainers to maintain tooth position. The usual retainer period is one half of the amount of time it took for the tooth to reach the desired location. The appliance that was used to create the movement is often used as the retainer. The types of retentive measures are determined by the number of teeth moved, rapidity of correction, periodontal health of the tissues, distance the teeth moved, occlusal harmony, and age of the patient [16,28].

Ancillary services related to orthodontics

The clinician needs to be able to produce good-quality impressions and models for study, appliance design, and as a guide for laboratory fabrication of appliances. These models also serve as teaching tools so that the client can acquire an appreciation for the way the therapy evolves (Fig. 16). Photographic and radiographic documentation of the presenting, interme- diate, and final stages of therapy logs the process for archival purposes.

At the end of therapy, removal of the appliances requires particular care so as not to damage the teeth on which they were anchored. Bands, brackets, and buttons, which require bonding techniques to attach them, also require careful removal to prevent damage to the enamel. To prevent

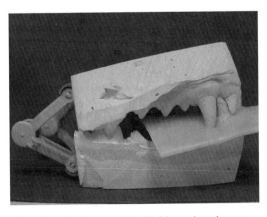

Fig 16. Articulated model with bite registration wax.

tooth discoloration, it is best to apply an unfilled resin after etching, especially when light cured acrylics are used and after removal of appliances, where the process of smoothing the enamel would result in an increased affinity for staining.

Although esthetics is not the primary objective in veterinary orthodontics, it is pleasing when the teeth involved in the process have a good finish. The use of white stones, finishing disks, and fine pumice produces an acceptable end result.

References

[1] Harvey CE, Emily PP. Function formation and anatomy of oral structures. In: Small animal dentistry. St. Louis: Mosby–Year Book; 1993. p. 1–18.
[2] Wiggs B, Lobprise H. Basics of orthodontics. In: Veterinary dentistry principles and practice. Philadelphia: Lippincott-Raven; 1997. p. 435–81.
[3] Harvey CE, Emily PP. Occlusion, occlusive abnormalities and orthodontic treatment. In: Small animal dentistry. St. Louis: Mosby–Year Book; 1993. p. 266–96.
[4] Hale F. Orthodontic correction for breeding and show dogs—an ethical dilemma. J Vet Dent 1991;8(3):14.
[5] Kertesz P. Dental development and abnormalities. In: A colour atlas of veterinary dentistry and oral surgery. Aylesbury, United Kingdom: Wolfe Publishing, Mosby–Year Book; 1993. p. 51–72.
[6] Hennet P. Orthodontics in small carnivores. In: Crossley DA, Penman S, editors. Manual of small animal dentistry. 2nd edition. Gloucestershire, United Kingdom: British Small Animal Veterinary Association; 1995. p. 182–92.
[7] Holmstrom SE, Frost Fitch P, Eisner ER. Orthodontics. In: Veterinary dental techniques for the small animal practitioner. 3rd edition. Philadelphia: WB Saunders; 2004. p. 499–558.
[8] Roberts WE. Bone physiology, metabolism, and biomechanics in orthodontic practice. In: Graber TM, Vanarsdall RL Jr, editors. Orthodontics, current principles and techniques. 3rd edition. St. Louis: Mosby–Year Book; 2000. p. 193–257.
[9] Schroeder HE. Periodontal ligament. In: Oral structural biology. New York: Thieme; 1991. p. 209–30.
[10] Ten Cate R. Physiologic tooth movement: eruption and shedding. In: Oral histology development structure and function. 5th edition. St. Louis: Mosby–Year Book; 1998. p. 289–314.
[11] Profit WR, Fields HW. The biological basis of orthodontic therapy. In: Reinhardt RW, editor. Contemporary orthodontics. 2nd edition. St. Louis: Mosby–Year Book; 1993. p. 266–88.
[12] Profit WR, Fields HW. Mechanical principles in orthodontic force control. In: Contemporary orthodontics. 2nd edition. St. Louis: Mosby–Year Book; 1993. p. 289–315.
[13] Ross DL. Orthodontics for the dog. Treatment methods. Vet Clin N Am Small Anim Pract 1986;16(5):939–54.
[14] McLaughlin R, Bennett J, Trevisi H. A brief history and overview of treatment mechanics. In: Systemized orthodontic treatment mechanics. St. Louis: Mosby–Year Book; 2001. p. 3–24.
[15] Surgeon TW. Surgical exposure and orthodontic extrusion of an impacted canine tooth in a cat: a case report. J Vet Dent 2000;17(2):81–5.
[16] Thilander B, Rygh P, Reitan K. Tissue reactions in orthodontics. In: Graber TM, Vanarsdall RL Jr, editors. Orthodontics, current principles and techniques. 3rd edition. St. Louis: Mosby–Year Book; 2000. p. 117–91.

[17] Hale FA. Orthodontic correction of lingually displaced canine teeth in a young dog using light- cured acrylic resin. J Vet Dent 1996;13(2):69–73.

[18] Verhaert L. A removable orthodontic device for the treatment of lingually displaced mandibular canine teeth in young dogs. J Vet Dent 1999;16(2):69–75.

[19] Burstone CJ. Application of bioengineering to clinical orthodontics. In: Graber TM, Vanarsdall RL Jr, editors. Orthodontics, current principles and techniques. 3rd edition. St. Louis: Mosby–Year Book; 2000. p. 259–92.

[20] Anusavice KJ. Wrought base metal and gold alloys. In: Philips' science of dental materials. 10th edition. Philadelphia: WB Saunders; 1996. p. 631–54.

[21] McLaughlin R, Bennett J, Trevisi H. Arch form. In: Systemized orthodontic treatment mechanics. St. Louis: Mosby–Year Book; 2001. p. 71–85.

[22] Rossouw PE, Tortorella A. Enamel reduction procedures in orthodontic treatment. J Can Dent Assoc 2003;69:378–83.

[23] Goldstein GS. The diagnosis and treatment of orthodontic problems. In: Manfra Maretta S, editor. Problems in veterinary medicine—dentistry. Philadelphia: Lippincott; 1990. p. 195–219.

[24] Ross DL. Orthodontics for the dog. Bite evaluation, basic concepts, and equipment. Vet Clin N Am Small Anim Pract 1986;16(5):955–66.

[25] Kavanagh T. Orthodontic diagnosis and treatment planing. In: Proceedings of the 1993 Veterinary Dental Congress. Auburn, AL. 1993. p. 97–100.

[26] Seleuk B, Evren U, Mete C, et al. Reconstruction of a large mandibular defect by distraction osteogenesis: a case report. J Oral Maxillofac Surg 2000;58:1425–8.

[27] Takato T, Harii K, Hirabayashi S, et al. Mandibular lengthening by gradual distraction: analysis using accurate skull replicas. Br J Plast Surg 1993;46:686–93.

[28] Joondeph DR. Retention and relapse. In: Graber TM, Vanarsdall RL Jr, editors. Orthodontics, current principles and techniques. 3rd edition. St. Louis: Mosby–Year Book; 2000. p. 985–1012.

ELSEVIER
SAUNDERS

Vet Clin Small Anim
35 (2005) 891–911

VETERINARY
CLINICS
Small Animal Practice

Gingivostomatitis

Kenneth F. Lyon, DVM

Arizona Veterinary Dentistry and Oral Surgery, 86 West Juniper Avenue,
Gilbert, AZ 85233, USA

Gingivostomatitis (GS) or recurrent oral ulceration (ROU) is found in veterinary patients with increasing frequency. Severe inflammation of the oral cavity is often seen in feline patients. GS is also seen with increasing incidence in canine patients. Histopathologic examination has been used to make a diagnosis by characterizing the reactive cells in the oral mucosa. This has led to chronic unrelenting oral disease, which is called by various descriptive names, including lymphoplasmacytic stomatitis (LPS), lympho-cytic plasmacytic gingivitis stomatitis (LPGS), plasmacytic stomatitis (PS), chronic ulcerative paradental stomatitis (CUPS), plasma cell gingivitis-stomatitis-pharyngitis, chronic ulcerative stomatitis, necrotizing stomatitis, feline chronic GS, and chronic gingivitis-stomatitis–faucitis. The use of the term *gingivostomatitis* is recommended when describing the general inflammation of the gingiva and oral cavity [1–9].

The pathogenesis of these oral diseases is not well defined but is becoming clearer. The histopathologic characteristics of gingivitis and periodontitis indicate that an immunologic response occurs in the pathogenesis of these diseases. The involvement of the oral cavity and the inflammation of the gingiva underscore the description of these oral diseases as GS. Clinical signs and symptoms of these diseases can overlap, creating confusion about choosing appropriate therapy. Abnormalities in the immune system alter the individual patient's response and lead to opportunistic infections, which contribute to the chronic nature of GS.

Oral pathologic findings

Oral pathologic findings are often overlooked as an evaluation for recurrent oral disease, and it becomes important to enhance our diagnostic skills through the use of differential diagnostic considerations. An

E-mail address: Lyon2THVet@aol.com

doi:10.1016/j.cvsm.2005.02.001
vetsmall.theclinics.com

appreciation of the significance of all possible diagnostic entities helps to prevent needless delay or haste in treatment and helps to eliminate the expense of unnecessary laboratory tests and consultations.

It is important to understand the inflammatory cell response to determine the differential diagnosis of GS. An understanding of the immune mechanism's role in GS allows us to evaluate the effects of the suppressed immune system. In chronic diseases of metabolic or endocrine origin, the immune system is suppressed. Viral diseases, such as feline leukemia virus (FeLV), feline immunodeficiency virus (FIV), calicivirus, feline infectious peritonitis (FIP), herpes virus, and panleukopenia virus, present with signs of oral inflammation. Nutritional disorders may also contribute to oral diseases. There is evidence that some breeds are more commonly affected, indicating a probable genetic predisposition as is seen in people with a hereditary factor in recurrent aphthous stomatitis (RAS) [10–12].

Calicivirus and herpes 1 virus have been evaluated in cats with GS, and there is evidence of high titers, indicating active shedding of calicivirus in these patents. Furthermore, when the GS is controlled, there seems to be a decrease in the virus shedding [13–24].

Gingivitis always precedes periodontitis, and periodontitis is always accompanied by gingivitis. As gingivitis becomes more severe, the gingival tissue loses integrity and ulceration of the gingival sulcus occurs, allowing bacteria and their byproducts to enter deeper periodontal structures. If the immune system is suppressed, this progression from gingivitis to perio-dontitis can be rapid and may even appear in young animals. Subsets of GS can be related to the presence of periodontal disease and resorptive lesions.

The immune system responds to chronic inflammation with the production of antibodies. The mature plasma cells are the primary source of these immunoglobulins. A monoclonal gammopathy may be seen [25]. Immunoglobulin-coated bacteria indicate that some of these immunoglo-bulins are specific for oral microorganisms. GS in veterinary patients is similar to those syndromes seen in human patients, especially erythema multiforme (EM).

Biopsy of oral inflammatory diseases should be emphasized. Chronic GS, eosinophilic granuloma complex, and neoplasia can look similar on physical examination (Fig. 1). Two distinct inflammatory patterns are seen on histopathologic examination of biopsy samples from cats with GS. One is an uncommon diffuse inflammatory syndrome primarily of leukocytic exo-cytosis and may indicate an immunocompromised patient that requires immunostimulation medication. The other more common pattern is an interface (lichenoid) dermal-epidermal inflammatory reaction primarily of plasma cells. This indicates an immunoreactive, often overresponsive, immune reaction, and these patients require immunosuppression medica-tion. In fact, plasma cell infiltrates respond best to corticosteroids. If the etiology of GS can be determined, focused treatment should eliminate the stimulus for the immune system response.

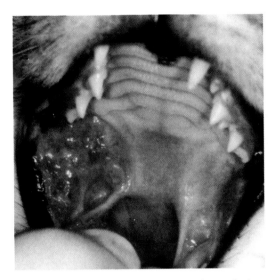

Fig. 1. Eosinophilic granuloma in a cat, which is presented as a gingivostomatitis patient.

A common pathologic finding is often described as a submucosal infiltrate primarily of plasma cells but with neutrophils, lymphocytes, and macrophages. Plasma cell–secreting potential as a diagnostic test is used to evaluate the prognosis in human patients with GS [26]. Elevated serum and salivary immunoglobulins are often evident. Immune response is measured by T-lymphocyte subsets, and these CD4/CD8 ratios are often low because of high CD8 levels, confirming the aggressive immune response. Cytokine gene expression in cats shows elevated interleukin 4 (IL-4) levels. There are also viral associations with calicivirus, herpesvirus, FIV, and FeLV. Gene transfer is a likely factor in these diseases [27,28]. Plasminogen activators from mast cells activate metalloproteinases, which are active in tissue responses to inflammation [16,29–32].

The etiology of GS is often unknown, and a multifactorial infection has been described, which includes bacteria, virus, genetics, nutrition, environment, and domestication in general. An increased level of immunoglobulins, including γ-globulin, often confirms the exaggerated immune response. Infections organisms like *Bartonella henselae* have been linked to chronic GS in cats, but focus treatment, which eliminates this organism, does not often result in resolution of the GS [33].

It is becoming more evident that bacterial persistence is contributing to ROU. Experimental and clinical evidence supports the concept that bacteria that are difficult to culture and dormant bacteria are involved in latency of infection and that these persistent bacteria may be pathogenic. A series of experimental studies involving host-bacterium interactions illustrates the probability that most bacteria exposed to a deleterious host environment can assume a form quite different from that of a free-living bacterium. Data on the basic biology of persistent bacteria are correlated with expression of disease, particularly the mechanisms of latency and chronicity that typify certain infections.

For example, in certain streptococcal and nocardial infections, it has been clearly established that wall-defective forms can be induced in a suitable host. These organisms can survive and persist in a latent state within the host, and they can cause pathologic responses compatible with disease. There are a series of cases illustrating idiopathic conditions in which cryptic bacteria have been implicated in the expression of disease. These conditions include nephritis, rheumatic fever, aphthous stomatitis, idiopathic hematuria, Crohn's disease, and *Mycobacterium* infections. By using polymerase chain reaction (PCR), previously nonculturable bacilli have been identified in patients with Whipple's disease and bacillary angiomatosis. Koch's postulates may have to be redefined in terms of molecular data when dormant and nonculturable bacteria are implicated as causative agents of mysterious diseases, such as GS [34].

Other oral inflammatory syndromes have been reported in animal and human patients and include eosinophilic granuloma complex, EM, toxic epidermal necrolysis (TEN), Steven-Johnson syndrome (SJS), Sjögren's syndrome, Marshall's syndrome (syndrome of periodic fever, aphthous stomatitis, pharyngitis, and cervical adenitis [PFAPA]), paraneoplastic pemphigus, mucous membrane pemphigoid, Behçet's disease, stomatitis glandularis, burning mouth syndrome (BMS), Waldenström's macroglobulinemia (monoclonal), linear gingival erythema (LGE), and oral lichen planus (OLP) with angular cheilitis. Some of these conditions are rare and illustrate the complex interactions involved in immune modulation of these diseases [35–37].

As described in human beings, EM is an acute inflammatory disease with an autoimmune pathogenesis clinically expressing a wide variety of mucocutaneous illnesses. It is usually described in a minor form (Von Hebra's syndrome) characterized by classic cutaneous lesions and in major form (SJS) involving mucosal damage, whereas a clinical type restricted to the oral mucosa is described in oral pathologic findings. A considerable number of factors of a different nature have been reported as etiologic agents of EM, but most of them are not well documented; however, a certain relation with EM is recognized for different classes of systemic drugs. One article describes a case of SJS with initial oral involvement, in which the precipitating factor was attributable to the administration of systemic glucocorticoids prescribed for the therapeutic treatment of an erosive form of OLP [36].

EM is a reactive mucocutaneous disorder in a disease spectrum that comprises a self-limited, mild, exanthematic, and cutaneous variant with minimal oral involvement (EM minor) to a progressive, fulminating, and severe variant with extensive mucocutaneous epithelial necrosis (SJS and

TEN). Significant differences exist among EM minor, EM major, SJS, and TEN with regard to severity and clinical expression; however, all variants share two common features: typical or less typical cutaneous target lesions and satellite-cell or more widespread necrosis of the epithelium [35].

The involvement of the oral cavity with a recurrent oral disease, GS, is what these diseases and syndromes have in common. Stomatitis glandularis is an unusual chronic inflammatory condition of the minor salivary glands mainly affecting the lower lip [38]. Two rare cases are reported in people, one of which was progressive and affected the glands of both cheeks as well as the lips. After confirmation of the clinical diagnosis by histopathologic appearance, treatment was by excision of the suppurating areas as staged procedures. The basic surgical tenet of wound debridement is important to consider when evaluating treatment options for GS.

Patient evaluation

A detailed history is important in evaluating all aspects of the pet's lifestyle to find clues that may lead to a causative factor for the recurrent oral disease. Questions should be asked about the pet's diet (eg, type, canned versus dry, changes, deficiencies), age at onset of first clinical signs, association of events at onset of signs (eg, vaccine, new food, new home, new floor cleaner, cosmetics), course and duration of clinical signs, activity pattern (eg, chronic licker or chewer, indoor or outdoor pet), environmental hazards (eg, pesticides, cleansers, toxins), chronic illness (eg, dermatitis, anal sacculitis, otitis, hairballs), other systemic illness (eg, gastrointestinal, upper respiratory, urinary tract infection, liver or kidney disease), vaccination history, and exposure to other pets.

Systemic causes should be ruled out. These include lupus erythematosus, pemphigus, adverse food reactions, viral processes, bacterial infections and hypersensitivity, hypothyroidism and hyperthyroidism, and immunodeficiency.

A thorough physical examination is extremely important. Do not take a quick look in the mouth and make a diagnosis (Figs. 2–4). A complete laboratory evaluation is also important. This should include a complete blood cell count (persistent neutropenia), serum chemistry profiles (eg, diabetes, azotemia), thyroid hormone profiles, fecal profiles (Giardia), toxoplasmosis, malabsorption and/or maldigestion (pancreatic exocrine insufficiency, trypsin-like immunoreactivity [TLI]), viral profiles (eg, FeLV, FIP, FIV, calicivirus, herpesvirus), immune profiles (eg, antinuclear antibody), and serum protein electrophoresis (monoclonal or polyclonal elevation in γ-globulin) [25,39].

A bacteriology evaluation may be indicated [40,41]. These cultures of the oral cavity may not be rewarding, and an appropriate laboratory test should be selected. Anaerobic culture of the gingival sulcus should be submitted using a sterile filter paper placed directly into anaerobic media. Some

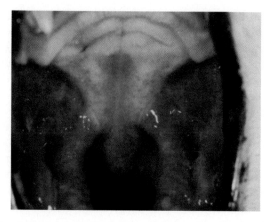

Fig. 2. Chronic gingivostomatitis in a cat—inflammation of palatoglossal folds.

laboratories may have PCR or enzyme-linked immunosorbent assay (ELISA) tests for antibody titers to various oral bacteria serotypes. Occasionally, fungal cultures may be necessary, especially in endemic areas, but fungal titers are preferred.

Radiographic examination is essential for evaluation of the entire tooth structure for evidence and extent of periodontal disease, evaluation of root resorption, nature of endodontic involvement, neoplastic destruction, pre- and postextraction evaluation, and evaluation of missing teeth. Nasal passages and sinuses can also be evaluated with radiographs.

Possible pathogenesis

Most diseases of the oral cavity have a basis in immunologic events taking place in the gingival sulcus and involving the complex interactions of the

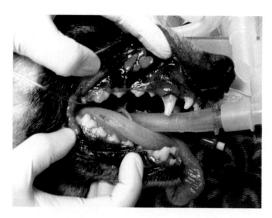

Fig. 3. Dog with gingivostomatitis—buccal view.

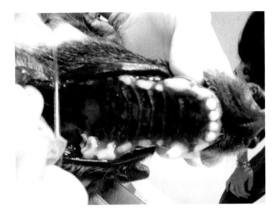

Fig. 4. Dog with gingivostomatitis—palatal view.

host immune system and various antigens. The inflammation in the gingiva is activated to some extent by the host's response to the continuous bacterial antigen exposure and to the direct effects of bacterial products from the dental plaque microorganisms.

The perspective on periodontal inflammation includes evidence about the interactions between the bacterial plaque and the host. Periodontal disease results from an imbalance between the host and the microbes. The imbalance may occur when the quantity or quality of bacteria changes or when the individual's level of immunity is altered or affected by environmental factors. Plaque bacteria are obviously the cause of chronic periodontal disease. The focus in understanding recurrent oral disease is on determining the impact of these bacteria on the immune response and the interaction of the host's defense mechanisms. The response of each site to a specific plaque composition is regulated by the individual immune system. A good immune response results in no evidence of progressive disease despite the presence of calculus and plaque. A patient with a faltering immune status and less extensive plaque may have generalized or localized evidence of disease [42,43].

The focus in treatment is on the nature of the host's immune response. The days of treating each patient identically are gone, and it is realized that each patient's characteristics and immune response are critical determinants in designing therapeutic interventions. The development of ways to boost the patient's immune response so as to promote and maintain gingival health is the focus for the new millennium.

In gingivitis, the cells necessary to activate immune responses are present. These are plasma cells, which produce immunoglobulins that play a role in immediate hypersensitivity and immune complex disease; lymphocytes, including T cells responsible for cell-mediated immunity and B cells responsible for antibody-mediated reactions; mast cells; polymorphonuclear neutrophils; and macrophages.

When the host's defense mechanism is activated in the form of inflammation to localize and destroy foreign material, the host's own tissues may also be destroyed in the inflammatory process.

It is important to understand the inflammatory cell response to determine the differential diagnosis of recurrent oral disease. An understanding of the immune mechanism's role in gingivitis allows us to evaluate the effects of the suppressed immunologic system. In chronic diseases of metabolic or endocrine origin, the immune system is suppressed. Viral diseases, nutritional disorders, and, sometimes, breed predilection also have effects on the immune system.

A possible pathogenesis of recurrent oral disease is evident when mucosal damage has occurred and oral antigens are released from the damaged mucosa. Antibody production begins in response to these new oral antigens. This leads to further mucosal damage as antibodies are produced against the host's own oral mucosa.

Because vasculitis plays a role in the ROU of GS, investigation of autoantibodies associated with vasculitis can provide for treatment recommendations directed at these inflammatory mediators. Two autoantibodies, raised antiendothelial cell autoantibodies (AECAs) and antineutrophil cytoplasmic autoantibodies (ANCAs), have been associated with vasculitis. AECAs target as yet unidentified antigens on the endothelial cell surface and have been identified in patients with vasculitic disorders and inflammatory conditions with a vasculitic component. ANCAs target specific neutrophil-associated proteins that are detected in specific vasculitic and chronic inflammatory disorders. AECA levels are highest during active inflammation in ROU; however, ANCAs are not associated with the vasculitis of ROU. The presence of raised levels of AECAs lends support to the hypothesis that a vasculitic process may underlie ROU. Modulation of this autoantibody is influenced by tumor necrosis factor-α (TNFα) and interferon-γ (IFNγ). Endothelial cell expression of AECA target antigens is increased by TNFα stimulation and decreased by IFNγ stimulation [44].

Another possible pathogenesis occurs when the host is exposed to a new antigen. This new antigen is processed by the oral epithelium. T-suppresser cells respond by downregulating the response to this antigen, or T-activator cells activate the immune response (T cells). An immunologically mediated reaction to a protein allergen (food) possibly precipitated by mucosal disruption (viral) activates the cascade of immunologic events that may create and perpetuate recurrent oral diseases.

Some patients may have a defect in their cell-mediated immune response. Helper and/or inducer (T_4) lymphocytes may be seen focally in the early stages of disease. Basal cells in these areas also express antigens early, suggesting a role for these cells as well. Because basal cell antigens are required for antigen presentation to immunocompetent cells, it could be speculated that these cells are presenting autoantigens to the infiltrating T_4 cells, leading to eventual basal cell destruction.

In human patients, lymphocyte blast transformation studies have shown that when lymphocytes from affected patients are incubated with mucosal homogenates, blast transformation occurs, thus indicating T-cell sensitization. Leukocyte migration inhibition has also been observed. T lymphocytes from human oral ulceration patients have been shown to be cytotoxic to cultured gingival epithelial cells but not to other epithelial cells.

From these studies, even though some of the evidence has been conflicting, it seems likely that human aphthous ulcers result from a focal immune dysfunction in which T lymphocytes play a significant role. The nature of the initiating stimulus remains a mystery. The causative agent could be endogenous (autoimmune) antigen or exogenous (hyperimmune) antigen, or it could be a nonspecific factor, such as trauma, in which chemical mediators may be involved.

Other causes of feline oral inflammation include uremic gingivitis, feline eosinophilic granuloma complex, food allergy, squamous cell carcinoma, foreign body reactions, and autoimmune disease (eg, pemphigus vulgaris, systemic lupus erythematosus).

Treatment

Treatment of GS begins with treatment of periodontal disease, with the emphasis on treating the periodontal infection. The term *periodontal debridement* describes "the treatment of gingival and periodontal inflammation through mechanical removal of tooth and root surface irritants to the extent that the adjacent soft tissues maintain or return to a healthy, noninflamed state." *Periodontal bacterial ultrasonic debridement* (Perio-BUD) is a term used to describe this treatment. Periodontal debridement is performed with ultrasonic or hand instruments, and the focus is on bacterial plaque and the byproducts that are toxic to periodontal tissues. Calculus removal is considered secondary to the debridement procedure. Calculus does contribute to periodontal disease because of its plaque-retentive effects and must be removed, but the focus of "grooming" the teeth is now a procedure from the past.

Periodontal debridement should focus on three areas. The first is supragingival debridement, which is the removal of all accessible plaque, plaque byproducts, and plaque retentive calculus located on the crown of the tooth above the gingival margin. The purpose is to facilitate the pet owner's personal plaque control efforts and to support the maintenance of healthy gingival tissues. The second area is subgingival debridement, which is the removal of accessible plaque, plaque byproducts, and plaque-retentive calculus located in inflamed periodontal pockets below the gingival margin. The purpose is to supplement supragingival plaque control by removing or disrupting bacterial plaque and toxic plaque byproducts that are inaccessible to the pet owner and are promoting inflammation of periodontal tissues.

Professional subgingival debridement also involves removal of plaque-retentive surfaces and deposits, including calculus, which may promote or contribute to plaque formation and retention. The final focus in periodontal debridement is on deplaquing, which is the removal or disruption of bacterial plaque and its byproducts within the gingival sulcus or periodontal pocket as a means of maintaining periodontal health. Antimicrobial rinses and pastes are useful for deplaquing, but the destruction of bacteria by sonication using ultrasonic scalers cannot be overemphasized.

Intraoral dental radiographs should be evaluated to diagnose any teeth with significant attachment loss or resorptive lesions. These teeth should be extracted, because they are contributing to the chronic nature of the GS.

In spite of active attempts to control GS by periodontal therapy, including deplaquing, the chronic inflammation often persists. Because GS is related to an immunologic defect, treatment logically includes drugs that can manipulate or regulate immune responses. Some forms of treatment can provide significant control (but not necessarily cure) of this disease. Systemic steroids are appropriate for severe disease but should not be used unless the veterinarian has experience in this treatment area or is working with a knowledgeable consultant.

Many medications have been reported in treating GS, including gold salts (aurothioglucose), azathioprine (Imuran), chlorambucil (Leukeran), vincristine (Oncovin), 5-fluorouracil, lactoferrin, azithromycin, glucocorticoids, metronidazole, sulodexide, tacrolimus topical, thalomide, zinc sulfate, colchicine, IFNα (interferon Alfa-2A, human recombinant), and cyclosporine [45–51].

These medications have varying toxicities, and familiarity with the drugs is recommended. It is obvious from a review of the literature that most treatments for oral diseases, such as OLP, pemphigoid, and pemphigus, are based on case reports, anecdotes, and small uncontrolled studies. Efforts must be made to perform more controlled studies to evaluate the efficacy of new treatments. Relatively low doses of azathioprine, cyclophosphamide, and cyclosporine could then be added for the treatment of severe or recalcitrant diseases.

Novel therapeutics used in human oral mucosal diseases include pentoxifylline, etretinate, dapsone, thalidomide, IFNγ, and a range of inhibitors of cytokine and growth factor action (ie, tacrolimus, sirolimus, leflunomide) [50,52,53].

Other treatments have been recommended, including paramunization, which was recommended in 1991 as a treatment option for chronic GS in cats [54]. Also, IFNα, which has antiviral, antiproliferative, and immunomodulation effects, can reduce the disease effects in virus-affected patients and can have an impact on bacteria. Interferon is used to treat cats infected with calicivirus and FeLV. Interferon is poorly absorbed after oral administration. In cats, 30 IU given orally once daily for 7 days on a 1-week-on–1-week-off cycle is recommended. Efficacy has not been proven [55–57].

Oral surgery

Oral surgery (exodontics or extractions) must be considered when damaged teeth are present or significant periodontal disease compounds the GS. All tooth remnants must be removed. Multirooted teeth should be sectioned, elevated, and extracted. Alveoloplasty is completed to remove any sharp bony margins. Complete extraction procedures should be confirmed with dental radiographs. All grossly evident periodontium or inflammatory tissue should be debrided. The postextraction care of these usually debilitated animals must center on supportive and corrective therapy until extraction sites are healing. Transabdominal gastrotomy or pharyngostomy tube feeding should be considered. Appropriate analgesic medications are indicated in most cases.

In an evaluation of response to extractions, it was found that 60% of the cats had complete remission of clinical disease and another 20% had remission with only mild flare-ups not requiring treatment. In the remaining cats, 13% still required medical management and 7% were unresponsive to surgical or medical management (Table 1). This illustrates that removal of plaque-retentive dentition and periodontium can have a positive effect on controlling GS [58].

Tonsillectomy

In human beings, tonsillectomy has been recommended with mixed success. In one study, the patients showed improvement, and in another study, no improvement was seen [59,60]. Tonsillectomy has not been evaluated in veterinary patients as a therapy for GS.

Laser thermoablation

Laser thermoablation is another option for cytoreduction of chronic proliferation of oral mucosa. Multiple treatments with a carbon dioxide laser have been recommended to control proliferative tissue. After laser

Table 1
Results of treatment of stomatitis 11–24 months following extraction of teeth in 30 cats

Clinically cured (no visible lesions, no oral clinical signs)	18/30	60%
Significant improvement (no continuing treatment other than plaque control)	6/30	20%
Little improvement	4/30	13%
No improvement	2/30	7%

Data from Hennet P. Chronic gingivo-stomatitis in cats: long-term follow-up of 30 cases treated by dental extractions. J Vet Dent 1997;14(1):15–21.

thermoablation, scar tissue forms in the re-epithelialization process. Because scar tissue has less blood supply, this tissue may be less reactive to immunologically related damage. Laser treatment offers an option to extraction of teeth. Histopathologic evaluation of oral mucosa after laser treatment shows no change in the underlying disease after laser treatment. The carbon dioxide laser has long been a favorite instrument of oral surgeons because of its wavelength's ready absorption into water (soft tissue). Although many of the reports indicate its use for the treatment of intraoral pathologic conditions, the carbon dioxide laser is still commonly used for a variety of surgical procedures on otherwise healthy tissue in the mouth. Similar to the carbon dioxide laser, the neodymium:yttrium-aluminum-garnet (Nd:YAG) laser has become a favorite among clinicians for intraoral soft tissue surgery because of its excellent coagulation ability, flexible fiberoptic delivery system, ease of use, and precision. The value of adjunctive lasing is in the enhanced bacterial reduction. Removal of proliferative oral tissues by lasing removes the tissue that may be producing tissue antigens and an area where bacteria are sequestered. Therapeutic success is achieved when there is elimination of proliferative tissue and inflammation, cessation of attachment loss, improvement of gingival contours, stabilization of mobile teeth, and proper patient oral hygiene maintenance. Laser thermoablation combined with cyclosporine therapy gives good results without extraction of teeth (Figs. 5–8).

Antimicrobials

Antimicrobial mouth rinses containing chlorhexidine gluconate are also beneficial. The mechanism for clinical improvement is related to the

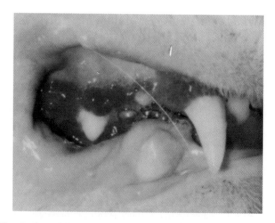

Fig. 5. Cat with gingivostomatitis—pretreatment buccal view.

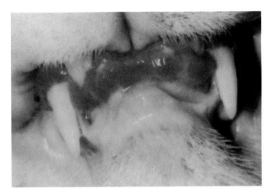

Fig. 6. Cat with gingivostomatitis—pretreatment anterior view.

diminishing the oral bacterial load and possibly to the binding to free nerve endings and epithelial cells. Antimicrobials for systemic application include amoxicillin and/or clavulanate, cephalexin, clindamycin, doxycycline, enrofloxacin, and metronidazole. Combination therapy with enrofloxacin (5 mg/kg q 12 h) and metronidazole (15 mg/kg q 12 h) is synergistic and has shown positive results on long-term administration.

Reoccurring infections indicate that bacteria have been eliminated during treatment but that once the treatment was stopped, a new infection occurred. This usually is indicative of chronic changes in local immune functions, rendering the site prone to colonization. Long-term therapy (months) may be indicated in relapsing infections but not in reoccurring infection. Infection management success is dependent on ensuring there is not an active infection present. If infections are reoccurring within 30 days after stopping antimicrobial treatment, pulse therapy can be effective. The goal is to prevent colonization, the first step to infection. The antimicrobial

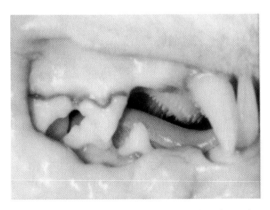

Fig. 7. Cat with gingivostomatitis 9 months after laser and cyclosporine treatment—buccal view.

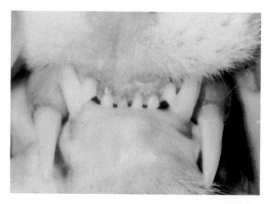

Fig. 8. Cat with gingivostomatitis 9 months after laser and cyclosporine treatment—anterior view.

of choice is administered at a normal dose but is given for 3 to 4 days, followed by 1 to 2 weeks without the drug and then another 3 to 4 days of treatment. This can continue indefinitely if needed. Periodically, the treatment may be stopped to determine if local factors have improved and if infection reoccurs. Remember that you are managing an infection rather than curing it. It is critical that active infection is not present or that other treatable factors are not involved in the reoccurrence of infection. Otherwise, infection occurs and becomes resistant to the antibiotic. Choosing another antibiotic and repeating this procedure would be a grave mistake.

Continuous low-dose therapy is another consideration. Usually, the low end of a dose is given once daily or every other day. Again, it is crucial that an active infection is not present. This is designed to prevent colonization only rather than for treating an infection. Some patients remain on antibiotics for their lifetime. Resistance is not a major concern as long as active infection is not present. It is best to use antibiotics with low resistance rates, such as amoxicillin and/or clavulate, clindamycin, or a fluoroquinolone.

Management options

Anti-inflammatory medications

For immediate control of GS in most cases, a low to moderate dose of prednisone or prednisolone over a short period is recommended. A daily dose (2–4 mg/kg) for 1 week followed by administration of half the initial dose for another week is typical. Maintenance doses are (0.5–1 mg/kg every 48 hours) generally lower once control has been established.

Methylprednisolone acetate can be given in cats and some dogs (20 mg SQ every 2 weeks) for three to six treatments and then reduced or given as needed.

Azathioprine can also be used and may allow for a reduction in the prednisone or prednisolone dosage if used concurrently. For cats, a tablet (50 mg) is pulverized and mixed in 15 mL of multivitamin syrup, and the dosage is 0.3 mg/kg administered once every 48 hours. (In cats, give 0.33 mL every 48 hours for an average 5-kg cat). For dogs, administer 2.2 mg/kg orally every other day and then reduce to 1 mg/kg every other day. Prednisone or prednisolone can be given on the alternate day if necessary. Azathioprine is a potent bone marrow suppression drug, and hemograms should be closely monitored [45].

Topical steroids or sublesional injections, if used judiciously, can be relatively efficacious and safe in the treatment of mild to moderate disease. The science of topical steroid use in dentistry is relatively primitive when compared with its use in dermatology. For mucosal diseases, it has not been established whether more potent topical compounds are significantly more effective than less potent compounds or whether more frequent application is more effective. Commercially available topical steroids have been recorded related to dermatologic use, with the most potent being clobetasol propionate (Temovate cream 0.05%), halcinonide (Halog cream 0.1%), fluocinonide (Lidex cream 0.05%) and desoximetasone (Topicort cream 0.25%). "Supertopical" glucocorticoids have high tissue binding and potency (15–100 times), and these are "first-pass" steroids with topical affinity, which then go to the liver, where they are rapidly removed, thereby reducing the systemic effects.

Pentoxifylline (Trental) administered at 400 mg once daily to every other day has been used primarily to treat ulcerative dermatosis in Shelties and Collies, and because of its ability to reduce the negative endotoxic effects of cytokine mediators, it has been used to treat GS in dogs. Gastrointestinal irritation is a common side effect.

Synthetic prostaglandin E_1 analogues, such as misoprostol (Cytotec), have important cytoprotective effects on mucosa, including promotion of increased blood flow. Their primary use is in the treatment of gastric erosions or ulcerations. Sulcralfate (Carafate) dissolved into a slurry has also been used to treat oral, esophageal, and gastrointestinal ulceration. It may stimulate prostaglandins E_2 and E_1, providing for a cytoprotective effect.

Plasmapheresis

Plasmapheresis has been use to treat chronic relapsing aphthous stomatitis in human patients and may have a future role in the treatment of animals with GS. Plasmapheresis improved the general status of the patients, accelerated epithelialization of the buccal mucosa, helped to attain prolonged remissions, and ameliorated the homeostasis parameters [61].

Human immunoglobulin

Human immunoglobulin has been used successfully in a dog with severe mucocutaneous ulceration consistent with SJS. A single intravenous infusion of human immunoglobulin at a rate of 0.51 g/kg was given and resulted in resolution of clinical signs. By blocking ligand interactions, human immunoglobulin is thought to prevent keratinocyte apoptosis. It also binds to immunoglobulin G receptors, inhibiting cell activation and cytokine synthesis; neutralizes autoantibodies and immune complexes; blocks complement activity; is antimicrobial; and increases colloid osmotic pressure. It has been used to treat EM in a cat and TEN in a dog [62].

Cyclosporine

Cyclosporine is a drug that alters the immunologic response. Cyclosporine is a medication that blocks T-helper cells. This is a specific and reversible inhibitor of immunocompetent lymphocytes, and T lymphocytes are preferentially inhibited. The T-helper cell is the main target, but T-suppresser cells may also be suppressed. Also, lymphokine production and release are inhibited, including IL-2 or T-cell growth factor (TCGF). Side effects include hepatic dysfunction, impaired renal function, and anemia. Oral absorption during chronic cyclosporine use is erratic. The doses of cyclosporine vary, and it is essential that these patients have blood levels evaluated to avoid toxicity (high levels). The risk increases with increasing dose and duration of cyclosporine therapy. Cyclosporine takes time to be beneficial, with some benefit seen by 4 weeks and the maximum benefit seen by 8 weeks. The absorption rates also vary with the form of this medication. The rate of oral cyclosporine absorption was less than expected, and there was substantial individual variation. Therapeutic drug monitoring strategies for cyclosporine in cats should be evaluated [63]. Sandimmune and Neoral are not bioequivalent and cannot be used interchangeably. In liver transplant patients treated with Neoral, peak levels were 40% to 106% greater than in those treated with Sandimmune. Sandimmune (Schering-Plough) has an expected absorption rate on oral administration of approximately 30%, and Neoral (Novartis) has an expected absorption rate on oral administration of approximately 60%. The higher absorption rates are related to the microemulsion form of the cyclosporine, with generics having the lowest absorption. The recommended dosage is 2 mg/kg administered twice daily up to 7.5 mg/kg administered twice daily.

Using Neoral oral solution (Novartis) is recommended because of better absorption and lower dosages—2 mg/kg administered orally twice daily. If Sandimmune is used, 7.5 to 15 mg/kg administered orally twice daily may be indicated. Most compounded cyclosporine solutions have poor absorption and response. Dosage adjustments may be necessary based on clinical response and given time to be effective (4–6 weeks). Serum levels are evaluated at 4 to 6 weeks, and Antech Diagnostics (Irvine, California) and IDEXX Laboratories, Inc, (Westbrook, Maine) run these tests. Dosage adjustments are made based on these levels. Some cats can be reduced to once-daily doses. We have seen no toxicity reactions even at above recommended doses. We have seen gingival hyperplasia, which we believe is related to the cyclosporine. The cats that have been treated eventually receive once-daily doses or alternate-day doses of cyclosporine, and some are maintained on once-weekly dosages. Clinical response is the only factor in our decision to decrease the dosage, which is subjective. There are some patients that still require cortisone.

Cyclosporine is not approved for veterinary use in cats. In the treatment of GS or chronic PS, there are no published reports of appropriate dosage schedules for this disease. There are some publications listed for veterinary patients with dermatology and ophthalmology use. We are still trying to establish the response to therapy and recommendations for dosage schedules. We think that evaluation of serum levels gives us the best indication of absorption. Adjunctive therapy with corticosteroids is recommended in some patients.

In human beings, in three open trials and one double-blind study, a topical formulation of this drug produced significant improvement in OLP. Cyclosporine blood levels were generally low in these studies, and no abnormalities of laboratory values resulted during use. Of six patients with oral bullous diseases treated with topical cyclosporine, four showed a decrease in erythema, partial healing of ulcerations, and a reduction in pain. Three patients relapsed shortly after cyclosporine was discontinued. Four of eight patients with persistent aphthous stomatitis remained virtually free of ulcers during 8 weeks of topical cyclosporine therapy. These results indicate that topical cyclosporine is beneficial as a therapy for OLP and possibly other mucosal diseases [36,49,53,63–69].

Summary

GS with various patterns of disease may require antiviral therapy, steroids, laser fulguration, immunomodulation drugs, or nonsteroidal anti-inflammatory drugs. The use of cyclosporine as an immunomodulation drug has long-term benefits in reduction of the immunologic events that contribute to GS. Whole-mouth extraction or partial extraction (premolars and molars), with radiographic conformation that all root remnants have been removed, may be the most viable option in nonresponsive and or intractably painful stomatitis in noncompliant cats or dogs. Oral inflammation subsided after extraction without the need for further medication in approximately 70% of the cats from two studies with previously chronic unrelenting oral disease. The combination of immunomodulation with cyclosporine together with laser resection of proliferative tissue should be recommended if extraction of teeth is not desired. Removal of proliferative oral tissues by lasing (carbon dioxide laser) removes the tissue that may be producing tissue antigens and the area where bacteria are sequestered. The use of anti-inflammatory medications is recommended in the management of GS. Therapeutic success is achieved when there is elimination of proliferative tissue and inflammation.

References

[1] Diehl K, Rosychuk RA. Feline gingivitis-stomatitis-pharyngitis. Vet Clin N Am Small Anim Pract 1993;23(1):139–53.

[2] White SD, Rosychuk RA, Janik TA, et al. Plasma cell stomatitis-pharyngitis in cats: 40 cases (1973–1991). J Am Vet Med Assoc 1992;200(9):1377–80.

[3] Rubel GH, Hoffmann DE, Pedersen NC. Acute and chronic faucitis of domestic cats. Vet Clin N Am Small Anim Pract 1992;22(6):1347–60.

[4] Pedersen NC. Inflammatory oral cavity diseases of the cat. Vet Clin N Am Small Anim Pract 1992;22(6):1323–45.

[5] Williams CA, Aller MS. Gingivitis/stomatitis in cats. Vet Clin N Am Small Anim Pract 1992; 22(6):1361–83.

[6] Lyon KF. The differential diagnosis and treatment of gingivitis in the cat. Probl Vet Med 1990;2(1):137–51.

[7] Harvey CE. Oral inflammatory diseases in cats. J Am Anim Hosp Assoc 1991;27:585–91.

[8] Johnessee JS, Hurvitz AI. Feline plasma cell gingivitis-stomatitis. J Am Anim Hosp Assoc 1983;19:179–81.

[9] Gaskell RM, Gruffyd-Jones TJ. Intractable feline stomatitis. Vet Annu 1977;17:195–7.

[10] Curran MA, Kaiser SM, Achacoso PL, et al. Efficient transduction of nondividing cells by optimized feline immunodeficiency virus vectors. Mol Ther 2000;1(1):31–8.

[11] Hofmann-Lehmann R, Berger M, Sigrist B, et al. Feline immunodeficiency virus (FIV) infection leads to increased incidence of feline odontoclastic resorptive lesions (FORL). Vet Immunol Immunopathol 1998;65(2–4):299–308.

[12] Greenberg MS, Pinto A. Etiology and management of recurrent aphthous stomatitis. Curr Infect Dis Rep 2003;5(3):194–8.

[13] Addie DD, Radford A, Yam PS, et al. Cessation of feline calicivirus shedding coincident with resolution of chronic gingivostomatitis in a cat. J Small Anim Pract 2003;44(4):172–6.

[14] Poulet H, Brunet S, Soulier M, et al. Comparison between acute oral/respiratory and chronic stomatitis/gingivitis isolates of feline calicivirus: pathogenicity, antigenic profile and cross-neutralisation studies. Arch Virol 2000;145(2):243–61.

[15] Lommer MJ, Verstraete FJ. Concurrent oral shedding of feline calicivirus and feline herpesvirus 1 in cats with chronic gingivostomatitis. Oral Microbiol Immunol 2003;18(2):131–4.

[16] Waters L, Hopper CD, Gruffydd-Jones TJ, et al. Chronic gingivitis in a colony of cats infected with feline immunodeficiency virus and feline calicivirus. Vet Rec 1993;132(14): 340–2.

[17] Knowles JO, McArdle F, Dawson S, et al. Studies on the role of feline calicivirus in chronic stomatitis in cats. Vet Microbiol 1991;27(3–4):205–19.

[18] Tenorio AP, Franti CE, Madewell BR, et al. Chronic oral infections of cats and their relationship to persistent oral carriage of feline calici-, immunodeficiency, or leukemia viruses. Vet Immunol Immunopathol 1991;29(1–2):1–14.

[19] Knowles JO, Gaskell RM, Gaskell CJ, et al. Prevalence of feline calicivirus, feline leukaemia virus and antibodies to FIV in cats with chronic stomatitis. Vet Rec 1989;124(13):336–8.

[20] Geissler K, Schneider K, Platzer G, et al. Genetic and antigenic heterogeneity among feline calicivirus isolates from distinct disease manifestations. Virus Res 1997;48(2):193–206.

[21] Harbour DA, Howard PE, Gaskell RM. Isolation of feline calicivirus and feline herpesvirus from domestic cats 1980 to 1989. Vet Rec 1991;128(4):77–80.

[22] Hargis AM, Ginn PE. Feline herpesvirus 1–associated facial and nasal dermatitis and stomatitis in domestic cats. Vet Clin N Am Small Anim Pract 1999;29(6):281–90.

[23] Veir JK, Lappin MR, Foley JE, Getzy DM. Feline inflammatory polyps: historical, clinical, and PCR findings for feline calicivirus and feline herpes virus-1 in 28 cases. J Feline Med Surg 2002;4(4):195–9.

[24] Dawson S, McArdle F, Bennett M, et al. Typing of feline calicivirus isolates from different clinical groups by virus neutralisation tests. Vet Rec 1993;133(1):13–7.

[25] Lyon KF. Feline lymphoplasmacytic stomatitis associated with monoclonal gammopathy and Bence-Jones proteinuria. J Vet Dent 1994;11(1):25–7.

[26] Symeonidis A, Kouraklis-Symeonidis A, Grouzi E, et al. Determination of plasma cell secreting potential as an index of maturity of myelomatous cells and a strong prognostic factor. Leuk Lymphoma 2002;43(8):1605–12.

[27] Song JJ, Lee B, Chang JW, et al. Optimization of vesicular stomatitis virus-G pseudotyped feline immunodeficiency virus vector for minimized cytotoxicity with efficient gene transfer. Virus Res 2003;93(1):25–30.

[28] Akkina RK, Walton RM, Chen ML, et al. High-efficiency gene transfer into CD34+ cells with a human immunodeficiency virus type 1-based retroviral vector pseudotyped with vesicular stomatitis virus envelope glycoprotein G. J Virol 1996;70(4):2581–5.

[29] Harley R, Gruffydd-Jones TJ, Day MJ. Salivary and serum immunoglobulin levels in cats with chronic gingivostomatitis. Vet Rec 2003;152(5):125–9.

[30] Harley R, Helps CR, Harbour DA, et al. Cytokine mRNA expression in lesions in cats with chronic gingivostomatitis. Clin Diagn Lab Immunol 1999;6(4):471–8.

[31] Kohmoto M, Uetsuka K, Ikeda Y, et al. Eight-year observation and comparative study of specific pathogen-free cats experimentally infected with feline immunodeficiency virus (FIV) subtypes A and B: terminal acquired immunodeficiency syndrome in a cat infected with FIV petaluma strain. J Vet Med Sci 1998;60(3):315–21.

[32] English RV, Nelson P, Johnson CM, et al. Development of clinical disease in cats experimentally infected with feline immunodeficiency virus. J Infect Dis 1994;170(3):543–52.

[33] Ueno H, Hohdatsu T, Muramatsu Y, et al. Does coinfection of Bartonella henselae and FIV induce clinical disorders in cats? Microbiol Immunol 1996;40(9):617–20.

[34] Domingue GJ, Woody HB. Bacterial persistence and expression of disease. Clin Microbiol Rev 1997;10(2):320–44.

[35] Ayangco L, Rogers RS III. Oral manifestations of erythema multiforme. Dermatol Clin 2003;21(1):195–205.

[36] Femiano F, Gombos F, Scully C. Oral erosive/ulcerative lichen planus: preliminary findings in an open trial of sulodexide compared with cyclosporin (ciclosporin) therapy. Int J Dermatol 2003;42(4):308–11.

[37] Perry HO. Idiopathic gingivostomatitis. Dermatol Clin 1987;5(4):719–22.

[38] Cannell H, Kerawala C, Farthing P. Stomatitis glandularis—two confirmed cases of a rare condition. Br Dent J 1997;182(6):222–5.

[39] Olivry T, Chan LS, Xu L, et al. Novel feline autoimmune blistering disease resembling bullous pemphigoid in humans: IgG autoantibodies target the NC16A ectodomain of type XVII collagen (BP180/BPAG2). Vet Pathol 1999;36(4):328–35.

[40] Mallonnee DH, Harvey CE, Venner M, et al. Bacteriology of periodontal disease in the cat. Arch Oral Biol 1988;33:677–83.

[41] Norris JM, Love DN. Serum responses of cats with periodontal/gingival disease to members of the genus Porphyromonas. Clin Infect Dis 1995;20(Suppl 2):S314–6.

[42] Sims TJ, Moncla BJ, Page RC. Serum antibody response to antigens of oral gram-negative bacteria by cats with plasma cell gingivitis-pharyngitis. J Dent Res 1990;69(3):877–82.

[43] Harvey CE, Thornsberry C, Miller BR. Subgingival bacteria—comparison of culture results in dogs and cats with gingivitis. J Vet Dent 1995;12:147–50.

[44] Healy CM, Carvalho D, Pearson JD, et al. Raised anti-endothelial cell autoantibodies (AECA), but not anti-neutrophil cytoplasmic autoantibodies (ANCA), in recurrent oral

ulceration: modulation of AECA binding by tumour necrosis factor-alpha (TNF-alpha) and interferon-gamma (IFN-gamma). Clin Exp Immunol 1996;106(3):523–8.

[45] Tiede I, Fritz G, Strand S, et al. CD28-dependent Rac1 activation is the molecular target of azathioprine in primary human CD4+ T-lymphocytes. J Clin Invest 2003;111(8):1133–45.

[46] Yamauchi K, Wakabayashi H, Hashimoto S, et al. Effects of orally administered bovine lactoferrin on the immune system of healthy volunteers. Adv Exp Med Biol 1998;443: 261–5.

[47] Sato R, Inanami O, Tanaka Y, et al. Oral administration of bovine lactoferrin for treatment of intractable stomatitis in feline immunodeficiency virus (FIV)-positive and FIV-negative cats. Am J Vet Res 1996;57(10):1443–6.

[48] Femiano F, Gombos F, Scully C. Recurrent aphthous stomatitis unresponsive to topical corticosteroids: a study of the comparative therapeutic effects of systemic prednisone and systemic sulodexide. Int J Dermatol 2003;42(5):394–7.

[49] Popovsky JL, Camisa C. New and emerging therapies for diseases of the oral cavity. Dermatol Clin 2000;18(1):113–25.

[50] Kaliakatsou F, Hodgson TA, Lewsey JD, et al. Management of recalcitrant ulcerative oral lichen planus with topical tacrolimus. J Am Acad Dermatol 2002;46(1):35–41.

[51] Orbak R, Cicek Y, Tezel A, et al. Effects of zinc treatment in patients with recurrent aphthous stomatitis. Dent Mater J 2003;22(1):21–9.

[52] Masucci G. New clinical applications of granulocyte-macrophage colony-stimulating factor. Med Oncol 1996;13(3):149–54.

[53] Vaden SL. Cyclosporine and tacrolimus. Semin Vet Med Surg (Small Anim) 1997;12(3): 161–6.

[54] Mayr B, Deininger S, Buttner M. Treatment of chronic stomatitis of cats by local paramunization with PIND-ORF. Zentralbl Veterinarmed B 1991;38(1):78–80.

[55] Bukholm G, Degre M, Whitaker-Dowling P. Interferon treatment reduces endocytosis of virus and facultatively intracellular bacteria in various cell lines. J Interferon Res 1990;10(1): 83–9.

[56] Mochizuki M, Nakatani H, Yoshida M. Inhibitory effects of recombinant feline interferon on the replication of feline enteropathogenic viruses in vitro. Vet Microbiol 1994;39(1–2): 145–52.

[57] Baldwin SL, Powell TD, Sellins KS, et al. The biological effects of five feline IFN-alpha subtypes. Vet Immunol Immunopathol 2004;99(3–4):153–67.

[58] Hennet P. Chronic gingivo-stomatitis in cats: long-term follow-up of 30 cases treated by dental extractions. J Vet Dent 1997;14(1):15–21.

[59] Berlucchi M, Meini A, Plebani A, et al. Update on treatment of Marshall's syndrome (PFAPA syndrome): report of five cases with review of the literature. Ann Otol Rhinol Laryngol 2003;112(4):365–9.

[60] Parikh SR, Reiter ER, Kenna MN, et al. Utility of tonsillectomy in 2 patients with the syndrome of periodic fever, aphthous stomatitis, pharyngitis, and cervical adenitis. Arch Otolaryngol Head Neck Surg 2003;129(6):670–3.

[61] Borisova OV, El'kova NL, Shcherbachenko OI, et al. The use of plasmapheresis in treating recurrent aphthous stomatitis. Stomatologiia (Mosk) 1997;76(3):23–5.

[62] Nuttall TJ, Malham T. Successful intravenous human immunoglobulin treatment of drug-induced Stevens-Johnson syndrome in a dog. J Small Anim Pract 2004;45(7):357–61.

[63] Mehl ML, Kyles AE, Craigmill AL, et al. Disposition of cyclosporine after intravenous and multi-dose oral administration in cats. J Vet Pharmacol Ther 2003;26(5):349–54.

[64] Eisen D, Ellis CN. Topical cyclosporine for oral mucosal disorders. J Am Acad Dermatol 1990;23(6 Pt 2):1259–63; discussion, 1263–4.

[65] Robson D. Review of the pharmacokinetics, interactions and adverse reactions of cyclosporine in people, dogs and cats. Vet Rec 2003;152(24):739–48.

[66] Robson D. Review of the properties and mechanisms of action of cyclosporine with an emphasis on dermatological therapy in dogs, cats and people. Vet Rec 2003;152(25):768–72.

[67] Robson DC, Burton GG. Cyclosporin: applications in small animal dermatology. Vet Dermatol 2003;14(1):1–9.

[68] Daigle JC. More economical use of cyclosporine through combination drug therapy. J Am Anim Hosp Assoc 2002;38(3):205–8.

[69] Bose S, Mathur M, Bates P, et al. Requirement for cyclophilin A for the replication of vesicular stomatitis virus New Jersey serotype. J Gen Virol 2003;84(Pt 7):1687–99.

ELSEVIER
SAUNDERS

Vet Clin Small Anim
35 (2005) 913–942

VETERINARY
CLINICS
Small Animal Practice

Update on the Etiology of Tooth Resorption in Domestic Cats

Alexander M. Reiter, Dipl Tzt, Dr Med Vet[a],*,
John R. Lewis, VMD[a], Ayako Okuda, DVM, PhD[b,c]

[a]*Department of Clinical Studies, School of Veterinary Medicine,
University of Pennsylvania, 3900 Delancey Street, Philadelphia, PA 19104–6010, USA*
[b]*Department of Anatomy, School of Veterinary Medicine,
Azabu University, Fuchinobe, Japan*
[c]*Vettec Dentistry, Tokyo, Japan*

Feline odontoclastic resorptive lesions (FORL) were first recognized and histologically differentiated from caries in the 1920s [1,2]. Some anecdotal reports describing caries-like lesions at the cervical region of feline teeth followed in the 1950s and 1960s, until two microscopic studies in the 1970s again revealed that FORL were not caries but a type of tooth resorption [3,4]. A recent study showed that cats with FORL have a significantly lower urine specific gravity and significantly higher serum concentration of 25-hydroxyvitamin D (25OHD) compared with cats without FORL [5], indicating that multiple tooth resorption in domestic cats could be the manifestation of some systemic insult rather than a local cause. In this article, the histologic and radiographic appearance of FORL and certain other peculiarities of feline teeth are reviewed. An attempt is then made to compare these findings with changes of the periodontium induced by administration of excess vitamin D or vitamin D metabolites in experimental animals.

Histologic and radiographic features of feline odontoclastic resorptive lesions

Tooth resorption is caused by *odontoclasts*. Their precursors derive from hematopoietic stem cells of bone marrow or spleen and migrate from blood vessels of the alveolar bone or periodontal ligament toward the external root

---

* Corresponding author.
E-mail address: reiter@vet.upenn.edu (A.M. Reiter).

0195-5616/05/$ - see front matter © 2005 Elsevier Inc. All rights reserved.
doi:10.1016/j.cvsm.2005.03.006   *vetsmall.theclinics.com*

surface, where mononuclear cells fuse with other cells to become multinucleated mature odontoclasts [6,7]. One important fact to understand is that FORL develop anywhere on the root surface and not just close to the cementoenamel junction [8]. Resorption of enamel as the initial event is only rarely observed [9]. Resorption may also start on the same tooth at various root surfaces simultaneously, progressing from cementum coronally into crown dentin as well as apically into root dentin. As the resorption progresses into crown dentin, the enamel often becomes undermined and a pink discoloration may be observed at the crown surface [10].

FORL that emerge at the gingival margin were originally referred to as *neck lesions* (Fig. 1) [4]. Exposure to periodontal inflammation, which is caused and maintained by bacterial infection, results in the formation of highly vascular and inflamed granulation tissue [11–16]. These defects may be painful and bleed easily when probed with a dental instrument [10]. One characteristic feature of *inflammatory root resorption* is that the alveolar bone adjacent to the tooth defect is also resorbed [17]. Such root lesions have been categorized as *type I root lesions* if unaffected root areas are surrounded by a radiographically visible periodontal space (Fig. 2) [18]. Although pulp involvement may be seen in advanced stages of FORL [19,20], the cervical root resorption in human beings typically proceeds laterally and in an apical and coronal direction, surrounding a thin shell of dentin and predentin, and envelops the root canal, leaving an apple core appearance of the cervical area of the tooth [21].

It has been demonstrated in several studies in human beings that superficial external resorption is common and usually self-limiting [22]. Spontaneously repaired defects of cementum and superficial dentin are called *surface resorptions*, in which the anatomic contour of the root surface is restored [17]. Most clinically evident FORL appear histologically to be in resorptive and reparative phases simultaneously [14]. Although attempts at repair can be noted by production of bone, cellular cementum, and bone-cementum [12–14,19,20,23], tooth resorption in cats is usually progressive

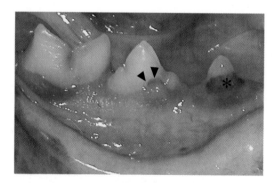

Fig. 1. Classic "neck lesions" at the right lower third (*) and fourth premolar teeth (*arrowheads*).

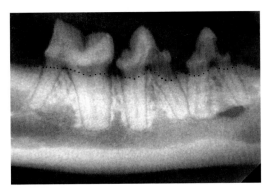

Fig. 2. Radiograph of teeth in Fig. 1; note that inflammatory root resorption is associated with adjacent alveolar bone resorption (*dotted line* outlining the alveolar margin).

and continues until the roots are completely resorbed or the crown breaks off, leaving root remnants behind [10].

Most previous research focused on FORL emerging at the gingival margin. The commonly observed fusion of roots of feline teeth with alveolar bone (*dentoalveolar ankylosis*) has not received the same investigative attention. It has previously been reported that the periodontal space is quite narrow in mandibular premolars and molars of adult cats [24]. In a recent histologic study, clinically and radiographically healthy teeth from cats with FORL on other teeth were evaluated. These apparently "healthy" teeth showed hyperemia, edema, and degeneration of the periodontal ligament, with marked fiber disorientation, increased osteoid formation along alveolar bone surfaces (*hyperosteoidosis*), gradual narrowing of the periodontal space, and areas of ankylotic fusion between the tooth and alveolar bone (Fig. 3) [25]. These findings demonstrate events that occur before resorption and suggest that the early FORL may be noninflammatory in nature [25]. Ankylosed roots are at risk of being incorporated into the normal process of bone remodeling, and the tooth substance is gradually resorbed and replaced by bone (*replacement resorption*) (Fig. 4) [10]. Ankylosed roots and those with replacement resorption have been categorized radiographically as *type II root lesions* [18].

Peculiarities of feline permanent teeth

It has previously been suggested that there is a need for further microscopic research to differentiate histopathologic findings of FORL from normal anatomy of feline teeth [26]. Several peculiarities can be noted in permanent teeth of cats that could represent separate pathologic entities or be associated with FORL.

Cementum is an avascular bone-like tissue covering the roots of mammalian teeth. It normally covers the cervical root surface as a thin

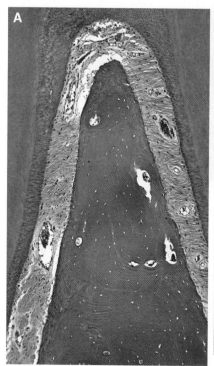

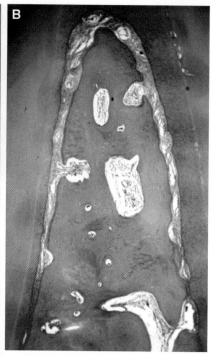

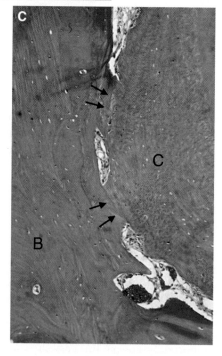

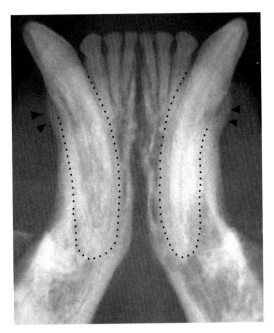

Fig. 4. Radiograph of dentoalveolar ankylosis and root replacement resorption of mandibular canine teeth (*dotted line* outlining original root contour); also note the bulbous enlargement of crestal alveolar bone (*arrowheads*).

layer that gradually becomes wider apically. Two types of cementum (acellular and cellular) are usually recognized, which can be further subdivided depending on the presence and origin of collagen fibers (afibrillar, intrinsic, or extrinsic). Cementum formation beyond physiologic deposition is called *hypercementosis* and can commonly be observed in teeth of cats with FORL [12]. In one study, hypercementosis was demonstrated in all investigated feline teeth [14]. Excessive amounts of cellular cementum are deposited particularly at apical and midroot surfaces, sometimes causing bulbous root apices (Fig. 5), whereas an abnormal thickening of acellular cementum can be found on cervical root surfaces (Fig. 6) [25]. In other species, hypercementosis has been observed in unerupted, hypofunctional, and extruding teeth without opposing antagonists [27–30] and in certain conditions, such as hyperthyroidism [31], hyperpituitarism [32–34], Paget's

Fig. 3. Histopathologic pictures of a feline premolar tooth with a normal furcation area (*A*) and a premolar tooth of a cat with feline odontoclastic resorptive lesions on other teeth showing degeneration of the periodontal ligament, narrowing of the periodontal space, and dentoalveolar ankylosis (*B*). Close-up of apical area of tooth root showing periodontal ligament degeneration and two areas of ankylotic fusion (*arrows*) between cementum (*C*) and alveolar bone (*B*).

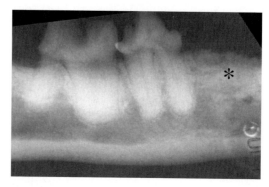

Fig. 5. Radiograph showing bulbous root apices of the right lower fourth premolar and first molar in a cat; note the missing third premolar tooth (*).

disease [35–37], and vitamin A deficiency [38,39]. It has also been demonstrated that occlusal trauma does *not* lead to hypercementosis [40,41].

Some cats seem to exhibit abnormal extrusion of teeth, referred to as *supereruption* [10]. Supereruption is most commonly observed in maxillary

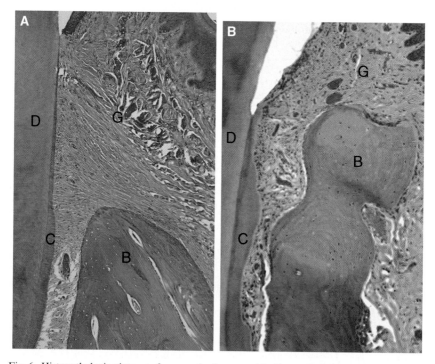

Fig. 6. Histopathologic pictures of a premolar in a cat with thin cervical cementum and normal biologic width (*A*) and a premolar of a cat with feline odontoclastic resorptive lesions on other teeth showing cervical hypercementosis, bulbous enlargement of crestal alveolar bone, and loss of biologic width (*B*). B, alveolar bone; C, cementum; D, dentin; G, gingival connective tissue.

canine teeth, leading to exposure of the root surface (Fig. 7). Normally, active eruption of brachyodont teeth does not cease when they meet their opposing teeth but continues throughout life; ideally, the rate of eruption keeps pace with tooth wear, preserving the vertical dimension of the dentition [42]. It has been speculated that supereruption in cats may be the result of hypercementosis [43] or increased osteoblastic activity of periapical alveolar bone [44]. Another peculiarity found in cats is a distinct thickening of bone along the alveolar margin or the surfaces of the alveolar plates, alone or in combination with supereruption. This *alveolar bone expansion* is commonly seen in maxillary canine teeth but occurs with less intensity around other teeth as well (Fig. 8) [10]. In human beings, a similar condition is called "peripheral buttressing" and is believed to be a result of the body's attempt to compensate for lost bone during the reparative process associated with trauma from occlusion. The condition may present as shelf-like thickening of the alveolar margin, referred to as "lipping", or as a pronounced bulge in the contour of the alveolar bone [45].

Unusual dentin formation has been described in feline teeth. In one study, *osteodentin* could be demonstrated in most feline premolars and molars, particularly in furcation areas of root dentin close to the root canal [13]. In osteodentin, cellular inclusions (remnants of odontoblasts) can be found between randomly running dentinal tubules. FORL were observed in areas of the tooth in which osteodentin was most typically found [13]. *Vasodentin* was found in 3 of 10 control teeth and in 6 of 49 teeth with FORL and was most often observed in the outer third of circumpulpal dentin [46]. In vasodentin, dentinal tubules run randomly, with penetration of canals that may contain vascular-like tissue. Another study found vasodentin almost equally in teeth with or without FORL, although the

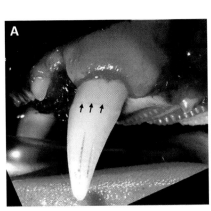
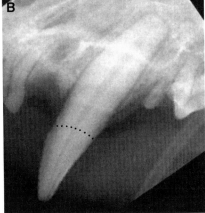

Fig. 7. Clinical picture (*A*) and radiograph (*B*) of the left upper canine tooth showing supereruption (*arrows* and *dotted line* outlining the cementoenamel junction).

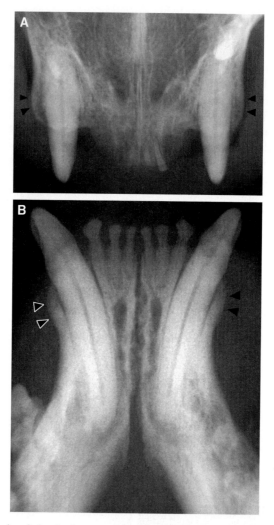

Fig. 8. Radiographs of alveolar bone expansion (*arrowheads*) of upper (*A*) and lower canine teeth (*B*) in cats with missing teeth and feline odontoclastic resorptive lesions on other teeth.

locations of vasodentin and FORL differed [13]. Furcation canals connecting the pulp chamber and the periodontal ligament were found in deciduous premolar teeth in kittens as well as in teeth of adult cats [47,48]. After experimental pulp injury, changes in the periodontal ligament at the opening of the furcation canal and resorption of dental tissues and alveolar bone in the furcation area took place [48]. In a more recent study, patent furcation canals were found in 27% of permanent carnassial teeth in adult cats [49].

Irregularities in dentin formation are generally considered to be evidence of deficient mineralization during dentinogenesis [50]. The inclusion of odontoblasts or pulp tissue into dentin may also be attributable to times of rapid mineralization of newly formed dentin matrix, however. This view is supported by the observation that the layer of predentin appeared extremely thin or was not present in teeth of cats with FORL [51].

Increased vitamin D activity in cats with feline odontoclastic resorptive lesions

Although FORL may have occurred more than 800 years ago [52], retrospective studies of zoologic collections of feline skulls showed a low prevalence of FORL before the 1960s [53,54]. It was suggested that the increased prevalence of FORL might be associated with aspects of domestication, such as altered feeding practices, vaccination, and neutering programs [10].

Unlike bone that undergoes resorption and apposition as part of a continual remodeling process, the roots of permanent teeth are normally not resorbed because of resorption-inhibiting characteristics of unmineralized layers on external and internal root surfaces (eg, periodontal ligament, cementoblasts and cementoid, odontoblasts and predentin) [10,17]. Odontoclasts may be attracted only to, or can attach only to, mineralized tissue. It has been postulated that removal or mineralization of the organic matrix of the root covering would make it possible for odontoclasts to recognize the mineral component [10,17].

Measurement of biochemical markers of bone turnover, bone alkaline phosphatase (BAP) and deoxypyridinoline (DPD), did not show significant differences between cats with and without FORL [55]. It has recently been demonstrated that cats with FORL expressed a significantly higher mean serum concentration of 25OHD compared with cats without FORL, however [5]. Furthermore, the mean serum concentrations of blood urea nitrogen and phosphorus were significantly higher and the mean urine specific gravity and mean calcium-phosphorus ratio were significantly lower in cats with FORL compared with cats without FORL [5]. Although the mean values of renal parameters remained within physiologic range, the results suggest the possibility of gradual impairment of renal function in cats with FORL. Using a human radioimmunoassay not yet validated for use in cats, calcitonin was significantly more often detected in blood sera of cats with FORL, which may be an expression of protective secretion during times of transient mild hypercalcemia [5]. It was also demonstrated that cats with FORL vomited significantly more often than cats without FORL [5,56].

The diet represents the only source of vitamin D in cats because they are unable to produce vitamin D in the skin [57]. Based on feeding studies in the 1950s, the National Research Council proposed a minimum vitamin D requirement for growing kittens of 500 IU/kg of dietary dry matter [58]. Later studies demonstrated that kittens given a diet with vitamin D_3 per kilogram of dry matter at a rate of 250 or 125 IU did not show clinical signs

Table 1
Changes in dental and periodontal tissues of experimental animals receiving excess vitamin D or vitamin D metabolites

Reference no.	Species	Age/weight at start of experiment	Type of vitamin D	Dose	Route of administration	Additional methods	Diagnostic tools
[103]	Rats	127–182 g	Vit D (nfd)	307,000–1,860,000 IU (once); killed after 48 h	SC	n/a	H
[108]	Dogs	39 d	irrad D2 or D3	10,000 IU/kg BW × 9.5 mo	Food	Some dogs also given excess vit A	R + H
[109,119]	Dogs	29 or 34 d	irrad D2	450,000 IU (once); killed at 2.5, 4, or 9 mo of age	PO	n/a	R + H
[110,114]	Dogs	2 mo	D2 or D3	10,000 IU/kg BW/d × 6 mo (intermittently) (total 1,270,000 and 1,450,000 IU); killed after additional 5 mo of "recovery period"	Food	n/a	R + H
[105]	Rats	21 d (∼100 g)	D2	500,000 IU (once); killed after 6 d	P	n/a	R + H (I + M)
[97]	Rats	40–50 g	D2	100,000 IU on 1st, 4th, 7th, 10th, and 14th d; killed on 15th d	IP	Some rats also given a collagen-damaging lathyrogen	H (M)
[121]	Rats	50–150 g	D2	50,000–200,000 IU × 2–4/wk; sacrifice after 1–12 wk	PO	n/a	H (LM + EM)
[111]	Rats	154 g	D2	1.25 mio IU/kg of diet × 6 wk	Food	n/a	H (M)
[112]	Hamsters	4 mo	D2	5,000 IU twice/wk × 8 wk	IP	n/a	H (M)
[102]	Pigs	5 d	D3	45,000–162,000 IU/d × 17–48 d	PO	n/a	H

Pulp/dentin	Cementum	Periodontal ligament	Gingival connective tissue	Alveolar bone	Comments
Calciotraumatic line on inner edge of dentin, followed by hypomineralized layer, wide hypermineralized zone, and ↓width of predentin	n/r	n/r	n/r	n/r	Formation of dentin proceeded at same rate as that of control rats but MIN was accelerated
DEG; pulp stones in permanent C + M	HC	MIN; ANK	MIN	Initial OP, followed by OS with ↓lumen of ES in younger dogs; less OS in older dogs	↓changes in dogs given vit D from tuna or halibut liver oil than irrad D2; ↓changes in dogs given excess vit A
DEG; MIN	HC; resorption	MIN	n/r	OP	n/a
Pulp stones	HC	Development of granulation tissue in furcation and interdental areas; MIN; ANK	MIN	Increased vascularity; granulation tissue formation; ↑periodontitis in dog given D3	OP was predominant
Hemorrhage, odontoblast DEG, accelerated dentin formation, MIN in M	n/r	n/r	n/r	n/r	n/a
n/r	n/r	MIN	MIN	n/r	↑changes in rats given the lathyrogen
n/r	Intracellular MIN of cementoblast-like cells; HC	DEG; MIN of fibers close to cemental surface ("sunburst" pattern)	MIN	OP followed, by HO and OS; alveolar crest raised to CEJ	n/a
n/r	HC	FD; ↓PS; MIN; ANK	MIN with 'sunburst' pattern near transeptal fibers	OP followed, by HO and OS; alveolar crest raised to CEJ; marrow spaces filled with young connective tissue	n/a
n/r	Cemental spurs	↓PS; MIN; ANK	n/r	Thinning of cortical bone and endosteal resorption, followed by HO	n/a
DEG and hyperemia; MIN; osteodentin formation	Resorption of cementum and dentin with pulp exposure	Hyperemia; MIN; ANK	n/r	OP, followed by HO	n/a

(continued on next page)

Table 1 (*continued*)

Reference no.	Species	Age/weight at start of experiment	Type of vitamin D	Dose	Route of administration	Additional methods	Diagnostic tools
[101]	Rabbits	15 d (~150 g)	D3	600,000 IU/kg BW once/wk × 4 wk; killed 30, 45, or 60 d after initial injection	IM	n/a	R + H
[106]	Rats	n/r	D3	10,000 IU/d × 1-4 wk	TGT	n/a	H (I + M)
[107]	Rats	8 or 12 wk (35–271 g)	D3	200,000 IU/d (on 6 d/wk) × up to 2 mo	TGT	n/a	H (I + M)
[122]	Rats	100 g	DHT	50 µg/d × 17 d	TGT	n/a	H (M)
[123]	Rats	140–150 g	DHT	50 µg/d × 31 or 62 d	TGT	Some rats also given FD	H (M)
[120]	Rats	~220 g	DHT	50 µg/d × 50 d	TGT	n/a	H
[91]	Rats	215 g	DHT	50 µg/d × 50 d	PO	Some rats also given FD	H (M)
[98]	Rats	200 g	DHT	50 µg/d × 7–50 d	TGT	Some rats also given FD	H
[95]	Rats	~100 g	DHT	50 µg/d × 40 d	TGT	Some rats also given TS	H (M)

Pulp/dentin	Cementum	Periodontal ligament	Gingival connective tissue	Alveolar bone	Comments
n/r	n/r	FD; MIN	n/r	OP, followed by HO and OS	n/a
Pulp stones in I	HC	MIN; ANK in M	n/r	HO and OS	n/a
↓width of predentin; DEG of odontoblasts; pulp stones (primarily in I of young and older rats)	HC (most intense in apical areas of young rats); resorption of cementum and dentin in nearly all M of rat fed longest with D3	↓PS; MIN; ANK in M	n/r	OP, followed by HO and OS (predominantly in young rats); ↓lumen of ES; ↑crestal alveolar bone (predominantly in young rats)	n/a
Hyperemia, hemorrhage, and separation of odontoblasts	HC	DEG, edema, and hemorrhage; FD; MIN; ANK	n/r	HO; ↓lumen of ES; edema of bone marrow	n/a
Edema, hyperemia, hemorrhage, and reticular atrophy; pulp stones	HC; "club"-shaped root apices; resorption of cementum and dentin, particularly in furcation areas	DEG, edema, and hemorrhage; FD; ↓PS; MIN; ANK	n/r	HO; ↓lumen of ES; bulbous enlargement of alveolar plates; edematous marrow tissue	↓changes in rats given FD
n/r	HC; "club"-shaped root apices; resorption of cementum and dentin with ingrowth of connective tissue cells into resorptive defects	FD; ↓PS; MIN; ANK	MIN with 'sunburst' pattern near transeptal fibers	Rapid and progressive resorption, followed by HO and OS	n/a
n/r	HC	DEG; FD; ANK	MIN with 'sunburst' pattern near transeptal fibers	HO and OS; ↓lumen of ES; bulbous enlargement of alveolar plates	↓changes in rats given FD; most severe changes in furcation areas
n/r	HC ("club"-shaped root apices)	DEG, hyperemia, and edema; ↓PS; MIN; ANK	MIN with 'sunburst' pattern near transeptal fibers	HO and OS; bulbous enlargement of alveolar plates causing coronal displacement of transeptal fibers; hyperemia and progressive fibrosis of bone marrow	↓changes in rats given FD; most severe changes in furcation areas
Hemorrhage; pulp stones	HC	DEG, hyperemia, and edema; ↓PS; ANK	n/r	HO; ↓lumen of ES; fibrosis of bone marrow; enlargement of buccal and lingual bone at areas of muscle insertion	↓changes in rats given TS

(continued on next page)

Table 1 (*continued*)

Reference no.	Species	Age/weight at start of experiment	Type of vitamin D	Dose	Route of administration	Additional methods	Diagnostic tools
[96]	Rats	~260 g	DHT	1 mg/100 g BW (once); killed after 10, 17 or 31 d	TGT	Gingival wound created 3 d after DHT was given	H (M)
[125]	Rats	40 d	DHT	50 μg/d × 50 d	TGT	n/a	H (M)
[99]	Rats	~100 g	DHT	50 mg/d × 1–7 wk	TGT	Some rats had all L max M extracted	H (M)
[117]	Rats	100 g	D2 or DHT	10,000 IU (D2)/d or 50 μg (DHT)/d × 50 d	SC (D2) or TGT (DHT)	Some rats also given TS or ED	H (M)
[116]	Rats	100 g	DHT	50 μg/d × 7–35 d	TGT	n/a	H (M)
[100]	Rats	180–220 g	DHT	50 μg/100 g BW/d × 28 d	TGT	Traumatic occlusion induced in some rats	H (M)
[118]	Rats	5 wk	DHT	50 μg/100 g BW/d × 28 d	TGT	Some rats also given SF	H (M)
[124]	Rats	140 g	DHT	50 μg/100 g BW/d × up to 20 d	TGT	n/a	
[115]	Rats	6 wk	DHT	25 or 50 μg/d × 1–4 wk	TGT	n/a	H (M)
[104]	Rats	4 wk	1,25(OH)2D3	0.075 μg/d × 5 wk	SC	n/a	H + R (I + M)

Abbreviations: ANK, ankylosis; BW, body weight; C, canine teeth; CEJ, cementoenamel junction; d, days; D2, vitamin D_2; D3, vitamin D_3; DEG, degeneration; DHT, dihydrotachysterol; ED, estradiol; EM, electron microscopy; FD, ferric dextran; h, hours; H, histology; HC, hypercementosis; HO, hyperosteoidosis; I, incisor teeth; IM, intramuscular junction; IP, intraperitoneal injection; irrad; irradiation; L, left; LM, light microscopy; M, molar teeth; max, maxillary; MIN, mineralization; mio, million; mo, months; nfd, not further defined; n/a, not applicable; n/r, not reported; 1,25(OH)2D3, 1,25-dyhydroxyvitamin D_3; OP, osteoporosis; OS, osteosclerosis; P, parenteral; PO, per os; PS, periodontal space; R, radiography; SC, subcutaneous; SF, sodium fluoride; TGT, transoral gastric tube; TS, testosterone; vit, vitamin; wk, weeks.

Pulp/dentin	Cementum	Periodontal ligament	Gingival connective tissue	Alveolar bone	Comments
n/r	HC	ANK	n/r	HO; new bone formation at alveolar crest below the injury	n/a
↓number of pulp cells; MIN; ↓lumen of pulp cavity	HC	DEG and FD; ↓PS; MIN	n/r	HO and OS; ↓lumen of ES; bulbous enlargement of alveolar plates	n/a
n/r	HC	DEG and FD; ↓PS	n/r	HO and OS; ↓lumen of ES; fibrosis of bone marrow; bulbous enlargement of alveolar plates	↓changes in male rats and teeth without opposing antagonists
n/r	HC	DEG, hyperemia, and FD; ↓PS; MIN	n/r	HO; ↓lumen of ES	↓changes in rats given D2; when given DHT, ↑changes in female rats; ↓changes in rats given DHT when also given sexual hormones
n/r	HC	DEG and FD; MIN; ANK	n/r	HO	n/a
n/r	HC	FD; ↓PS	n/r	HO	↑changes in rats with traumatic occlusion
n/r	HC	FD; ↓PS	n/r	HO	↓changes in rats given FD
n/r	HC	DEG and FD; ↓PS; ANK	n/r	HO	n/a
n/r	HC	DEG; ↓PS; ANK	n/r	HO; ↓lumen of ES; fibrosis of bone marrow	Progeria-like changes
↓width of predentin; DEG of odontoblasts and fibroblasts; formation of irregular dentin and osteodentin	HC	ANK of M	n/r	HO	n/a

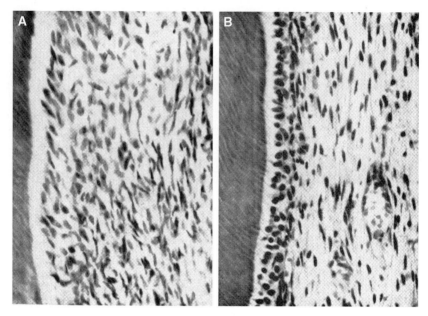

Fig. 9. Histopathologic pictures of pulp from molar teeth of a control rat (*A*) and pulp from a molar tooth of a rat given dihydrotachysterol showing increased activity of odontoblasts, fluid accumulation in the odontoblastic layer, and reticular atrophy with hyperemia and edema (*B*). (*From* Ratcliff PA, Itokazu H. The effect of dihydrotachysterol on the teeth and periodontium. J Periodontol 1964;35:324; with permission.)

of vitamin D deficiency [59,60]. Furthermore, it was found that one third of commercial cat foods contained vitamin D_3 in excess of current maximal allowances (>10,000 IU/kg of dietary dry matter), and a direct linear relation was demonstrated between 25OHD serum concentrations and dietary intake of vitamin D [61]. Therefore, higher 25OHD serum concentrations in cats with FORL suggest that they had ingested larger amounts of vitamin D or vitamin D metabolites compared with cats without FORL [5]. Three separate incidences of fatal hypervitaminosis D were reported in cats in Japan after consumption of commercial cat foods prepared from fish [62–64]. Clinical, laboratory, and histopathologic findings in these cats included vomiting, hypercalcemia, hyperphosphatemia, azotemia, proteinuria, calciuria, phosphaturia, decreased urine specific gravity, and mineralization of various body tissues, particularly the kidneys and walls of large blood vessels [62]. One may speculate as to whether there is indeed a predisposition to impairment of renal function in cats with FORL, because results of experimental studies on cats fed diets high in vitamin D_3 (15,000–33,840 IU/kg of dry matter) were contradictory, ranging from no evidence of detrimental effects on feline health to a high prevalence of renal dysfunction and mortality [65].

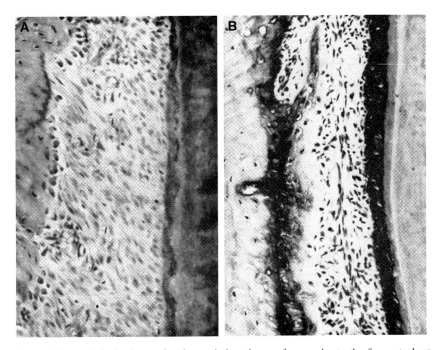

Fig. 10. Histopathologic picture showing periodontal space from molar teeth of a control rat (*A*) and a rat given dihydrotachysterol showing periodontal ligament fiber disorientation, edema, hyperemia, hypercementosis, hyperosteoidosis with bone spur formation, and narrowing of the periodontal space (*B*). (*From* Ratcliff PA, Itokazu H. The effect of dihydrotachysterol on the teeth and periodontium. J Periodontol 1964;35:323; with permission.)

Vitamin D and vitamin D metabolites are important regulators of osteoclastic bone resorption [66]. Serum calcium concentration is maintained within a normal range through the primary action of 1,25-dihydroxyvitamin D_3 [1,25$(OH)_2D_3$], which increases intestinal absorption of dietary calcium and recruits hematopoietic stem cells to become osteoclasts. Osteoclasts, in turn, mobilize calcium stores from bone into the circulation. Osteoclasts do not possess receptors for 1,25$(OH)_2D_3$, however [66]. Receptors for 1,25$(OH)_2D_3$ are located on osteoblasts that produce factors stimulating osteoclasts, such as receptor activator of nuclear factor-κB ligand (RANKL), which plays an important role in osteoclastogenesis [67] and osteoclast activation [68].

Role of local trauma

The occlusal stress (tooth flexure) theory was created in an attempt to explain *noncarious cervical lesions*, an overall term for tooth wear (not resorption) at the cervical portion of human teeth [69–71]. Repeated compressive and tensile forces attributable to tooth flexure during

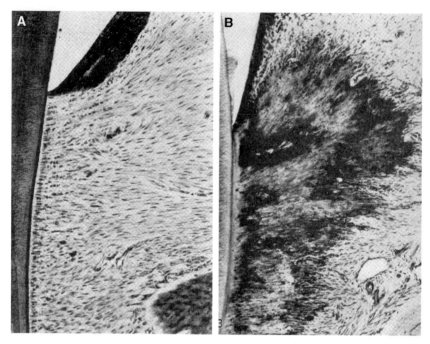

Fig. 11. Histopathologic pictures of cervical portion from teeth of a control dog (*A*) and a dog given excessive amounts of vitamin D showing abnormal thickening of cervical cementum (*B*). (*From* Becks H. Dangerous effects of vitamin D overdosage on dental and paradental structures. J Am Dent Assoc 1942;29:1960; with permission.)

mastication and malocclusion may disrupt the bonds between enamel rods and between enamel and dentin, resulting in abfraction of enamel, exposure of dentin, and cervical hypersensitivity [72,73]. Although FORL are clearly resorptive in nature and develop on any tooth and any root surface (not just on those exposed to occlusal or shearing forces), occlusal stress caused by eating large dry kibbles has been suggested to be associated with FORL [18,74,75]. A different approach for a possible role of occlusal stress in the development of FORL is presented in this article.

Surface resorption of cementum and superficial dentin may develop in response to normal masticatory stress [76] and excessive occlusal force [77–80]. Apical root resorption has been linked with bruxism in human beings, although the apical defect in that case report could also have resulted from endodontic disease [81]. Traumatic occlusion from maloccluding teeth may cause resorption of roots in rats and people, with the apical area being affected most often [22,82–86]. Root resorption has been demonstrated after experimental intrusion of teeth in people [87] and long-standing occlusal trauma in dogs and monkeys [88,89]. Subsequent repairs could eventually result in ankylosis [90].

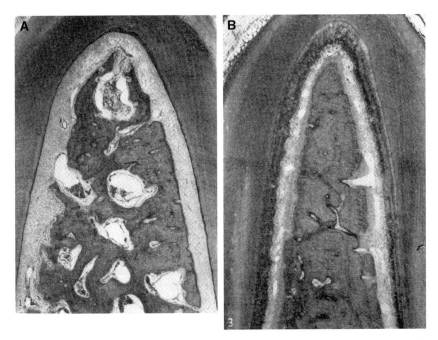

Fig. 12. Histopathologic pictures of furcation area from teeth of a control dog (*A*) and a dog given excessive amounts of vitamin D showing hypercementosis, hyperosteoidosis, and narrowing of the periodontal space (*B*). (*From* Becks H. Dangerous effects of vitamin D overdosage on dental and paradental structures. J Am Dent Assoc 1942;29:1951; with permission.)

Calciphylaxis is a condition of induced local or systemic hypersensitivity in which tissues respond to appropriate challenging agents with precipitous, sometimes evanescent, local mineralization of various tissues and organs [91,92]. Substances that predispose the organism to calciphylaxis are known as *sensitizers*. Sensitizers are systemically administered agents that promote mineralization of tissues and include vitamin D and vitamin D metabolites, parathyroid hormone, and sodium acetylsulfathiazole among many other calcium salts and phosphates [91]. Agents that precipitate the calciphylaxis phenomenon are known as *challengers*. Challengers may be direct or indirect. Direct challengers include mechanical trauma and various chemical agents (eg, salts of iron, chromium, aluminum, zinc, manganese, cesium) that cause mineralization at the site of application and may elicit some form of systemic calciphylaxis when administered intravenously or intraperito-neally. Indirect challengers have little or no effect at the site of application and produce diverse systemic syndromes of mineralization and sclerosis [91].

Experiments in dihydrotachysterol (DHT)-sensitized rats indicated that functional stress and topical trauma can produce local calcium deposits in various parts of the body [91,93,94]. In rats given DHT, enlargement of

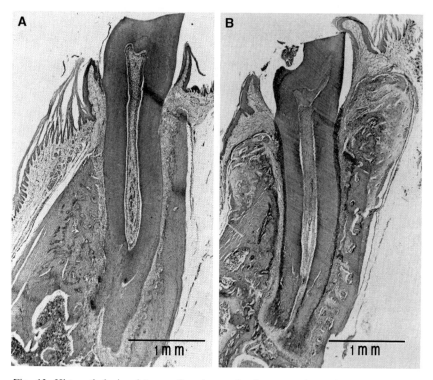

Fig. 13. Histopathologic pictures of molar teeth of a control rat (*A*) and a rat given dihydrotachysterol showing hypercementosis, hyperosteoidosis, narrowing of the periodontal space, and bulbous enlargement of crestal alveolar bone with loss of biologic width (*B*). (*From* Glickman I, Selye H, Smulow JB. Reduction by calciphylaxis of the effects of chronic dihydrotachysterol overdosage upon the periodontium. J Dent Res 1965;44:735–6; with permission.)

buccal and lingual bone occurred most notably at muscle insertions [95]. Alveolar bone formation at the site of a gingival injury took place more rapidly and was more evident in experimentally injured than noninjured rats that also received DHT [96]. Similarly, mineralization of the periodontal ligament and gingival connective tissue was enhanced when a collagen-damaging agent was given to rats receiving intraperitoneal injections of vitamin D_2 [97]. In rats given DHT, degeneration of the periodontal ligament, hypercementosis, hyperosteoidosis, narrowing of the periodontal space, and ankylosis were markedly more pronounced in furcation areas [91,98] and teeth that were in occlusion [99] or subjected to traumatic occlusion [100]. Daily masticatory stress could be the reason why chronic increased vitamin D intake manifests sooner and is more pronounced in periodontal tissues compared with other soft tissues, and FORL may therefore occur before or without obvious signs of vitamin D–induced systemic disease.

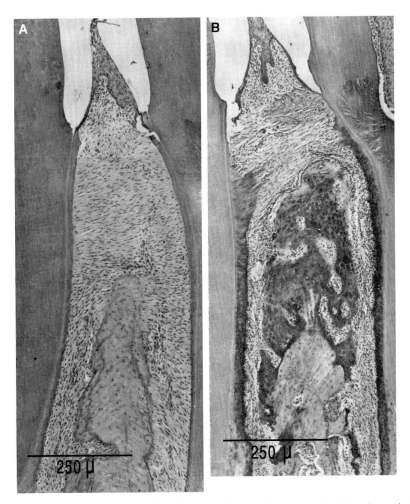

Fig. 14. Histopathologic pictures of interdental area from teeth of a control rat (*A*) and a rat given dihydrotachysterol showing hypercementosis, hyperosteoidosis, edematous degeneration of the periodontal ligament, narrowing of the periodontal space, bulbous enlargement of crestal alveolar bone, coronal displacement of transeptal fibers, and reduction of biologic width (*B*). (*From* Glickman I, Selye H, Smulow JB. Reduction by calciphylaxis of the effects of chronic dihydrotachysterol overdosage upon the periodontium. J Dent Res 1965;44:738; with permission.)

Experimental studies with vitamin D and vitamin D metabolites

Numerous reports describe the effects of excess vitamin D and vitamin D metabolites on the pulp-dentin complex and periodontium in experimental animals (rodents, lagomorphs, pigs, and dogs) (Table 1).

In the pulp-dentin complex, pulpal hyperemia and degeneration, decreased width of the predentin layer, and formation of osteodentin and

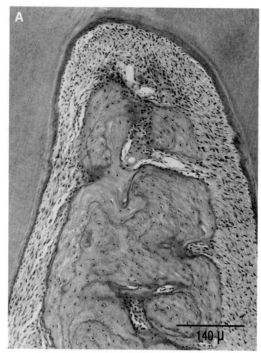

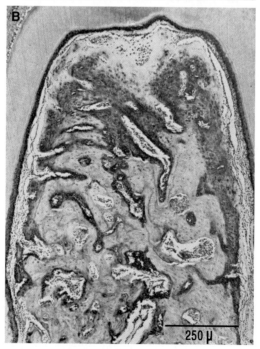

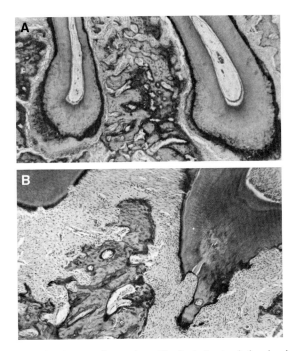

Fig. 16. Histopathologic pictures of rats given dihydrotachysterol showing bulbous enlargement of root apices (A) and resorption of cementum, dentin, and alveolar bone (B). (*From* Moskow BS, Baden E. The effect of chronic dihydrotachysterol overdosage on the tissues of the periodontium. Periodontics 1964;2:279–80; with permission.)

irregular dentin containing small vascular canals (Fig. 9) have been reported [101–107].

In the periodontium, periodontal ligament hyperemia, edema, and degeneration with fiber disorientation; mineralization of Sharpey's fibers; hypercementosis with abnormal thickening of cervical cementum and a bulbous appearance of root apices; hyperosteoidosis along periosteal and endosteal surfaces; reduced endosteal lumina; bone marrow fibrosis; bulbous enlargement of alveolar plates with coronal displacement of transeptal fibers at the alveolar margin; narrowing of the periodontal space; dentoalveolar ankylosis; granulation tissue formation; irregular resorptive lacunae in cementum and dentin; and a mixed pattern of osteoporosis and osteosclerosis (Fig. 10–16) have been reported [91,95–102,104,106–125].

Fig. 15. Histopathologic pictures of furcation area of molar teeth in a control rat (A) and a rat given dihydrotachysterol showing hypercementosis, hyperosteoidosis, degeneration of the periodontal ligament, and narrowing of the periodontal space (B). (*From* Glickman I, Selye H, Smulow JB. Reduction by calciphylaxis of the effects of chronic dihydrotachysterol overdosage upon the periodontium. J Dent Res 1965;44:743–4; with permission.)

Extrapolating these findings to the domestic cat should be done with caution, however, because the results of these experimental studies are not uniform. Furthermore, the ages, sizes, and species of animals; the character of their diets; the varying forms, quantities, and routes of administration of vitamin D and vitamin D metabolites; and the duration of the experiments differed. Nevertheless, there are distinct similarities between the changes in dental and periodontal tissues induced by administration of excess vitamin D and vitamin D metabolites in experimental animals and radiographic and microscopic features that can be found in teeth from cats with FORL (eg, thin predentin layer, irregular dentin formation, periodontal ligament degeneration and fiber disorientation, hypercementosis, hyperosteoidosis, thickening of crestal alveolar bone, narrowing of the periodontal space, dentoalveolar ankylosis, root resorption, mixed pattern of osteoporosis and osteosclerosis). Vitamin D–induced thickening of cervical cementum and abnormal apposition of osteoid at the alveolar crest and other periosteal surfaces causing bulbous enlargement of alveolar plates and coronal displacement of transeptal fibers could result in reduction of the biologic width (the dimension of space occupied by junctional epithelium and gingival connective tissue) and loss of gingival attachment. Supereruption of teeth in cats with increased vitamin D activity may actually be an attempt to maintain or re-establish normal biologic width.

Certain findings are worthy of additional discussion, including (a) differences in effects of vitamin D and vitamin D metabolites between continuously growing and continuously erupting teeth and between young and adult animals and (b) apparent alleviation of the detrimental effects of vitamin D and vitamin D metabolites by concurrent administration of other agents. In rats, pulpal mineralization and pulp stones occurred more commonly in incisors than in molars and more commonly in younger than in older animals [107], which may be an indication that vitamin D activity is more influential on "young" or continuously renewing tissue. Although pulpal mineralization has not been reported in permanent teeth of cats with FORL, pulp stones have been demonstrated in experimental vitamin D studies in puppies [108,110,114]. Young animals (dogs and rats) showed initial alveolar bone resorption and osteoporosis followed by hyperosteoidosis and osteosclerosis with a narrowing of endosteal spaces, whereas alveolar bone resorption and osteoporosis were predominant in adult or older animals [107,108]. Studies investigating the appearance of alveolar bone in younger and older FORL-affected cats have not yet been conducted. Effects of vitamin D or vitamin D metabolites were less severe or could be reduced in animals given various amounts of vitamin A [108,114], sexual hormones [95,117], ferric dextran [91,98,123], or sodium fluoride [118], in addition to excess administration of vitamin D or vitamin D metabolites. This may be of interest when considering future research that focuses on prevention of FORL.

Summary

The following conclusions can be drawn:

1. Cats depend on dietary vitamin D intake because they are not able to produce vitamin D in the skin.
2. Some commercial cat foods contain vitamin D concentrations in excess of current maximal allowances.
3. Cats with FORL have significantly higher serum concentrations of 25OHD compared with cats without FORL, indicating that cats with FORL must have ingested higher concentrations of dietary vitamin D.
4. Cats with FORL have significantly decreased urine specific gravity compared with cats without FORL.
5. Experimental studies on laboratory animals have shown that excess administration of vitamin D or vitamin D metabolites causes changes to dental and periodontal tissues that resemble many characteristics of teeth from cats with FORL.
6. Clinical and experimental studies have shown that excess administration of vitamin D or vitamin D metabolites can lead to soft tissue mineralization and various degrees of renal disease.

Dietary intake of excess vitamin D over several years may lead to periodontal ligament degeneration, narrowing of the periodontal space, dentoalveolar ankylosis, and root replacement resorption. If such a process occurs close to the gingival margin, an inflammatory component may join the disease. Further histologic and experimental studies are required to determine the role of daily masticatory stresses on the development of FORL and to verify relations between FORL, vitamin D, and renal insufficiency.

References

[1] Hopewell-Smith A. The process of osteolysis and odontolysis, or so-called "absorption" of calcified tissues: a new and original investigation. Dental Cosmos 1930;72:1036–48.
[2] Reiter AM. Feline "odontolysis" in the 1920s: the forgotten histopathological study of feline odontoclastic resorptive lesions (FORL). J Vet Dent 1998;15:35–41.
[3] Kerebel B, Daculsi G. Histologie et histopathologie dentaires du chat. Sci Rech Odonto-stomatol 1971;7(5):29–32.
[4] Schneck GW, Osborn JW. Neck lesions in the teeth of cats. Vet Rec 1976;99:100.
[5] Reiter AM. The role of calciotropic factors in the etiology of feline odontoclastic resorptive lesions (FORL) [thesis]. Vienna: University of Veterinary Medicine Vienna; 2004.
[6] Reiter AM. Biology of alveolar bone and tooth resorbing cells. In: Proceedings of the 12th Annual Veterinary Dental Forum. New Orleans, 1998. p. 225–7.
[7] Sahara N, Toyoki A, Ashizawa Y, et al. Cytodifferentiation of the odontoclast prior to the shedding of human deciduous teeth: an ultrastructural and cytochemical study. Anat Rec 1996;244:33–49.
[8] Harvey CE, Orsini P, McLahan C, et al. Mapping the radiographic central point of feline dental resorptive lesions. J Vet Dent 2004;21:15–21.

[9] Eriksen T, Koch R, Nautrup CP. Microradiography of the feline marginal periodontium with a microfocal high-resolution x-ray system. Scand J Dent Res 1994;102:284–9.

[10] Reiter AM, Mendoza K. Feline odontoclastic resorptive lesions. An unsolved enigma in veterinary dentistry. Vet Clin N Am Small Anim Pract 2002;32:791–837.

[11] Keinath G. Tierzahnheilkunde bei Katzen unter besonderer Beruecksichtigung der Aetiologie und Therapie von "Neck-Lesions" [thesis]. Munich: Munich University, Faculty of Human Medicine; 1997.

[12] Ohba S, Kiba H, Kuwabara M, et al. A histopathological study of neck lesions in feline teeth. J Am Anim Hosp Assoc 1993;29:216–20.

[13] Okuda A, Harvey CE. Etiopathogenesis of feline dental resorptive lesions. Vet Clin N Am Small Anim Pract 1992;22:1385–404.

[14] Reichart PA, Dürr U-M, Triadan H, et al. Periodontal disease in the domestic cat. A histopathologic study. J Periodont Res 1984;19:67–75.

[15] Roes F. Pathogenese, Diagnostik und Therapie bei "neck lesions" der Katze unter Verwendung von Glas-Ionomer-Zementen [thesis]. Berlin: Free University of Berlin, Faculty of Veterinary Medicine; 1996.

[16] Steinberg S. Histologische Untersuchungen zu Fruehveraenderungen der Felinen Odonto-klastischen Resorptiven Laesionen (FORL) an klinisch gesunden Zaehnen [thesis]. Berline: Free University of Berlin, Faculty of Veterinary Medicine; 2002.

[17] Trope M, Chivian N. Root resorption. In: Cohen S, Burns RC, editors. Pathways of the pulp. 6th edition. St. Louis: Mosby-Year Book; 1994. p. 486–512.

[18] DuPont GA, DeBowes LJ. Comparison of periodontitis and root replacement in cat teeth with resorptive lesions. J Vet Dent 2002;19:71–5.

[19] Berger M, Schawalder P, Stich H, et al. "Neck Lesion" bei Grosskatzen; Untersuchungen beim Leoparden (Panthera pardus). Kleintierpraxis 1995;40:537–49.

[20] Schlup D, Stich H. Epidemiologische und morphologische Untersuchungen am Katzengebiß. II. Mitteilung: Morphologische Untersuchungen der "neck lesions". Kleintierpraxis 1982;27:179–88.

[21] George DI, Miller RL. Idiopathic resorption of teeth. A report of three cases. Am J Orthod 1986;89:13–20.

[22] Henry JL, Weinmann JP. The pattern of resorption and repair of human cementum. J Am Dent Assoc 1951;42:270–90.

[23] Shigeyama Y, Grove TK, Strayhorn C, et al. Expression of adhesion molecules during tooth resorption in feline teeth: a model system for aggressive osteoclastic activity. J Dent Res 1996;75:1650–7.

[24] Forsberg A, Lagergren C, Lönnerblad T. The periodontal tissue of mandibular premolars and molars in some mammals. A comparative anatomical study. Svensk Tandlakare-Tidskrift 1969;62(Suppl 1):1–54.

[25] Gorrel C, Larsson A. Feline odontoclastic resorptive lesions: unveiling the early lesion. J Small Anim Pract 2002;43:482–8.

[26] Reiter AM. Etiopathology of feline odontoclastic resorptive lesions (FORL). In: Proceedings of the 12th Annual Veterinary Dental Forum. New Orleans, 1998. p. 228–34.

[27] Blackwood HJJ. Resorption of enamel and dentine in the unerupted tooth. Oral Surg Oral Med Oral Pathol Oral Radiol Endod 1958;11:79–85.

[28] Boyle PE. Cementum—changes with age, function, and infection. In: Kronfeld's histopathology of the teeth and their surrounding structures. Philadelphia: Lea & Febiger; 1955. p. 258–72.

[29] Stafne EC, Austin LT. Resorption of embedded teeth. J Am Dent Assoc 1945;32:1003–9.

[30] Zemsky JL. Hypercementosis in relation to unerupted and malposed teeth. A preliminary report. J Dent Res 1931;11:159–74.

[31] Kupfer IJ. Correlation of hypercementosis with toxic goiter. A preliminary report. J Dent Res 1951;30:734–6.

[32] Farmer ED, Lawton FE. The effects of endocrine disorders on the jaws and teeth. In: Stones' oral and dental diseases. Aetiology, histopathology, clinical features and treatment. 5th edition. Baltimore: Williams & Wilkins; 1966. p. 30–48.

[33] Gardner BS, Goldstein H. The significance of hypercementosis. Dent Cosmos 1931;73: 1065–9.

[34] Schour I, Massler M. Endocrines and dentistry. J Am Dent Assoc 1943;30:595–603.

[35] Rushton MA. The dental tissues in osteitis deformans. Guys Hosp Rep 1938;88:163–71.

[36] Smith NHH. Monostotic Paget's disease of the mandible presenting with progressive resorption of the teeth. Oral Surg Oral Med Oral Pathol Oral Radiol Endod 1978;46: 246–53.

[37] Stafne EC. Paget's disease involving the maxilla and the mandible: report of a case. J Oral Surg 1946;4:114–5.

[38] Farmer ED, Lawton FE. Cementum: abnormalities associated with its formation. In: Stones' oral and dental diseases. Aetiology, histopathology, clinical features and treatment. 5th edition. Baltimore: Williams & Wilkins; 1966. p. 447–67.

[39] King JD. Dietary deficiency, nerve lesions and the dental tissues. J Physiol 1937;88:62–77.

[40] Kellner E. Das Verhaeltnis der Zement- und Periodontalbreiten zur funktionellen Beanspruchung der Zaehne. Z Stomatol 1931;29:44–62.

[41] Kronfeld R. Die Zementhyperplasien an nicht funktionierenden Zaehnen. Z Stomatol 1927;25:1218–27.

[42] Itoiz MA, Carranza FA. The gingiva. In: Newman MG, Takei HH, Carranza FA, editors. Carranza's clinical periodontology. 9th edition. Philadelphia: WB Saunders; 2002. p. 16–35.

[43] Black GV. The periosteum and peridental membranes. Dent Rev 1887;1:233–43, 353–65.

[44] Lyon KF. Subgingival odontoclastic resorptive lesions. Classification, treatment and results in 58 cats. Vet Clin N Am Small Anim Pract 1992;22:1417–32.

[45] Carranza FA, Camargo PM. Periodontal response to external forces. In: Newman MG, Takei HH, Carranza FA, editors. Carranza's clinical periodontology. 9th edition. Philadelphia: WB Saunders; 2002. p. 371–83.

[46] Lukman K, Pavlica Z, Juntes P. Prevalence patterns and histological survey of feline dental resorptive lesions. In: Proceedings of the 8th Annual Scientific Meeting of the British Veterinary Dental Association. Birmingham, 1996.

[47] Boling LR. Blood vessels of the dental pulp. Anat Rec 1942;82:25–37.

[48] Winter GB, Kramer IRH. Changes in periodontal membrane and bone following experimental pulpal injury in deciduous molar teeth in kittens. Arch Oral Biol 1965;10: 279–89.

[49] Negro VB, Hernandez SZ, Maresca BM, et al. Furcation canals of the maxillary fourth premolar and the mandibular first molar teeth in cats. J Vet Dent 2004;21:10–4.

[50] Okuda A, Habata I. Lacunae or tubular structures in dentin of feline teeth. J Anim Res Found 1993;2(1):7–14.

[51] Okuda A, Harvey CE. Histopathological findings of features of odontoclastic resorptive lesions in cat teeth with periodontitis. In: Proceedings of the 5th Annual Veterinary Dental Forum. New Orleans, 1991. p. 141–4.

[52] Berger M, Stich H, Schaffner T, et al. Testimony from a silent late medieval witness—what can it tell us about FORL? In: Proceedings of the 13th European Congress of Veterinary Dentistry. Krakow, 2004. p. 17–8 (plus addendum).

[53] Dobbertin F. Zur Pathologie der Zahn- und Zahnbetterkrankungen bei *Felis silvestris forma catus* [thesis]. Hamburg: Hamburg University, Faculty of Human Medicine; 1993.

[54] Harvey CE, Alston WE. Dental diseases in cat skulls acquired before 1960. In: Proceedings of the 4th Annual Veterinary Dental Forum. Las Vegas, 1992. p. 41–3.

[55] DeLaurier A, Jackson B, Ingham K, et al. Biochemical markers of bone turnover in the domestic cat: relationships with age and feline osteoclastic resorptive lesions. J Nutr 2002; 132(Suppl):1742S–4S.

[56] Clarke DE, Cameron A. Feline dental resorptive lesions in domestic and feral cats and the possible link with diet. In: Proceedings of the 5th World Veterinary Dental Congress. Birmingham, 1997. p. 33–4.

[57] How KL, Hazewinkel AW, Mol JA. Dietary vitamin D dependance of cat and dog due to inadequate cutaneous synthesis of vitamin D. Gen Comp Endocrinol 1994;96:12–8.

[58] National Research Council. Nutrient requirements of cats. Washington, DC: National Academy Press; 1986. p. 4, 15, 16, 23, 56.

[59] Morris JG, Earle KE. Growing kittens require less dietary calcium than current allowances. J Nutr 1999;129:1698–704.

[60] Morris JG, Earle KE, Anderson PA. Plasma 25-hydroxyvitamin D in growing kittens is related to dietary intake of cholecalciferol. J Nutr 1999;129:909–12.

[61] Morris JG. Vitamin D synthesis by kittens. Vet Clin Nutr 1996;3(3):88–92.

[62] Haruna A, Kawai K, Takaba T, et al. Dietary calcinosis in the cat. J Anim Clin Res Found 1992;1(1):9–16.

[63] Morita T, Awakura T, Shimada A, et al. Vitamin D toxicosis in cats: natural outbreak and experimental study. J Vet Med Sci 1995;57:831–7.

[64] Sato R, Yamagishi H, Naito Y, et al. Feline vitamin D toxicosis caused by commercially available cat food. J Jpn Vet Med Assoc 1993;46:577–81.

[65] Sih TR, Morris JG, Hickman MA. Chronic ingestion of high concentrations of cholecalciferol in cats. Am J Vet Res 2001;62:1500–6.

[66] Holick MF. Vitamin D: photobiology, metabolism, mechanism of action, and clinical applications. In: Favus MJ, editor. Primer on the metabolic bone diseases and disorders of mineral metabolism. 4th edition. Philadelphia: Lippincott Williams & Wilkins; 1999. p. 92–8.

[67] Itonaga I, Sabokbar A, Murray DW, et al. Effect of osteoprotegerin and osteoprotegerin ligand on osteoclast formation by arthroplasty membrane derived macrophages. Ann Rheum Dis 2000;59:26–31.

[68] Burgess TL, Qian Y-X, Kaufman S, et al. The ligand for osteoprotegerin (OPGL) directly activates mature osteoclasts. J Cell Biol 1999;145:527–38.

[69] Braem M, Lambrechts P, Vanherle G. Stress-induced cervical lesions. J Prosthet Dent 1992; 67:718–22.

[70] Lee WC, Eakle WS. Possible role of tensile stress in the etiology of cervical erosive lesions of teeth. J Prosthet Dent 1984;52:374–80.

[71] Lee WC, Eakle WS. Stress-induced cervical lesions: review of advances in the past 10 years. J Prosthet Dent 1996;75:487–94.

[72] Bevenius J, L'Estrange P, Karlsson S, et al. Idiopathic cervical lesions: in vivo investigation by oral microendoscopy and scanning electron microscopy. A pilot study. J Oral Rehabil 1993;20:1–9.

[73] Goel VK, Khera SC, Ralston JL, et al. Stresses at the dentinoenamel junction of human teeth. J Prosthet Dent 1991;66:451–9.

[74] Burke FJT, Johnston N, Wiggs RB, et al. An alternative hypothesis from veterinary science for the pathogenesis of noncarious cervical lesions. Quintessence Int 2000;31:475–82.

[75] Johnston N. Acquired feline oral cavity disease. Part 2: feline odontoclastic resorptive lesions. In Pract 2000;22:188–97.

[76] Orban B. Resorption and repair on the surface of the root. J Am Dent Assoc 1928;15: 1768–77.

[77] Chipps HD. Two cases of root resorption. Dental Cosmos 1928;70:461–2.

[78] Coolidge ED. The reaction of cementum in the presence of injury and infection. J Am Dent Assoc 1931;18:499–525.

[79] Wood P, Rees JS. An unusual case of furcation external resorption. Int Endod J 2000;33: 530–3.

[80] Yusof WZ, Ghazali MN. Multiple external root resorption. J Am Dent Assoc 1989;118: 453–5.

[81] Rawlinson A. Treatment of root and alveolar bone resorption associated with bruxism. Br Dent J 1991;170:445–7.

[82] Harris EF, Robinson QC, Woods MA. An analysis of causes of apical root resorption in patients not treated orthodontically. Quintessence Int 1993;24:417–28.

[83] Itoiz ME, Carranza FA, Cabrini RL. Histologic and histometric study of experimental occlusal trauma in rats. J Periodontol 1963;34:305–14.

[84] Kameyama Y. Histopathologic and autoradiographic studies of the changes of the rat peri-odontium in experimental traumatic occlusion. Bull Tokyo Med Dent Univ 1968;15:339–57.

[85] Orban B. Tissue changes in traumatic occlusion. J Am Dent Assoc 1928;15:2090–106.

[86] Ramfjord SP, Kohler CA. Periodontal reaction to functional occlusal stress. J Periodontol 1959;30:95–112.

[87] Mjör IA, Stenvik A. Microradiography and histology of decalcified human teeth following experimental intrusion; with emphasis on resorption. Arch Oral Biol 1969;14:1355–64.

[88] Bhaskar SN, Orban B. Experimental occlusal trauma. J Periodontol 1955;26:270–84.

[89] Lefkowitz W, Waugh LM. Experimental depression of teeth. Am J Orthod Oral Surg 1945; 31:21–36.

[90] Boyle PE. Tooth resorption. In: Kronfeld's histopathology of the teeth and their surrounding structures. Philadelphia: Lea & Febiger; 1955. p. 273–96.

[91] Glickman I, Selye H, Smulow JB. Reduction by calciphylaxis of the effects of chronic dihydrotachysterol overdose upon the periodontium. J Dent Res 1965;44:734–49.

[92] Sindelka Z. Die Kalziphylaxie im Zahnmark. Stoma (Heidelb) 1968;21:101–9.

[93] Selye H, Grasso S, Padmanabhan N. Topical injury as a means of producing calcification at predetermined points with dihydrotachysterol (DHT). Proc Zool Soc 1960;13(1):1–3.

[94] Selye H, Jean P, Veilleux R. Role of local trauma in the production of cutaneous calcinosis by dihydrotachysterol. Proc Soc Exp Biol Med 1960;104:409–11.

[95] Ratcliff PA, Krajewski J. The influence of methyl testosterone on dihydrotachysterol intoxication as it affects the periodontium. J Oral Ther Pharmacol 1966;2:353–61.

[96] Stahl SS, Cohen C, Epstein B. The responses of injured and noninjured rat periodontal tissues to a single administration of dihydrotachysterol. Oral Surg Oral Med Oral Pathol Oral Radiol Endod 1967;23:531–7.

[97] Shoshan S, Pisanti S, Sciaky I. The effect of hypervitaminosis D on the periodontal membrane collagen in lathyritic rats. J Periodont Res 1967;2:121–6.

[98] Moskow BS, Baden E, Zengo A. The effects of dihydrotachysterol and ferric dextran upon the periodontium in the rat. Arch Oral Biol 1966;11:1017–26.

[99] Kojima M. Experimental study on the physio-pathological changes of periodontal tissues. Bull Stomatol Kyoto Univ 1969;9:101–40.

[100] Takano K, Watanabe Y, Fuzihashi H, et al. The histological changes of alveolar bone, cementum and periodontal fiber due to experimental progeria-like syndrome of the rat. J Jpn Assoc Periodontol 1981;23:357–66.

[101] Cai JJ. Effect of vitamin D overdosage on the tooth and bone development of rabbits. Chin J Stomatol 1992;27:296–9, 319.

[102] Daemmrich K. Experimentelle D$_3$-Hypervitaminose bei Ferkeln. Zentrabl Veterinarmed A 1963;10:322–49.

[103] Irving TJ, Weinmann JP, Schour I, et al. Experimental studies in calcification. VIII. The effect of large doses of calciferol on the dentin of the incisor in normal and nephrectomized rats. J Dent Res 1949;28:362–8.

[104] Pitaru S, Blauschild N, Noff D, et al. The effect of toxic doses of 1,25-dihydroxychole-calciferol on dental tissues in the rat. Arch Oral Biol 1982;27:915–23.

[105] Tempestini O. Nuove ricerche sugli effetti sperimentali della somministrazione di una alta dose di vitamina D$_2$ nei tessuti dentali e paradentali del ratto. Riv Ital Stomatol 1952;7: 373–410.

[106] Weinmann J. Experimentelle Untersuchung ueber die Wirkung grosser Dosen Vigantol auf Knochen und Zaehne. Klin Wochenschr 1929;8:841–2.

[107] Weinmann J. Untersuchungen an Knochen und Zaehnen der Ratte bei Verfuetterung grosser Dosen D-Vitamin. Dtsch Mschr Zahnheilk 1933;51:577–603, 625–54.

[108] Becks H. Dangerous effects of vitamin D overdosage on dental and paradental structures. J Am Dent Assoc 1942;29:1947–68.

[109] Becks H, Collins DA, Axelrod HE. The effects of a single massive dose of vitamin D_2 (D-stoss therapy) on oral and other tissues of young dogs. Am J Orthod Oral Surg 1946;32: 452–62.

[110] Becks H, Collins DA, Freytag RM. Changes in oral structures of the dog persisting after chronic overdoses of vitamin D. Am J Orthod Oral Surg 1946;32:463–71.

[111] Bernick S, Ershoff BH, Lal JB. Effects of hypervitaminosis D on bones and teeth of rats. Int J Vitam Nutr Res 1971;41:480–9.

[112] Fahmy H, Rogers WE, Mitchell DF, et al. Effects of hypervitaminosis D on the periodontium of the hamster. J Dent Res 1961;40:870–7.

[113] Harris LJ, Innes JRM. Mode of action of vitamin D. Biochem J 1931;25:367–90.

[114] Hendricks JB, Morgan AF, Freytag RM. Chronic moderate hypervitaminosis D in young dogs. Am J Physiol 1947;149:319–32.

[115] Hirukawa T. Effect of dihydrotachysterol on the periodontal tissues in rats. Aichi-Gakuin J Dent Sci 1990;28:367–87.

[116] Kondo M. The changes of parodontal tissues of rat, caused by the administration of dihydrotachysterol. Shigaku 1971;59:219–45.

[117] Mabuchi H. Experimental study on the effect of sexual hormones and calcification enhancing substances on growth of the alveolar bone. Bull Stomatol Kyoto Univ 1970;10: 31–60.

[118] Miwa Y, Watanabe Y. The effect of fluoride on the periodontal tissues of dihydrotachysterol administered rats. Bull Josai Dent Univ 1985;14:343–54.

[119] Morgan AF, Axelrod HE, Groody M. The effect of a single massive dose of vitamin D_2 on young dogs. Am J Physiol 1947;149:333–9.

[120] Moskow BS, Baden E. The effect of chronic dihydrotachysterol overdosage on the tissues of the periodontium. Periodontics 1964;2:277–83.

[121] Nomura H. Histopathological study of experimental hypervitaminosis D_2 on the periodontium of the rat. Shikwa Gakuho 1969;69:539–93.

[122] Ratcliff PA, Itokazu H. The effect of dihydrotachysterol on the teeth and periodontium. J Periodontol 1964;35:320–5.

[123] Ratcliff PA, Itokazu H. The effect of dihydrotachysterol and ferric dextran on the teeth and periodontium of the rat. J Oral Ther Pharmacol 1964;1:7–22.

[124] Takano K, Watanabe Y. The histological study on osteoid- and cementoid-like tissues of rats treated with dihydrotachysterol. Bull Josai Dent Univ 1987;16:307–22.

[125] Terai Y. Studies on experimental stimulation of ossification in the paradental tissues of rats and blood level of Ca, P and alkaline phosphatase in them. Bull Stomatol Kyoto Univ 1968; 8(4):191–244.

VETERINARY
CLINICS
Small Animal Practice

ELSEVIER
SAUNDERS

Vet Clin Small Anim
35 (2005) 943–962

Radiographic Evaluation and Treatment of Feline Dental Resorptive Lesions

Gregg A. DuPont, DVM*

Shoreline Veterinary Dental Clinic, Seattle, WA, USA

Dental resorptive lesions (RLs) are one of the most common oral problems experienced by cats today [1]. More than a dozen different names and acronyms have been used in the literature to refer to feline RLs. As we learn more about these lesions, we realize that terms like *cat caries, neck lesions,* and *cervical line lesions* are misnomers. The acronym FORL (feline odontoclastic resorption lesion) is now sometimes used. This nomenclature may create confusion in the literature because at this point, there is no reason to believe that feline RLs are any different from some types that occur in dogs, human beings, pigs, rats, mice, and marmosets [2]. The word "odontoclastic" also seems unnecessary, because odontoclasts are a component of most types of dental resorption, whether inflammatory, pressure, physiologic, replacement, traumatic, extracanal invasive, or internal [3].

The reporting of human RLs has experienced the same challenges that we have seen with feline RLs, where lack of information and understanding has resulted in more than a dozen different names for them in the literature as they are "rediscovered" or better understood [4–6]. People suffer from a number of different types of "noncarious cervical lesions." The most common are unrelated to feline RLs, such as abrasion from aggressive tooth brushing. One type seems to be similar to feline RLs in location, pathophysiology, and clinical progression, with localized gingival overgrowth or granulomatous tissue infiltration and aggressive progression [6]. Currently, these human lesions are most commonly called "extracanal invasive resorptions" and, more recently, "abfraction lesions" [7].

RLs were first described in domestic cats in detail more than 74 years ago [8]. They were also described in human beings as early as 1920; at that time, they were called (among other things) the "pink spot of Mummery" [4]. In spite of their extremely long history of recognition, and although several

* 16037 Aurora Avenue North, Seattle, WA 98133–5653, USA.
E-mail address: GatorGregg@aol.com

0195-5616/05/$ - see front matter © 2005 Elsevier Inc. All rights reserved.
doi:10.1016/j.cvsm.2005.03.008 *vetsmall.theclinics.com*

theories about the cause have been proposed, the cause of feline RLs has not been proved. Regardless of the cause or causes, a full evaluation and treatment are important for all affected teeth.

Diagnosis of feline resorptive lesions

RLs have been reported to cause anorexia, ptyalism, lethargy, depression, dysphagia, halitosis, and discomfort. It is likely that many of them cause no clinical signs, however. Much of our information about discomfort in animals comes from using human beings as a model. Although use of models is low-level evidence, for syndromes of minor or unapparent discomfort, we can obtain some helpful information by identifying similar syndromes in human beings. People who have dental RLs are often asymptomatic, and the RLs are typically discovered as incidental radiographic findings [5–7]. RLs that do not expose dentin to air or pressure gradients should not cause discomfort. Many RLs are subgingival or covered with gingiva or granulation tissue and may be relatively asymptomatic.

If this is true, relying on clinical signs would be of little use. RLs begin as a superficial (usually cemental) resorption of tooth substance, most frequently at or close to the cementoenamel junction (CEJ) or cervical area. They can also sometimes begin more apically on the root surface and become clinically apparent coronally on the crown as a "pink spot" caused by internal resorption (Fig. 1).

Surface lesions on the enamel of the crown are readily diagnosed clinically by direct visual observation. They may be difficult to see if covered by plaque and calculus, requiring dental scaling for complete evaluation. They often appear as a surface defect in the enamel, frequently beginning in the midbuccal area of premolar teeth [1]. Gingival tissue frequently grows into the lesion. Histologic examination shows tight adherence of a soft tissue

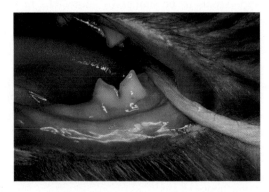

Fig. 1. The "pink spot" 2 mm above the gingival margin on the buccal aspect of a lower molar tooth indicates internal resorption.

granuloma with collagen infiltrating into the resorbing dentin [9]. This same gingival overgrowth is also seen in dogs and people [6]. Chronic lesions with these adherent tissues often appear as a seemingly quiet growth of gingiva up onto the crown of a tooth. These teeth may have no resorption exposed to the oral cavity, and the clinical crown may look otherwise normal. A radiograph of this type of tooth often shows advanced resorption of the roots, however (Fig. 2). Tissue upgrowth can sometimes be quite pronounced on the canine teeth (Fig. 3). Confirmation may require probing a suspected lesion with a sharp dental explorer to demonstrate the characteristic sharp enamel margin of an RL. The dentin lining the lesion is generally hard. It is not soft, as is characteristic of dental caries lesions. Localized marginal gingivitis, particularly on the midbuccal surface of premolars and canine teeth, should prompt further investigation with the dental explorer. When an affected area is probed with a fingernail or dental explorer, cats often react with an immediate jaw movement and a pain response. This reaction can also occur

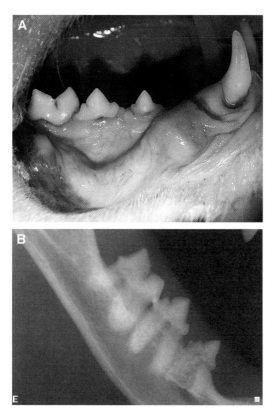

Fig. 2. (*A*) Lower third premolar tooth (just distal to canine tooth) has slight gingival upgrowth on the distal aspect of the crown. (*B*) Radiograph shows marked loss of root radiopacity compared with other roots, indicating advanced root resorption.

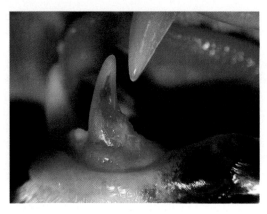

Fig. 3. Gingiva and granulomatous tissue have grown into a resorptive lesion coronally more than two thirds up the crown of the canine tooth.

in the absence of lesions, however, and is not a reliable test for their presence. The defect is generally concave and lined by odontoclasts. Cats often have lesions on multiple teeth. When a lesion is identified, special care should be taken to examine the other teeth fully.

If a lesion begins under the gingival margin in the "furcation area" of a premolar or molar (where a multirooted tooth's roots meet to form the crown), it may first present as an area of localized gingivitis. Reflecting the gingival margin with an instrument or a gentle flow of air exposes the lesion. As a lesion progresses, it eventually extends through the enamel to the dentin. As the lesion progresses, the crown is ultimately destroyed until little or none remains. When a lesion has progressed to its final stages with complete destruction of the crown and healing of the gingiva, it may appear as a raised area of gingiva with no clinical crown remaining above the gums (Fig. 4). Box 1 details the grading system that we prefer to use for RLs [10].

Early or suspected lesions should be examined further under general anesthesia to remove overlying or adjacent calculus. This also allows a more detailed examination with a dental explorer to determine the presence and severity of lesions. One must take care in natural furcation areas to avoid overdiagnosis. Inflammation in a root furcation can mimic an RL (and indeed may eventually cause an RL), but in the absence of an RL, the furcation does not have the characteristic irregular enamel lip (Fig. 5).

All teeth affected by clinical RLs should be evaluated with dental radiographs, because the supragingival lesion is often the "tip of the iceberg," representing only a small fraction of the pathologic change affecting that tooth. Some lesions may be completely subgingival and can be found only on radiographs. There is some evidence that taking full-mouth dental radiographs of cats, even in the absence of any clinical lesion, may be of value in identifying RLs of the root or within the pulp chamber [11]. When a cat is diagnosed with an RL, it becomes more important to

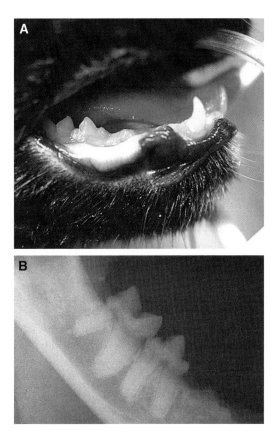

Fig. 4. (A) Lower third premolar is missing, and there is convex architecture in the edentulous area. This is typical of end-stage resorptive lesions. (B) Radiograph confirms that a tooth is still in the process of resorption and remodeling.

radiograph the other teeth, because that cat is more likely to be affected with subgingival RLs on teeth that are clinically normal [12].

Radiographic imaging of feline resorptive lesions

Radiographs routinely reveal a more severe lesion than is indicated on clinical examination. Well-positioned intraoral dental radiographs with high definition and detail are required for adequate evaluation of all teeth that are affected by RLs. Teeth with root resorption but no clinical crown involvement can only be identified through dental radiographs. Conventional radiography, digital radiography using charge-coupled device sensors, and digital storage phosphor systems can all provide high-quality radiographs for diagnosing RLs. Conventional radiography may be inadequate for diagnosing small root resorptions [13]. The digital systems provide the

---

Box 1. Grading system for resorptive lesions

- Stage 1: incipient or extremely early lesions involving a small area of enamel
- Stage 2: a lesion that extends into the dentin but does not involve the pulp
- Stage 3: a lesion that involves the pulp
- Stage 4: a lesion that has destroyed enough crown to weaken the tooth significantly
- Stage 5: no remaining supragingival crown, gingiva completely covers the site

---

advantages of shorter exposure times, image enhancement ability, and negative image evaluation, all of which may improve the ability to identify early lesions [14]. Some investigators have concluded that subtraction radiography techniques can further improve the sensitivity for diagnosing small root external resorptions in human teeth [15]. Inability to diagnose these early lesions may be clinically insignificant, however.

Radiographic evaluation includes assessing the integrity of the lamina dura surrounding the entire root of the tooth, including the periapical area. The lamina is the white line closely surrounding the root that represents the alveolar bone plate. It is separated from the root by a black line that represents the periodontal ligament (PDL). In cats, the PDL and lamina dura are not always visible. When they are identifiable, loss of their integrity can indicate resorption but can also result from ankylosis or focal inflammation. On radiographs, RLs can appear as a discreet radiolucent lesion on the root surface, as a diffuse decrease in radiodensity of the entire root

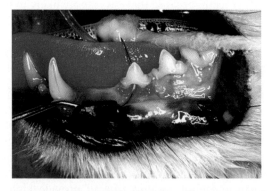

Fig. 5. Dental explorer passes through the furcation. The enamel at the cementoenamel junction is smooth and has a normal appearance. This tooth has periodontal disease with no resorption.

compared with the roots adjacent to it (Fig. 6), as a focal enlargement of the root canal (internal inflammatory resorption indicating a period of pulpitis and most commonly associated with a traumatically fractured tooth) (Fig. 7), as persistent roots missing their clinical crown (end-stage lesions), or as a slightly increased radiodensity compared with the surrounding alveolar bone with marginal convex bony ridge architecture in an edentulous area (end-stage RL that has been replaced by bone) (Fig. 8). Chemical contamination of the film can create an artifact that mimics dental resorption, but the surface film emulsion damage can be seen and the dark discoloration extends beyond the tooth image. Cervical burnout, the overexposure of the cervical area of teeth attributable to the different densities of the regional tissues, can also mimic dental resorption [16]. Other radiographic details to evaluate include pulp width, periapical radiolucency, alveolar bone quality and quantity, and root fractures.

Radiographs show that the roots of many teeth affected by RLs seem to "disappear," with loss of the PDL space, lamina dura, and, eventually, any evidence of the root itself. The radiopacity of the root decreases to match that of the surrounding alveolar bone. Many roots do not follow this course, however, and, other than focal lucencies, maintain their normal radiographic anatomy. Distinguishing between these two radiographic presentations allows treatment options that are more comfortable for selected patients and may also result in superior healing. For this reason, we label them as two separate "types," designating the type that shows normal root radiodensity as "type 1" lesions and the type with the roots becoming more radiolucent as "type 2" lesions.

Every tooth identified with an RL on the crown should be radiographed to determine the true extent of the lesion and the type of lesion. One study determined that radiographs of feline teeth affected with clinical RLs revealed additional information about the extent of the lesion in 98.4% of the teeth [11]. This study also showed that 8.7% of cats without clinical RLs

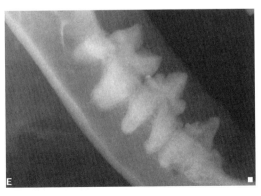

Fig. 6. Roots of the lower third premolar (tooth on the right) are radiolucent compared with the roots of adjacent teeth.

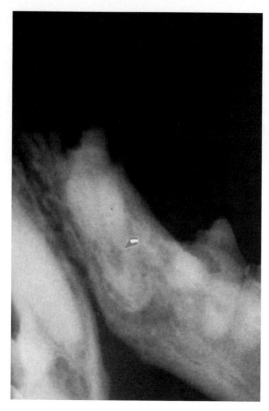

Fig. 7. Radiolucency one third of the way up the root is associated with the root canal. This indicates internal resorption and an episode of pulp inflammation.

revealed radiographic evidence of an RL. Much more importantly, however, a radiograph is the only way to decide on the best treatment as determined by whether the roots are being quietly resorbed or are affected by peri-radicular pathologic findings.

Clinically, type 1 lesions seem to be associated with the presence of inflammation from severe gingivitis or periodontitis or from endodontic disease causing apical periodontitis [17,18]. Lesions in patients with moderate to severe periodontal disease routinely manifest as cervical region resorptions with minimal or no general root resorption. Although the lesions may extend down onto the root, the remaining root does not give the appearance of "disappearing" in a radiographic image.

In contrast, inflammation seems to play a small role in type 2 lesions, and they are generally not associated with endodontic disease or periodontitis. Type 2 lesions frequently have only mild localized gingivitis or sometimes a hyperplastic gingiva or associated granuloma. In these lesions, the inflammation is minimal and gives the appearance of being a result rather than a cause of the resorption. They commonly show general root resorption on

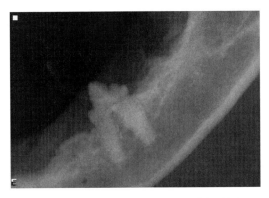

Fig. 8. Although there is no evidence of the tooth or roots of the third premolar (tooth on the left), the convex shape of the alveolar ridge shows that this is an end-stage resorptive lesion.

radiographs, as indicated by loss of radiopacity of the roots of the involved tooth when compared with those of adjacent teeth. When this radiographic appearance is evident, the root is being replaced by a cementum-like tissue that eventually converts to bone.

The peripulpal dentin of type 2 RLs is spared from the resorptive process until late in the syndrome. This is similar to the syndrome seen in human beings [4]. Even when the process has become advanced, pulp involvement does not result in pulpitis or necrosis; the pulp remains viable and healthy as the root is replaced by new bone [9,18,19]. Identifying RLs on radiographs requires searching for any irregularity in the PDL. Loss of integrity of the PDL may indicate an area of ankylosis or cemental breakdown and early resorption. More commonly, an area of radicular radiolucency is noted. When the lucency is superimposed over the pulp, taking an off-angled radiograph can differentiate an external resorption from an internal resorption. The tube shift causes an external root resorption to move in relation to the root canal, whereas an internal resorption retains its relation to the root canal. More commonly, the resorptive process progresses to affect the entire root. In these cases, the radiodensity of the roots is carefully evaluated and compared with that of adjacent teeth.

Both types of RLs can occur in a single patient (Fig. 9). Indeed, a multi-rooted tooth can have one root resorbing as a classic type 2 lesion and another root maintaining a normal radiopacity and PDL. It is possible that the type 1 root may be transitional in this case and, given time, would eventually become a type 2 root and resorb. We do not know whether the association of type 1 lesions with periodontitis might be related to inflammation as a cause of this type of lesion or possibly because the presence of inflammation interferes with the process of root replacement that would otherwise have resulted in the lesion becoming a type 2 lesion. There are still many unknowns.

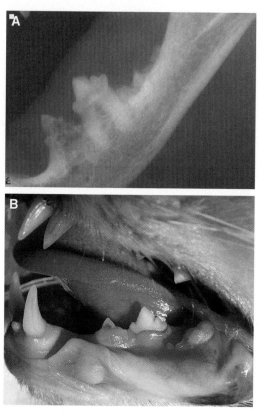

Fig. 9. (*A*) Lower third premolar (tooth on the left) is a type 2 lesion with roots seeming to "disappear" on the radiograph. The persistent root tips of the lower molar (area missing a tooth on the right) show an intact periodontal ligament, and the mesial root has slight periradicular lucency. The premolar is a type 2 lesion, whereas the molar is a type 1 lesion. (*B*) Clinical photograph shows little gingival inflammation affecting the third premolar, typical of a type 2 lesion. The area of the missing molar tooth has some associated inflammation and hyperplastic gingivitis caused by traumatic contact of the swollen tissue with the upper fourth premolar tooth.

Treatment of feline resorptive lesions

Previous recommendations for treatment of feline RLs have included fluoride treatment for stage 1 lesions, restoration for stage 2 lesions, restoration with root canal treatment for stage 3 lesions, and extraction of stage 4 and 5 lesions [20,21]. Other more exotic treatments have also been proposed and performed over the years. In 1992, the appropriate statement was made that "...the enthusiasm of 2 or 3 years ago for glass ionomer restorations and fluoride applications as a cure-all is now meeting the reality of less than satisfactory long-term results" [22]. One study showed that 65% of 154 glass ionomer restorations (72% of 58 cats) had further resorption at 6 to 37 months of follow-up [20]. This sounds similar to the experience of our counterparts in the human dental field, which has prompted statements like "Treatment of some types of resorption can be fraught with frustration and failure" as well as statements about the comparable type of resorption in human beings, "... this type of resorption has a high risk of recurrence, even after extensive repair" [5]. This high failure rate is not surprising, because the etiology has not been addressed.

Restorations are now infrequently placed, because their success rate is only 20% to 65% (study results vary) within a few years after placement; most clients do not choose this treatment, given the expected poor long-term clinical outcome. This failure rate is most likely attributable to the fact that restoration does not address the etiology; thus, the lesions continue, often progressing apically from the restoration. We sometimes place restorations in canine teeth to keep them functional and comfortable as long as possible. This gives them time to show what amount of root might resorb quietly and what portion must be removed (Fig. 10). The clients are advised of the poor long-term prognosis for saving the teeth, and the lesions are closely monitored clinically for recurrence or progression. Our choice for restorative material (in those rare instances when we restore an RL) is a glass ionomer.

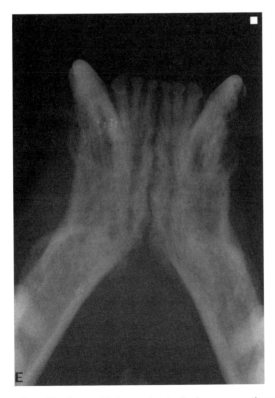

Fig. 10. Apical portion of both mandibular canine teeth shows resorption and replacement. The coronal aspects show expanded alveoli and associated radiolucency indicating pathologic changes that should be removed.

Glass ionomer bonds intrinsically to the tooth structure. It does not require a bonding agent, so it is relatively simple to place. Because it does not need a mechanical undercut, no additional tooth must be removed before placement. In addition, it more closely approximates the modulus of elasticity (flexibility) of the tooth than do other restorative materials, and it releases fluoride. The mixture ratio of glass ionomer components is precise and important. Therefore, products that are the easiest to use contain the premeasured components in a carpule that is activated to combine them into one chamber and then is cycled in an amalgamator to mix them. Placement is quite simple, involving the removal of any granulation or gingival tissue from the lesion, applying a conditioner to etch the dentin, drying and flowing the glass ionomer into the defect to form a slight overfill, and then finishing the restoration (after the initial 5-minute set time) to bring the material down to the defect margins for a smooth contoured finish. Controlling the field to prevent sulcular fluid from contaminating the material during placement and until after the initial 5-minute set can be challenging. Immediately after placement and then again after finishing, the restorative is covered with a surface coat of a varnish or an unfilled resin to prevent desiccation or moisture absorption during the set.

Some operators have reported success with pulpectomy and calcium hydroxide endodontic treatment for affected teeth, but significant studies have yet to be done. Generally, extraction remains the treatment of choice to speed the progress through the stages of potential discomfort. Our current treatment recommendations take a number of factors into account, as described in Box 2.

An important feature of type 2 RLs is that a simultaneous repair process accompanies the destructive process: odontoclasts and osteoblasts are active at the same time in the same lesion [9]. Further, the newly formed bone then experiences further osteoclastic resorption as it undergoes bone remodeling. In 1992, an enlightened individual wrote, "Further investigation of the result of leaving feline root structures in place needs to be completed…" [20]. This thought, along with personal clinical experience, prompted the author to investigate this concept. In a study completed in 1995, crown amputation with intentional root retention of type 2 lesions showed continued root resorption and replacement for up to 3 years of follow-up [23]. In these cats, the gingiva healed without incident and there was no evidence of gingivitis after healing, except in one cat that eventually developed ulcero-proliferative lesions of the mucosa between the upper and lower molar areas commonly called "feline stomatitis". Although crown amputation and full tooth extraction resulted in clinically normal gingiva with no apparent discomfort at the sites, the general radiographic pattern was of less alveolar ridge loss and smaller bony defects for teeth treated with crown amputation compared with those treated with extraction.

The author concluded that crown amputation is a superior alternative treatment to complete tooth extraction for lesions that are stage 2 through 4

Box 2. Factors that influence treatment of resorptive lesions

- Fluoride has not been shown to affect the progression of dental resorption. Fluoride converts dental enamel into a form that is resistant to acid demineralization and therefore more resistant to dental caries. Cats have not been shown to suffer from caries, however. The only possible benefit that fluoride might provide is desensitization, and some forms of fluoride have antibacterial action.
- Early lesions and subgingival lesions may be asymptomatic, making treatment nonemergent.
- Restorations are temporary.
- Type 2 RLs, given enough time, seem to resolve themselves by resorbing the roots and replacing them with bone.
- Type 1 lesions often have infection or inflammation associated with the roots, which do not resorb.
- No treatment has yet been shown to stop the progression of resorption reliably in the long term.

---

and are type 2 lesions. Their clinically weakened crowns and roots as well as ankylosis of the roots complicate extraction of teeth with advanced type 2 RLs. Extraction often requires a surgical approach and trauma to the periradicular tissues. Frequently, the roots fracture, requiring the operator to use a high-speed dental burr to remove the entire root, causing even more collateral damage to healthy bone and tissues. Patients with type 2 RLs are already quietly converting the roots into healthy bone. Crown amputation is a means of helping nature resolve the lesion in the least traumatic and least invasive fashion.

The procedure of crown amputation with intentional root retention is quick and simple; a limited envelope flap is developed, consisting only of minimal elevation of the gingiva from the tooth and marginal alveolar bone using a Pritchard PR3 or smaller periosteal elevator. The gingiva is reflected and protected with the flat end of the elevator. A number 1 round burr in a high-speed handpiece under a sterile water flush is used to remove the tooth to a level slightly below the alveolar crestal bone. Any sharp bony ridge projections are smoothed, and the gingiva is closed with a single 4-0 surgical gut suture. Gentle digital pressure is placed on the gingiva for 30 seconds to stabilize the clot and to adapt the gingiva to the new ridge shape. The entire procedure takes only a few minutes. When performed, the client must be advised that roots are being intentionally left behind and why.

Important caveats must be followed when deciding to amputate tooth crowns instead of fully extracting the teeth. It is vitally important that selected cases have no buried pathologic changes. Preprocedural radiographs are mandatory to determine that it is a type 2 lesion. Selected cases should not have periodontitis, tooth mobility, or radiographic evidence of endodontic disease or apical pathologic changes. The roots that can be retained are those that are already turning into normal healthy bone. Another important selection criterion is that there must be no clinical evidence of "feline stomatitis" ("plasmacytic-lymphocytic stomatitis"). These patients often need full extraction of all the premolars and molars in an attempt to cure or improve their "feline stomatitis". For them, it is critical that all fragments of all roots are completely removed as well as the associated PDL. A final selection criterion is that if the retrovirus status of the patient is known, roots should not be left behind on a patient that is positive for feline immunodeficiency virus (FIV) or feline leukemia virus (FeLV). Crown amputation should be rarely performed on canine teeth unless they are late in the process and clearly quietly resorbing the roots. Canine teeth more commonly have periodontal involvement and alveolar osteomyelitis, making them more likely to cause problems and infection if left behind. The current treatment protocol for RLs, based on all these considerations, is shown in Box 3.

Areas with missing teeth, particularly when there is no ridge loss, should be radiographed. End-stage (stage 5) type 2 lesions (see Fig. 4) require no intervention. End-stage type 1 lesions, even when the crown is completely missing, should be surgically approached and the roots removed, however (Fig. 11).

Box 3. Current treatment protocol for resorptive lesions

- Stage 1: debride all tissue from the defects, acid etch, and place dentin sealant.
- Stage 2, 3, or 4 on premolar and molar teeth
  Type 1 lesion (or type 2 that does not meet the selection criteria for crown amputation): complete extraction
  Type 2 lesion with no "feline stomatitis," no periodontitis, no endodontic disease, and not known to be retrovirus-positive: crown amputation
- Stage 2 or 3 on canine tooth: consider restoration until it becomes stage 4
- Stage 4 on canine tooth
  Type 1: extraction
  Type 2: crown amputation to the level of clear and quiet root replacement, removing all lucent dentin and bone
- Stage 5
  Type 1: extract root remnants
  Type 2: no treatment; advise and monitor radiographically

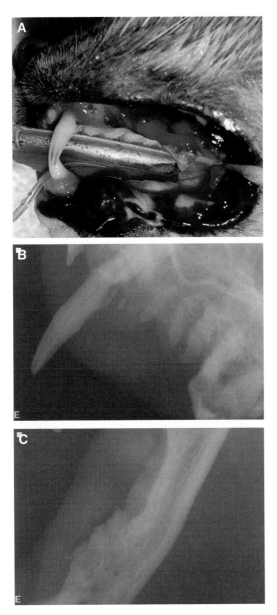

Fig. 11. (*A–C*) Clinical and radiographic appearance of a patient with multiple end-stage type 1 resorptive lesions with no clinical crowns and roots that are not resorbing, have intact periodontal ligaments, and have reactive bone.

Root canal treatment and restoration would generally be indicated in cats with type 1 RLs that have periapical inflammation and no other contra-indications. Caution is recommended, however, because the etiology may not have been addressed. In human beings, the same sparing of the pulp that is seen in cats has been noted in many RLs. Although root canal treatment stops internal resorption, it does not affect the progression of external resorption that is unrelated to lesions of endodontic origin [4]. The author has seen two cases in which root canal treatment was received for endodontic disease in canine teeth that, although they had no resorptive lesions visible clinically or radiographically, eventually went on to have the roots completely resorb, leaving the gutta percha clearly visible in the alveolar bone. Both of these cats had multiple resorptive lesions in other teeth, and one went on to lose all its teeth to resorptions, retaining only the crown of the endodontically treated tooth (Fig. 12).

Prevention

Until we can prove the cause, we cannot prevent RLs. Of those theories of etiology that still seem to have merit, the current most likely possibility is

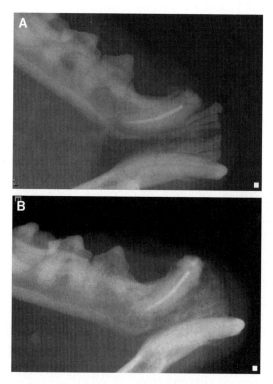

Fig. 12. (*A*) Lower canine tooth immediately after endodontic treatment. (*B*) Same patient at 7-year follow-up. The patient was being treated for other teeth that had resorptive lesions. The root of the canine tooth is losing detail and radiodensity. (*C*) Same patient at 8-year follow-up. The resorption has continued. Although there is no periapical lucency, the tooth was extracted because of periradicular coronal lucency and periodontal disease. (*D*) Root canal–treated tooth in an otherwise edentulous cat that lost all its teeth to resorptive lesions.

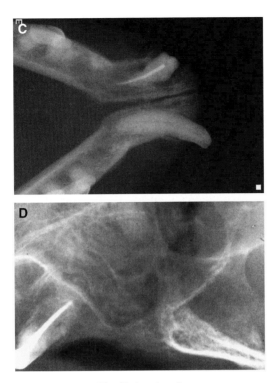

Fig. 12 (*continued*)

that there is an inciting cause (or more than one) that results in surface demineralization of the root. This is followed by a characteristic progression attributable to a peculiarity that may be inherent in certain cats or that is induced in them through diet (ie, vitamin D levels?) or some other extrinsic factor or factors.

Until we can prove the cause, we cannot prevent RLs. Preventing the initial inciting lesion would be ideal. Because periodontal inflammation is known to cause external root resorption, routine oral hygiene and prevention of plaque accumulation should always be recommended. The most common form of RL occurs in the absence of marked gingivitis, however, and the cause is not yet proven [12,18]. One good prospect for a cause of the initial cemental lesion in type 2 lesions is abfraction. Abfraction refers to the lesions caused when lateral flexural forces on the tooth crown are directed to the cervical area of the tooth. This region is a natural stress riser because of the free crown meeting the firmly supported root. Biting on hard foods would be expected to apply lateral forces on the crown as a result of a cat's sectorial dentition. If abfraction is indeed a contributing factor, feeding a diet with a consistency that does not flex the teeth during ingestion could help.

In addition to preventing the inciting cause we may be able to identify the factors that cause the lesions to progress rapidly and invasively in some individuals. It is theorized that all cats, similar to human beings, routinely develop small areas of cementum resorption on their roots [12]. These are repaired in unaffected cats, whereas in affected cats, the resorption leads to an RL. It has been proposed that a diet high in vitamin D may play a role in the rapid and invasive progression of radicular resorption once the initial lesion has damaged the cementum. This is based, in part, on a study reported at the Eighth World Veterinary Dental Congress in 2003 that showed a correlation between serum 25-hydroxyvitamin D level and presence of RLs [24]. The author also reported finding excessive levels of vitamin D in many commercial cat foods. This theory is similar to one in human beings hypothesizing that an initial physical injury to the root surface fails to repair in the normal fashion; thus, the affected individual develops a progressive resorption [6]. If research shows this to be true, reformulating cat foods that contain excessive vitamin D may slow this aspect of the pathophysiology of RLs in cats. In addition, we still need to address the origin of the initial injury, whether it is abfraction, inflammation, or something else.

Discussion

There is debate on whether or not to take routine full-mouth survey radiographs. There is some evidence that when this is done for all new patients, RLs that were not clinically suspected can be discovered. Although it is undoubtedly true that some cats with no clinical lesions show radiographic resorption, documenting this process may not affect treatment in any way. Radiographs that guide treatment or contribute to deciding whether intervention is indicated are important. Full-mouth radiographs would certainly provide additional information regarding future clinical RLs. Nevertheless, the question is whether finding possibly asymptomatic lesions in some cats justifies imposing the additional expense on all clients and the anesthesia time and radiation on all patients. Further, if radiographs would identify an additional 9% of affected cats but histopathology studies show that we are still missing a much larger percentage of early lesions that are not yet radiographically detectable, the question becomes "how much value is there to earlier detection, and how early matters" [11,12]. Intervention is not recommended when subgingival noninflammatory type 2 RLs are found on a radiograph of a tooth with no associated pathologic findings or clinical intraoral lesion. Therefore, we do not take routine full-mouth survey radiographs in patients that have no clinical lesions. There may be a stronger argument for full-mouth survey films on a cat with one or more clinical RLs, because there is a higher likelihood of finding additional affected teeth in these patients.

Summary

Dental RLs continue to affect a large number of our feline patients. Radiographs should be taken of every tooth that has clinical evidence of resorption. Lesions that are clinically apparent on the tooth crown should be treated to prevent possible patient discomfort. Restorations are considered temporary treatments. Extraction of affected teeth is a common treatment. For selected lesions meeting specific criteria, crown amputation offers an alternative that is less invasive, more comfortable, easier to perform, and faster to heal. This procedure cannot be performed without oral radiographs and strict adherence to the selection criteria, however. Ignoring these caveats could result in burying pathologic changes that might continue to cause discomfort, inflammation, and persistent infection in the patient.

References

[1] van Wessum R, Harvey CE, Hennet P. Feline dental resorptive lesions. Prevalence patterns. Vet Clin N Am Small Anim Pract 1992;22:1405–16.

[2] Reichart PA, Durr UM, Triadan H, et al. Periodontal disease in the domestic cat. J Periodontal Res 1984;19:67–75.

[3] Ten Cate AR. Hard tissue formation and destruction. In: Oral histology development, structure, and function. 4th edition. St. Louis: Mosby-Year Book; 1994. p. 111–9.

[4] Frank AL. Extracanal invasive resorption: an update. Compend Contin Educ Dent 1995; 16(3):250–4.

[5] Benenati FW. Root resorption: types and treatment. Gen Dent 1997;45(1):42–5.

[6] Patel K, Darbar UR, Gulabivala K. External cervical resorption associated with gingival overgrowth. Int Endod J 2002;35:395–402.

[7] Frank AL, Torabinejad M. Diagnosis and treatment of extracanal invasive resorption. J Endod 1998;24(7):500–4.

[8] Hopewell-Smith A. The process of osteolysis and odontolysis, or so-called "absorption of calcified tissues": a new and original investigation. The Dental Cosmos 1930:1036.

[9] Okuda A, Harvey CE. Etiopathogenesis of feline dental resorptive lesions. Vet Clin N Am Small Anim Pract 1992;22:1385–404.

[10] Wiggs RB, Lobprise HB. Domestic feline oral and dental disease. In: Veterinary dentistry: principles and practice. Philadelphia: Lippincott-Raven; 1997. p. 492.

[11] Verstraete FJ, Kass PH, Terpak CH. Diagnostic value of full-mouth radiography in cats. Am J Vet Res 1998;59(6):692–5.

[12] Gorrel C, Larsson A. Feline odontoclastic resorptive lesions; unveiling the early lesion. J Small Anim Pract 2002;43(11):482–8.

[13] Chapnik L. External root resorption: an experimental radiographic evaluation. Oral Surg Oral Med Oral Pathol Oral Radiol Endod 1989;67(5):578–82.

[14] Borg E, Källqvist A, Gröndahl K, et al. Film and digital radiography for detection of simulated root resorption cavities. Oral Surg Oral Med Oral Pathol Oral Radiol Endod 1998; 86(1):110–4.

[15] Kravitz LH, Tyndall DA, Bagnell CP, et al. Assessment of external root resorption using digital subtraction radiography. J Endod 1992;18(6):275–84.

[16] Mulligan TW, Aller MS, Williams CA. Acquired defects: caries and regressive changes. In: Atlas of canine and feline dental radiography. Trenton: Veterinary Learning Systems; 1998. p. 153–69.

[17] DuPont GA, DeBowes LJ. Comparison of periodontitis and root replacement in cat teeth with resorptive lesions. J Vet Dent 2002;19(2):71–5.

[18] Gengler W, Dubielzig R, Ramer J. Physical examination and radiographic analysis to detect dental and mandibular bone resorption in cats: a study of 81 cases from necropsy. J Vet Dent 1995;12(3):97–100.

[19] Lommer MJ, Verstraete FJ. Prevalence of odontoclastic resorption lesions and periapical radiographic lucencies in cats: 265 cases (1995–1998). J Am Vet Med Assoc 2000;217(12): 1866–9.

[20] Lyon KF. Subgingival odontoclastic resorptive lesions. Vet Clin N Am Small Anim Pract 1992;22:1417–32.

[21] Frost P, Williams CA. Feline dental disease. Vet Clin N Am Small Anim Pract 1986;16: 851–73.

[22] Harvey CE. Preface to feline dentistry. Vet Clin N Am Small Anim Pract 1992;22:1405–16.

[23] DuPont G. Crown amputation with intentional root retention for advanced feline resorptive lesions: a clinical study. J Vet Dent 1995;12:9–13.

[24] Reiter AM. Evaluation of serum concentration of calcitropic hormones in cats with feline odontoclastic resorptive lesion (FORL). In: Proceedings of Eighth World Veterinary Dental Congress. Kyoto, 2003. p. 186–7.

ELSEVIER
SAUNDERS

Vet Clin Small Anim
35 (2005) 963–984

VETERINARY
CLINICS
Small Animal Practice

Simple and Surgical Exodontia

Linda J. DeBowes, DVM, MS

*Shoreline Veterinary Dental Clinic, Veterinary Dental Referral Service of Puget Sound,
Seattle, WA, 98102, USA*

Preoperative considerations

Extractions are indicated for a number of reasons; some are simple extractions and others are surgical extractions. Appropriate client education regarding the extraction procedure, potential complications, other treatment options, and aftercare should be provided before the actual procedure. A plan for managing the pain associated with any existing dental disease and that associated with the extraction procedure should be formulated.

Surgical extractions (complicated extractions) are those that include some combination of tooth sectioning, mucoperiosteal flaps, and bone removal. An uncomplicated extraction can turn into a complicated one when the tooth root fractures during the procedure. It is especially difficult when the apical third of the root fractures (root tip fracture) [1].

Periodontal disease can result in significant attachment loss, and extraction may be the best treatment option. These extractions generally are not difficult and do not require the use of mucoperiosteal flaps or bone removal unless a complication occurs, such as breaking a root tip.

In general, teeth with a healthy periodontium and those with multiple roots are surgically extracted. A surgical extraction is recommended whenever there is any suspicion that the tooth or bone is likely to fracture when attempting a simple extraction.

Pain management

Pain can be physiologic (protective) or pathologic (tissue or nerve damage). The goal in managing pain associated with dental extractions is to decrease pathologic pain associated with the underlying dental problem and to decrease or eliminate acute pain after the extraction.

Pain management using multiple analgesic drugs acting on different portions of the pain pathway and by different mechanisms provides the best

E-mail address: ldebowes@aol.com

0195-5616/05/$ - see front matter © 2005 Elsevier Inc. All rights reserved.
doi:10.1016/j.cvsm.2005.03.004   *vetsmall.theclinics.com*

results. Commonly used drugs in managing and preventing dental pain include local anesthetic agents, opioids, nonsteroidal anti-inflammatory drugs (NSAIDs), N-methyl-D-aspartate (NMDA)–receptor antagonists, and α_2-receptor agonists.

Preemptive analgesia results in a decrease in the intensity and duration of postoperative pain. This is possible to attain when extracting a tooth that is not painful before the extraction. When pain from infection, inflammation, or nerve injury exists before the extraction, preventative pain management is our goal.

Tooth-related pain can originate in the pulp, dentin, or periodontal ligament (PDL) [2]. The pain associated with extractions varies with each patient and the procedure performed. A simple extraction of a mobile tooth with severe periodontal disease generally does not require gingival surgery or bone removal and does not cause significant postoperative pain. The surgical extraction of a large multirooted tooth requiring a flap and bone removal is painful after surgery.

The need to perform extractions should be anticipated, and preemptive pain management should be applied to these patients. Generally assume that if a procedure is painful in human beings, it must also be painful in other animals. Administer analgesics preemptively if there is any question that a procedure may induce pain in a patient. Surgical extractions result in pain secondary to inflammation and stimulation of peripheral nociceptors. Surgical extractions with gingival incisions, elevation of attached gingiva, and mucogingival flaps produce more postoperative pain than do simple extractions not involving the soft tissues [3,4]. The intensity of acute pain after a tissue insult is greatest within the first 24 to 72 hours after the insult.

The response to pain varies according to many factors, and these should be considered when developing a plan for managing pain for the dental patient. Factors to be considered include the patient's current status, age, and anticipated sensitivity to pain as well as potential drug effects. Young patients generally have a lower tolerance to acute pain but are less sensitive to emotional stress or anxiety associated with an anticipated painful procedure. Ill patients are less capable of tolerating pain than are healthy patients [5,6].

Regional nerve blocks using local anesthetics may be used along with other drugs in providing preemptive analgesia in patients having extractions. Local anesthetics block input from peripheral nociceptors and thus may result in decreased peripheral and central sensitization [7]. A regional nerve block is performed by the injection of a local anesthetic solution close to the nerve trunk. The advantage of this block is that it blocks sensation from a large portion of the anatomy with a single injection. This block is used extensively in the oral cavity. A potential disadvantage is the possibility of accidentally piercing an artery or vein that is located near the nerve trunk.

Bupivacaine is a commonly used local anesthetic in veterinary medicine for intraoral regional anesthesia nerve blocks [8–10]. Others that may be used include mepivacaine, ropivacaine, and lidocaine. The time to onset and duration of action vary for each local anesthetic.

Local anesthetics are relatively safe if administered correctly. Correct dosage calculations, especially for small dogs and cats, are important. Administration of an excessive dose and accidental intravenous administration are probably the most common causes of systemic toxicity [10]. Administering local anesthetics at a slow rate helps to prevent systemic toxicity if accidentally given in a vessel by means of its dilution with blood as it is slowly administered. Careful administration, aspirating for blood, and slowly administering the local anesthetic decrease the chances of systemic toxicity.

Additional drugs for providing preemptive analgesia include the anti-inflammatory drugs. NSAIDs have central analgesic actions as well as peripheral actions (anti-inflammatory). Peripheral opioid receptors are activated during the inflammatory process, and a synergistic action between the NSAIDs and opioids exists. NSAIDs are effective analgesics in the 4- to 24-hour postoperative period. If NSAIDs are given after surgery, there is a decreased likelihood of bleeding causing a problem. The potential risks associated with NSAID use include renal injury, bleeding secondary to platelet dysfunction, and gastric ulceration. The potential for renal injury is greater in the anesthetized patient because of the hemodynamic effects of general anesthesia. Hypotension and increased sympathetic tone are common effects of surgery and anesthesia [11]. At a mean arterial pressure (MAP) of 77 to 95 mm Hg, the kidneys in dogs are dependent on prostaglandins (PGs) to maintain the glomerular filtration rate (GFR) and renal blood flow [11]. The PGs necessary for this renal autoregulation are primarily cyclooxygenase (COX)-1 dependent, although some COX-2 PGs are also implied.

Opioids act supraspinally, spinally, and peripherally to produce analgesia, thereby reducing central and peripheral sensitization [12]. Opioid receptors are located on the afferent sensory nerves in the spinal dorsal horn. Stimulation of these receptors by an opioid agonist decreases the neurotransmitter released from the primary afferent fibers, thereby resulting in a decrease of pain sensation to the secondary afferent pain sensors in the spinal cord [12]. The μ-receptor agonists prevent the nociceptor sensitization caused by inflammatory mediators, such as PGE_2. After surgery, the combination of an NSAID and tramadol works well for severe pain management after extractions in dogs. Oral (buccal absorption) buprenorphine is effective for postoperative pain management in cats.

A large number of NMDA-receptors are located in the spinal cord and play an important role in the process of central sensitization [12–14]. A continuous rate infusion (CRI) of ketamine, an NMDA-receptor antagonist, during surgery is part of the preemptive analgesia plan in the author's clinic when performing extractions.

A potent analgesia response may be produced by stimulation of α_2-adrenergic receptors in the spinal cord and higher centers. The potency of the α_2-receptor agonists is increased by concomitant opioid administration [12]. A low dose of an α_2-receptor agonist may be added to the pain management plan as needed. This is especially useful in young or anxious patients.

Infection control

Antibiotic use should be considered for those patients with periapical infections, draining fistulae, and periodontal abscesses as well as those that are likely to have poor healing.

Equipment for simple and surgical (complicated) extractions

The correct instruments, equipment, and operating area greatly enhance the experience for the operator and patient. To aid in visualization, operating telescopes are recommended. These are beneficial when trying to visualize a small root tip at the apex of an alveolus in a cat. Lighting is also important, and having a high-speed handpiece with fiberoptics provides a light source directly on your surgery site.

Having the ability to take radiographs is essential if doing any extraction procedure. Intraoral dental radiographs are preferred, and standard dental film (sizes 2 and 4) or digital radiographs (sensor instead of film) may be used.

Instruments used in performing simple and complicated extractions include those employed for incising tissue, elevating mucoperiosteum, retracting soft tissues, controlling hemorrhage, grasping tissue, removing bone, removing soft tissue from bony defects, suturing mucosa, and loosening and removing teeth.

Incising tissue

A scalpel handle and blade can be used to make incisions around teeth and through the mucoperiosteum. A round or flat scalpel handle and number 15 scalpel blade are the most commonly used tools for this purpose. A number 12 blade may be useful when making an incision on the distal aspect of a tooth.

Elevating mucoperiosteum

A periosteal elevator is used to reflect the mucosa and periosteum as a single layer from the bone. A molt number 9 periosteal elevator (Fig. 1) has a sharp pointed end and a broader flat end that are used to elevate and reflect soft tissues. A double-ended molt periosteal elevator has a small end and a large end (Fig. 2) that are useful when working on a variety of different sized patients. The periosteal elevators are used with a prying motion or push stroke to separate the periosteum from the underlying bone.

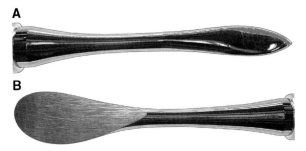

Fig. 1. Molt number 9 periosteal elevator: sharp pointed end (A) and broad flat end (B). (Courtesy of Cislak Manufacturing, Niles, IL; with permission.)

Retracting soft tissue

Soft tissue retraction is necessary for adequate visualization and access as well as to protect the soft tissues. The periosteal elevators may be used to retract the soft tissue flaps once the tissue has been reflected from the bone. A Pritchard PR 3 has a broad rectangular end that is useful for this purpose (Fig. 3).

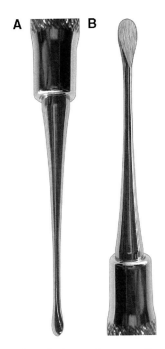

Fig. 2. Double-ended molt periosteal elevator has a small end (A) and a large end (B). (Courtesy of Cislak Manufacturing, Niles, IL; with permission.)

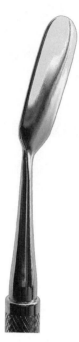

Fig. 3. Pritchard PR 3 has a broad rectangular end that is useful for protecting the soft tissues from trauma when sectioning teeth or removing alveolar bone. (Courtesy of Cislak Manufacturing, Niles, IL; with permission.)

Controlling hemorrhage

Controlling bleeding during surgery improves visibility and decreases postoperative clots within the wound. Clots inside the wound are an excellent culture medium, increasing the infection rate, interfering with blood flow to the area, and separating the periosteum from the bone [15]. When planning flap design, major vessels should be avoided and the incision should be over bone when closed so that direct pressure can be applied to help control bleeding.

When performing a full-thickness mucoperiosteal flap, the initial incisions made should be completely through the periosteum. The periosteal elevator should be placed in direct contact with the bone, and the full-thickness flap should be reflected carefully to avoid excessive bleeding. To avoid tearing the flap, start the elevation at the gingival margin or attached gingiva. Direct pressure on the extraction site with a gauze sponge may control bleeding. If not, an absorbable gelatin sponge (Gelfoam; Pfizer Animal Health, New York, New York) or microporous polysaccharide beads (Hemablock; Abbott Laboratories Animal Health, Abbott Park, Illinois) can be placed in the socket before suturing to enhance hemostasis.

Bleeding from the bone may occur as small vessels in bone rupture when reflecting a full-thickness mucoperiosteal flap. Bleeding from these vessels is usually minor and often can be controlled by burnishing the area with the sharp end of the periosteal elevator to compress bone over the bleeding canal.

Grasping tissues

Adson forceps are commonly used for gently holding tissue and stabilizing it during suturing.

Removing bone

The most common method for removing bone is with a burr and handpiece. The ideal handpiece is a high-speed one that does not exhaust air into the operative field. When air is exhausted into the wound, it may be forced into deeper tissues, producing tissue emphysema and possibly an air embolus. The high-speed turbine drills used by most veterinarians performing extractions do not fit this criterion; they do exhaust air into the operating area. There have not been significant complications of this technique reported in the veterinary literature or encountered by the author or other veterinary dental specialists. Nevertheless, when using this type of drill, one should be aware of these potential complications. Another method for removing bone is to use end- and side-cutting rongeur forceps.

Removing soft tissue from bony defects

Bone curettes can be used to remove soft tissue from the alveolus and periapical area before closing the extraction sites.

Suturing mucosal incisions

The suture material for closure of the extraction sites is chosen based on operator preference, the size of the patient, and the length of time the sutures need to remain. The author uses 4-0 chromic gut on a reverse cutting 0.375-inch needle (PS-1) for most extraction procedures. A cutting needle passes through tissue more easily than a tapered one.

Scissors

Suture scissors are used for cutting suture, and tissue scissors (eg, Iris scissors, Metzenbaum scissors) are used for cutting soft tissue.

Holding the mouth open

Bite blocks or ratchet type action mouth props are used to hold the mouth open. Exercise caution when using these, because prolonged use or excessive opening may cause postoperative temporomandibular joint (TMJ) and muscle discomfort. They are generally not needed except possibly when working deep in the back of the mouth.

Irrigation

When using a burr to remove bone, irrigation is essential to cool the burr and prevent bone-damaging heat buildup. With the high-speed turbine drills, water flows through the handpiece and provides the cooling irrigation. If using a handpiece without this feature, water flushed from a syringe is utilized to provide the cooling irrigation.

Dental elevators

Elevators are available in multiple designs and sizes, and each operator should choose elevators that fit his or her hand and are appropriate for the patient's size and tooth being worked on. Dental elevators are designed to loosen teeth and elevate them from the alveolus. Forces are applied with elevators by placing them between the alveolus and root surface and then gently rotating the instrument to apply force in a slow and deliberate fashion. Elevators may also be placed between crown portions of sectioned teeth or against crestal bone and the side of tooth and rotated to apply force.

A few of the author's most frequently used elevators are the 3-mm straight luxator from The Original Luxator Kit (JS Dental MFG, Inc., Ridgefield, Connecticut), a "bone preservation elevator" with a spade tip (style 63; A. Titan Instruments, Hamburg, New York), and the extremely narrow elevators recommended for cats (Cislak Manufacturing, Niles, IL) (Fig. 4).

Extraction forceps

A variety of extraction forceps are available for removing the tooth from the alveolus (Fig. 5). They should fit the operator's hand, the beaks should adapt well to the contours of the tooth root, and the applied force should be along the long axis of the tooth. Extraction forceps are standard instruments; depending on the size of the tooth, and possibly on the size of your hand, small-breed and large-breed extraction forceps are used. Root tip forceps are used to reach down into an alveolus and obtain a firm hold on a small loose root tip at the apex of the alveolus (Fig. 6).

Tooth extraction

The tooth is anchored in the alveolus by the PDL, which is attached to the cementum and to the alveolar bone. Perfectly conical teeth are maintained in place only by the PDL, and a simple extraction, with severing of the PDL, is all that is required to extract these teeth.

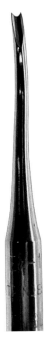

Fig. 4. A narrow elevator is recommended for cats. (Courtesy of Cislak Manufacturing, Niles, IL; with permission.)

Multirooted teeth and teeth with divergent roots are anchored by bone as well as by the PDL. These teeth require surgical extraction. Marked root curvature and bulbous roots also require surgical extraction.

General extraction principles include obtaining adequate access to the tooth root(s), creating an unimpeded path for root and/or tooth removal, and using controlled force.

Basic steps

Radiographs

Radiographs should be taken before performing an extraction. The radiographs are used to evaluate the tooth root(s) and surrounding structures for anomalies, pathologic findings, and fractures, which are all things that might affect the procedure time, difficulty, and/or approach (Fig. 7). Preprocedural radiographs also document pathologic findings present before the extraction so that there can be no question of iatrogenic trauma or problems developing as a result of the extraction procedure.

Coronal gingiva incised from tooth

The coronal attachment of gingiva can be incised with a scalpel blade, periosteal elevator, or sharp luxator and/or elevator.

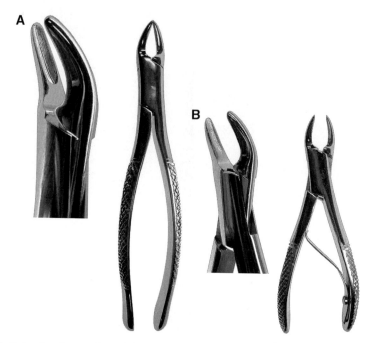

Fig. 5. Extraction forceps: large (*A*) and small (*B*). (Courtesy of Cislak Manufacturing, Niles, IL; with permission.)

Flaps (mucoperiosteal)

Flaps are created for the purposes of providing increased visualization and access to the underlying structures as well as to protect the tissue from iatrogenic trauma that might occur during bone removal or tooth sectioning. The flaps should be large enough to provide adequate visual and instrument access. When creating the flaps, major nerves or blood vessels should be avoided and the flaps should be full-thickness mucoperiosteal flaps.

A basic envelope flap is useful for allowing access to the furcation area of multirooted teeth and for exposing the coronal aspect of the buccal bone (Fig. 8). An envelope flap is a full-thickness flap created by a horizontal incision through the gingival attachment at the alveolar crest, followed by elevation of the attached gingiva with a periosteal elevator. The horizontal incision may be short to just expose the furcation area, or it may be extended beyond the tooth to be extracted to allow for greater flap reflection and tooth and/or root exposure.

The envelope flap can be modified for increased exposure by one vertical relaxing incision (Fig. 9). The papilla is included in the flap to make closure easier. If even more exposure is required, two vertical relaxing incisions can be made, creating a rectangular flap (Fig. 10). To provide adequate blood supply to the entire flap tissue, the base of the flap should not be narrower

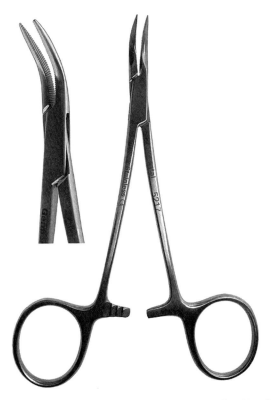

Fig. 6. Root tip forceps. (Courtesy of Cislak Manufacturing, Niles, IL; with permission.)

than the coronal aspect of the flap. The flap should be designed so that the vertical relaxing incisions are over bone when the flap is sutured closed.

Sectioning tooth and alveolar bone removal

Teeth are sectioned and bone is removed in a controlled manner so as to prevent fracture of the tooth root and alveolar process. Before sectioning multirooted teeth, it is helpful to look at a skull or model if you are not familiar with the normal anatomy of the tooth and surrounding structures (Fig. 11).

Multirooted teeth should be sectioned through the crown so that all crowns and associated roots are completely separated. If attempts to tear the PDL and elevate the tooth are made before complete sectioning of the crown, the tooth is likely to fracture (Fig. 12).

For difficult extractions, reflection of a mucoperiosteal flap and removal of some labial or buccal bone are usually required for adequate access. Removing alveolar bone decreases the attachment area, making it easier to luxate and elevate the tooth root. Bone is also removed to create a pathway for removal of enlarged or curved roots (Fig. 13).

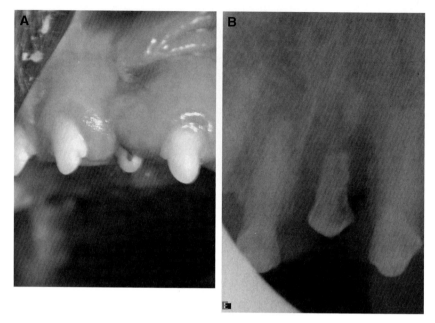

Fig. 7. (*A*) Incisor with a draining fistula. (*B*) Preprocedural radiograph shows a fractured root.

To section a tooth, the author generally uses a number 2 round burr on a high-speed handpiece with adequate water to prevent heating the tooth and surrounding bone. To avoid traumatizing the attached gingiva, an envelope flap is made and the gingiva is reflected in the area of the furcation.

The first step in sectioning a double-rooted tooth or in sectioning the mesial roots from the distal root of the upper fourth premolar is to remove bone at the furcation area. The burr is directed from the buccal side to the

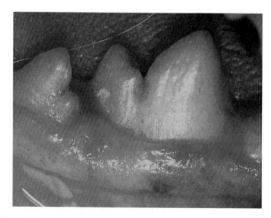

Fig. 8. Basic envelope flap, with the gingiva incised at the attachment to the tooth.

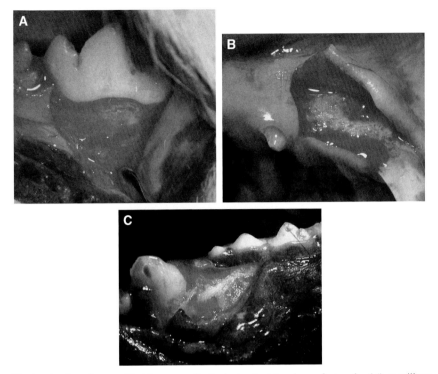

Fig. 9. Envelope flap modified by one vertical relaxing incision: lower first molar (*A*), maxillary canine (*B*), and mandibular canine (*C*).

palatal or lingual side. The burr is then used to section the crown, directing the burr from the furcation area toward the coronal aspect (Fig. 14). Using this technique, you can be assured of completely sectioning the crown. If sectioning from the crown toward the furcation area, it may be necessary in large dogs to use a surgical length burr to reach the furcation area.

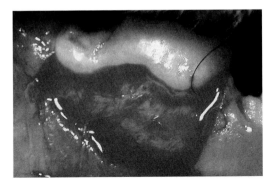

Fig. 10. Envelope flap modified into a rectangular flap by two vertical relaxing incisions.

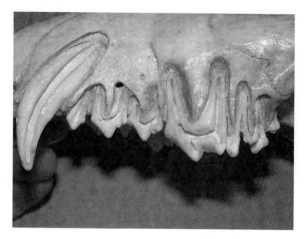

Fig. 11. Skull demonstrates the normal anatomy of the tooth and surrounding structures.

The mesial roots of the upper fourth premolar are sectioned between the palatal and buccal roots. This may be difficult to do with the crown in place; frequently, less experienced operators angle the burr and cut through the palatal root instead of between the two roots. It is helpful to remove the coronal aspect of the crown over the mesial roots, exposing the root canals of both roots so that the burr can be easily directed between the two mesial roots (Fig. 15).

The upper first molar in a dog is sectioned first between the one palatal root and two mesial roots and then between the two mesial roots (Fig. 16). Once the teeth are sectioned, the individual tooth roots and associated crown are elevated from the alveolus.

Tooth roots that are bulbous or enlarged at the apex may be loosened so that they are mobile but extraction with forceps is still not possible. In these

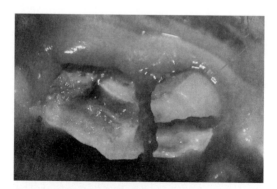

Fig. 12. Multirooted tooth (upper fourth premolar) is sectioned through the crown so that all crowns and associated roots are completely separated.

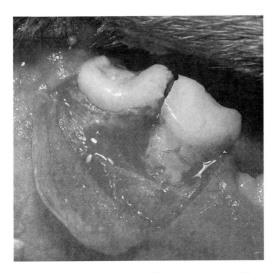

Fig. 13. Reflection of a mucoperiosteal flap and removal of buccal bone.

cases, remove bone around the root to alleviate the obstruction for extraction (Fig. 17).

Elevating, luxating, and removing tooth

A scalpel blade or sharp luxator can sever the coronal portion of the PDL. Controlled force is necessary when luxating and elevating teeth. Excessive force may result in fracture of the tooth or alveolar process. Patience is a must when trying to tear the PDL fibers and elevate the tooth root. To tear the PDL fibers, a steady force has to be applied, stretching the fibers until they fatigue and tear. To do this, a dental luxator or elevator is inserted between the tooth root and alveolar bone. Once in place, force is

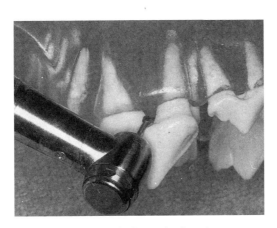

Fig. 14. Begin sectioning at the furcation area.

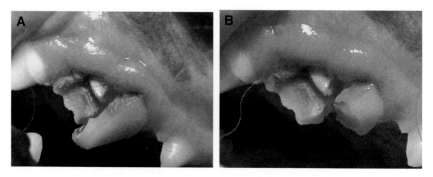

Fig. 15. Coronal aspect of the crown over the mesial roots of upper fourth premolar has been removed so that the burr can be easily directed between the two mesial roots.

applied apically while rotating the instrument blade slightly to apply tension on the PDL fibers. The tension has to be applied for a sufficient duration to cause tearing of the fibers. If you do not hold the tension, but instead wiggle the instrument back and forth, the PDL fibers just stretch and return to normal like a rubber band. As a general rule of thumb, once tension is applied to the PDL, it should be held for 30 to 60 seconds. When performing this step, the operator should place a finger close to the end of the blade to provide a "stop" in case the instrument slips (Fig. 18).

In a multirooted tooth, an instrument (elevator) can be placed between the sectioned pieces of crown and rotated to stretch the PDL. When doing this, great care should be taken not to apply enough force to break the crown or root. Fractured apical roots in these instances may be difficult to extract.

Once the tooth root has become mobile, extraction forceps can be used to extract the tooth carefully. The forceps should be placed at the crown root

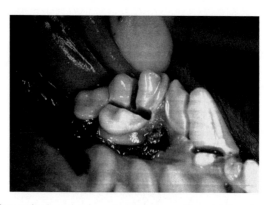

Fig. 16. Upper first molar in a dog is sectioned between the palatal root and the two mesial roots.

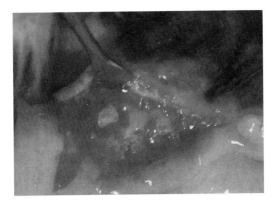

Fig. 17. Bone around the root has been removed to alleviate the obstruction for extraction.

junction or as far apically on the root as possible. If too much force is applied before the tooth is sufficiently loose, it is fairly easy to fracture the tip of the root.

When a root tip fracture occurs, the tooth may be difficult to extract; this turns the procedure into a complicated extraction procedure. If an infected root tip remains, it eventually causes a problem for the patient. If a root fractures during the extraction process, it is usually obvious because of the cracking sound made when it fractures as well as the fractured surface of the coronal portion of the extracted root. The root tip should be checked to be sure that the entire tip has been removed. The root tip should be smooth, rounded, and covered by the PDL, which is reddish in color (Fig. 19). The alveolus should be cleaned out after the extraction so that no debris, periapical granulation, or cystic material is left behind.

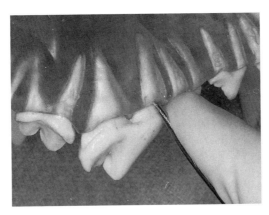

Fig. 18. Finger placed close to the end of the blade provides a "stop" in case the instrument slips.

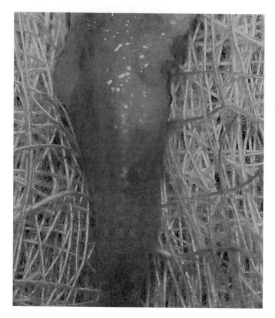

Fig. 19. Root tip should be smooth, rounded, and covered by the periodontal ligament, which is reddish in color.

Smoothing alveolar bone

Once the tooth has been extracted, the edges of the alveolar bone should be smoothed. This is generally done with a high-speed handpiece and round burr. This makes the patient more comfortable after surgery and enhances healing of the soft tissue over the extraction site.

Suturing flap

Mucoperiosteal flaps should be sutured using an absorbable suture material. Chromic gut or a synthetic suture material, such as polyglycolic or polylactic acid, is used. The suture size depends on the patient; generally, 3-0 or 4-0 suture is appropriate. A swaged-on cutting needle passes through the mucoperiosteum more easily and with less trauma than a tapered needle or suture threaded through a needle.

Specific extractions

Extraction of canine teeth

Extracting mandibular canine teeth in dogs can be difficult unless they are extremely mobile; even then, great care is recommended to prevent problems. The major complication associated with extracting a mandibular canine is fracturing the mandible. This is most likely to occur in smaller breeds with significant bone loss and when excessive force is used. The tongue hangs out to the side in dogs after extracting the mandibular canine, and some clients find this objectionable. These complications may be avoided by performing a root canal rather than an extraction on the mandibular canines.

Extracting a maxillary canine tooth in a dog may result in an apparent oronasal fistula. A single- or double-flap closure should be performed to close the fistula.

Cats that have a maxillary canine extracted may bite the upper lip with the lower canine tooth. In an attempt to avoid this, it is recommended to remove as little of the alveolar bone as possible.

Full-mouth extraction in cats

Extracting all premolars and molars is recommended for treating idiopathic chronic gingivostomatitis faucitis in cats. It is important to remove all teeth, including all the roots as well as the PDL. Persistent inflammation and oral discomfort remain when a portion of the root remains. Surgery is extensive, and the tissues are usually friable and bleed easily. The first step in each quadrant is incising the gingiva so that a full-thickness gingival flap can be created. Using a periosteal elevator, the attached gingiva is elevated on the lingual and/or palatal and buccal aspects. Once this has been done, the teeth are sectioned and a small amount of alveolar bone is removed. Sharp luxators and/or elevators with a narrow width (1 mm) are used to severe the PDL and rotated to stretch the PDL. These teeth may break with little applied force, especially if a portion of the tooth structure has been lost from a resorptive lesion. A root may become mobile but still cannot be removed because of a bulbous end at the apex. Removal of additional bone is necessary to remove these teeth. Once all teeth and roots have been extracted, the alveolus is curetted to remove any remaining remnants of the PDL. The alveolar bone is smoothed with a round burr to remove any spicules or infected bone. Simple interrupted sutures are placed.

Extracting roots and root pieces

Roots may be fractured during an extraction or from trauma. When a root is fractured deep within the alveolus, it may be difficult to place an instrument between the root and alveolar bone. It may also be difficult to visualize a small amount of root at the apex of a deep alveolus. A radiograph at this point is often helpful. If you can visualize the root within the alveolus, you can create a space with a small round burr surrounding the root. This provides a small space within which to place an elevator or luxator. It is important to insert the instrument next to the root before placing apical forces so as to avoid pushing the root tip beyond the alveolus. If a root is pushed into the nasal cavity or mandibular canal, it should be retrieved, and this may be difficult to do. If the potential for trauma is great, it may be better to leave the root tip instead of further attempting to remove it. The client should be advised of any retained roots. Referral to a more experienced veterinary dentist may also be an option.

Complications and precautions

Complications may occur during an extraction procedure and are related to the operator's experience and technique.

Orbital penetration by dental elevators may occur during an extraction of the upper fourth premolar or first molar (Fig. 20) [16–18]. The caudal maxillary tooth roots are close to the orbit, and if using an elevator incorrectly, it is possible to slip and penetrate the eye. This is most likely to occur when severe periodontal disease is present. Use proper extraction techniques to avoid accidental orbital penetration. Excessive force should be avoided. Hold the elevator down on the shaft of the instrument to minimize slippage of the instrument and iatrogenic trauma.

A potential complication of extracting mandibular teeth, especially the canines or first molars, is to fracture the mandible. This is more likely in smaller dogs with less mandibular bone and in those with extensive bone loss from periodontal disease (Fig. 21).

Home care follow-up

For the first 7 to 10 days after an extraction, the pet should be fed only soft foods. It should not be allowed to chew on toys, treats, or any object that might tear the sutures. If the animal has dermatologic problems, it may need to wear a collar or some other device to keep it from breaking down the incision and contaminating the extraction site with hair and debris.

Systemic or topical antimicrobials may be indicated if there is an abscess or generalized infection of the soft tissues. Topical chlorhexidine gel or rinse may be used for its topical antimicrobial effect.

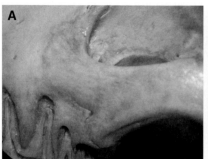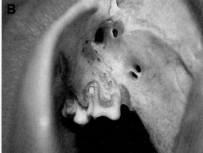

Fig. 20. Caudal maxillary tooth roots are close to the orbit.

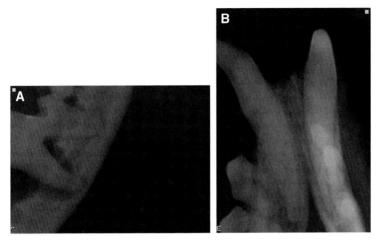

Fig. 21. Small dogs with loss of mandibular bone and the potential for fracture during extraction: (*A*) mandibular first molar and (*B*) mandibular canine.

Pain management is important, and the drugs used and duration of treatment vary depending on the individual patient and the type of oral surgery performed.

Summary

Preemptive and postoperative pain management is part of patient care when performing extractions. Simple extractions can become complicated when tooth roots are fractured. Adequate lighting, magnification, and surgical techniques are important when performing surgical (complicated) extractions. Radiographs should be taken before extractions and also during the procedure to assist with difficult extractions. Adequate flap design and bone removal are necessary when performing surgical extractions. Complications, including ocular trauma, jaw fracture, and soft tissue trauma, are avoided or minimized with proper patient selection and technique.

References

[1] Hooley JR, Golden DP. Surgical extractions. Dent Clin N Am 1994;38(2):217–36.
[2] Byers MR, Närhi MVO. Dental injury models: experimental tools for understanding neuroinflammatory interactions and polymodal nociceptor functions. Crit Rev Oral Biol Med 1999;10(1):4–39.
[3] Clauser C, Barone R. Effect of incision and flap reflection on postoperative pain after the removal of partially impacted mandibular third molars. Quintessence Int 1994;25(12):845–9.
[4] Shevel E, Koepp WG, Butow KW. A subjective assessment of pain and swelling following the surgical removal of impacted third molar teeth using different surgical techniques. SADJ 2001;56(5):238–41.

[5] Wolfe TM, Muir W. Local anesthetics: pharmacology and novel applications. Compend Contin Educ Prac Vet 2003;25(12):916–26.

[6] ACVA. ACVA position paper. Available at: www.acva.org/professional/position/pain.

[7] Dermot JK, Ahmad M, Brull SJ. Regional anesthesia and pain: preemptive analgesia II: recent advances and current trends. Can J Anesth 2001;48(11):1091–101.

[8] Carmichael DT. Using intraoral regional anesthetic nerve blocks. Veterinary Medicine 2004; 99(9):766–70.

[9] Lantz GC. Regional anesthesia for dentistry and oral surgery. J Vet Dent 2003;20(3):181–6.

[10] Lemke KA, Dawson SE. Local and regional anesthesia. Vet Clin N Am Small Anim Pract 2000;30(4):839–57.

[11] Crandell DE, Mathews KA, Dyson DH. Effect of meloxicam and carprofen on renal function when administered to healthy dogs prior to anesthesia and painful stimuli. Am J Vet Res 2004;65(10):1384–90.

[12] Kelly DJ, Ahmad M, Brull SJ. Preemptive analgesia I: physiological pathways and pharmacological modalities. Can J Anesth 2001;48(10):1000–10.

[13] Snijdelaar DG, Korean G, Katz J. Effects of perioperative oral amantadine on postoperative pain and morphine consumption in patients after radical prostatectomy; results of a preliminary study. Anesthesiology 2004;100(1):134–41.

[14] McCartney CJ, Sinha A, Katz J. A qualitative systematic review of the role of N-methyl-D-aspartate receptor antagonists in preventive analgesia. Anesth Analg 2004;98(5):1385–400.

[15] Ogle OE. Perioperative hemorrhage. In: Dym H, Ogle OE, editors. Atlas of minor oral surgery. Philadelphia: WB Saunders; 2001. p. 54–65.

[16] Smith MM, Smith EM, La Croix N, et al. Orbital penetration associated with tooth extraction. J Vet Dent 2003;20(1):8–17.

[17] Smith MM. Tooth extraction: complications—anticipation, avoidance, and alleviation. NAVC Clinician's Brief 2004;37–40.

[18] Ramsey DT, Manfra-Maretta S, Hamor RE, et al. Ophthalmic manifestations and complications of dental disease in dogs and cats. J Am Anim Hosp Assoc 1996;32(3):215–24.

ELSEVIER
SAUNDERS

Vet Clin Small Anim
35 (2005) 985–1008

VETERINARY
CLINICS
Small Animal Practice

Maxillofacial Fracture Repairs

Loïc Legendre, DVM

Northwest Veterinary Dental Services, 4037 Sunset Boulevard,
North Vancouver, British Columbia, Canada V7R 3Y7

Oral trauma remains a common presentation in a small animal practice. Most fractures are the result of vehicular accidents. Among other causes are falls, kicks, gunshots wounds, and encounters with various hard objects ranging from baseball bats and golf clubs to horse hooves and car doors. Next in popularity are dog fights, especially when a large dog and a small dog are involved, and fights with other animals [1]. With cats, falls from various heights are responsible for a large percentage of presentations.

Nontraumatic causes comprise periodontal disease, neoplastic processes, and metabolic abnormalities [2]. In dogs and cats, mandibular fractures are more common than maxillary fractures [2,3]. In dogs, mandibular fractures total 3% to 6% of all fractures [1].

Emergency, stabilization, and planning

Whatever the cause, the first priority is to stabilize the patient. Emergency medical care is described elsewhere and needs not be repeated here. A particular problem associated with maxillofacial fractures is to ensure that the animal can self-feed and, if not, to establish ways to get proper nutrition into it. Usually, this entails placing esophageal or gastrotomy feeding tubes (Figs. 1 and 2).

Repairs before dentistry

Fractures other than maxillofacial ones are a surgical problem. As such, the goal of repair is to fix the broken bone. To that end, the instruments used are pins, plates, and screws as well as external fixation devices, for example. These are proven techniques, and they would be more successful in

E-mail address: ledentiste@aol.com

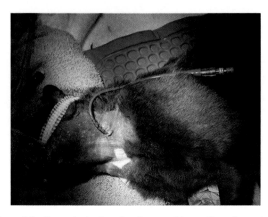

Fig. 1. The esophageal feeding tube is placed and sutured in to allow the maintenance of caloric intake without the patient using its mouth.

maxillofacial cases if it were not for the presence of special conditions existing in the oral cavity. First and foremost is the presence of teeth. Teeth interfere with the placement of any of these devices [1,4,5]. With the Kirschner-Ehmer apparatus and screws and plates, it is almost impossible not to perforate roots (Figs. 3 and 4) [1,4]. Intramedullary pins actually penetrate the mental canal, resulting in neurovascular damage (Fig. 5). If placed dorsally to the mental canal, they damage teeth [2].

Occlusion is the second specific oral condition to be respected when repairing maxillofacial fractures. Plates, unless well contoured, straighten bones that are naturally curved, resulting in malocclusion. Intramedullary pins share the same problem.

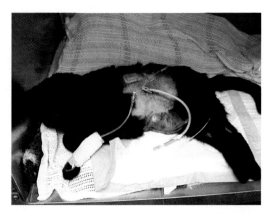

Fig. 2. The gastrotomy tube is another way of feeding the patient while protecting its oral cavity.

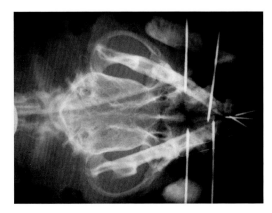

Fig. 3. A Kirschner apparatus with seven pins is driven at oblique angles through both bodies of the mandible, without any thought about the roots damaged in the process.

The third particularity of the mouth is that the jaw bones are not weight bearing. Rigid fixation is not necessary for healing. As long as vascularization is preserved and infection is controlled, mandibular fractures heal, even if some mobility remains [6].

The fourth particularity is that the mandible is covered by large muscles that make its exposure difficult.

The fifth particularity is the fact that the maxilla is composed of multiple thin bones, which are hard to manipulate and repair.

Because teeth are not part of a surgeon's training, they are ignored. Ignoring the teeth leads to endodontic trauma, chronic infection, osteomyelitis, and even pathologic fractures. There is then occlusion to be reckoned with; if the teeth are slightly displaced, the bone still heals but the patient is unable to prehend and chew correctly. This situation is not easy to remedy, because dentists are still far and few.

Modern veterinary dental techniques

With the advent of modern dentistry also came the realization that the biggest problem after a maxillofacial fracture is the loss of occlusion [2,4,6–10]. Therefore, in principle, when faced with a fracture of one or both jaws, strive to re-establish normal occlusion. To that effect, one has to concentrate on the position of the teeth. The teeth are set in bone; thus, realigning the teeth automatically realigns the bone. Occlusion becomes the crucial factor. If it is maintained, the bone heals correctly. The other concern is still to minimize dental trauma during repair. This is accomplished by using the crowns of the teeth to realign them by employing different dental equipment, such as wire and acrylic compounds, instead of pins, plates, and screws. Today, composite resins are used more commonly than acrylic. They have several advantages,

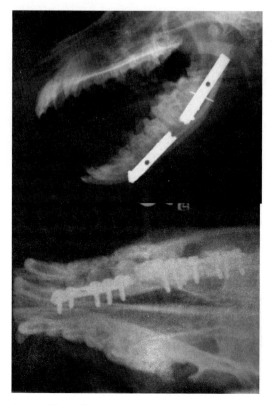

Fig. 4. Two parts of a mandibular fracture are repaired using two plates and several screws. As in Fig. 1, one can see that the screws perforate the roots while stabilizing the bone.

including ease of use, nonexothermic properties, no mixing necessary, no noxious fumes, improved bonding, and improved esthetics.

The tension side on the mandible and maxilla is the oral side. More stable repairs are achieved when working on the coronal end of teeth. Manipulating teeth and working on their crowns is less invasive than working on bone. Jaws do not bear weight; thus, bones do not need to be rigidly fixed, compression is not required, and coaptation is almost always sufficient. When necessary, wires are placed to reinforce the composite. Wires can be passed around teeth or through small drilled holes between roots (Fig. 6). Their flexibility makes them easier to use around teeth. Wires also prevent total failure of acrylic implants [2].

Symphyseal separation

Symphyseal separation is the most common oral trauma in cats, and 73% of oral trauma is related to the symphysis [4]. Fifteen percent of all feline

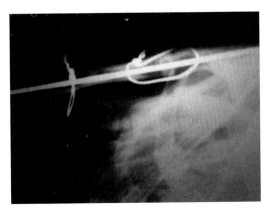

Fig. 5. An intramedullary pin is driven inside the mandibular canal in an attempt to repair a fracture of the mandibular body of an edentulous dog. No teeth were damaged in this process, but the neurovascular bundle running into the canal was destroyed.

fractures are mandibular symphyseal separations [6]. The symphysis is a true joint with a fibrocartilaginous disc stabilizing both halves. Stabilization is easily achieved using a wire entering and exiting through the chin, looping it around the bodies of the mandible between the canine teeth and the third premolars [2,4]. To increase stability and control the angle of the crowns of the canine teeth, a second wire can be shaped into a figure-of-eight or twisted around the base of the canine teeth (Fig. 7) [11]. A small amount of composite resin is added on the buccal surface of the canine teeth to cover the twisted end of the wire and to prevent it from slipping. A ball of composite can also be placed around the twisted end of the wire sticking under the chin to prevent it from catching on objects (Fig. 8). Another method consists of making a small incision in the skin of the chin and rolling

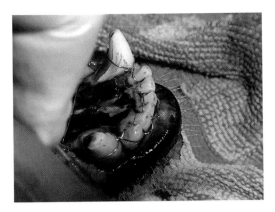

Fig. 6. Demonstration of the use of interdental wires to stabilize a fracture before applying composite resin to increase the rigidity of the splint.

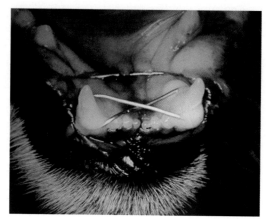

Fig. 7. A symphyseal separation is easily repaired with the help of a loop wire around the bodies of the mandible and a figure-of-eight wire around the canine teeth. Note that a small amount of composite resin was added to the base of the canine teeth to cover the ends of the wire, which can be irritating.

the end of the wire under the skin before stitching it closed [4]. The wire is kept in place for 6 weeks and then removed with the patient under sedation.

Mandibular body fracture

A mandibular body fracture occurs most commonly in dogs between the first premolars and second molars [6]. Most fractures are open and are seen in male dogs less than 1 year old (Fig. 9) [12]. Once again, the goal of repair is to appose the fragments. Compression is not necessary. Mandibular

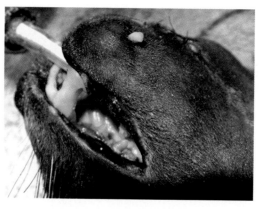

Fig. 8. The twisted ends of the loop wire exiting under the chin are covered with a bead of composite to prevent the animal getting them caught.

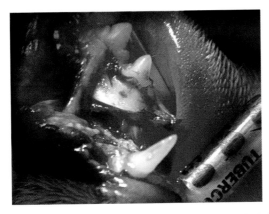

Fig. 9. Open diagonal fracture of the right body of the mandible in a cat.

fractures heal even with gaps as long as revascularization is encouraged and infection is prevented [6]. Three variations exist: vertical fractures (Fig. 10), favorable fractures (Fig. 11), and unfavorable fractures (Fig. 12). In favorable fractures, the fracture line runs in a ventrorostral direction such that the pull of the masticatory muscles on the distal fragment helps to keep the fragments apposed. In unfavorable fractures, the fracture line runs in a dorsorostral direction, and the pull of the masticatory muscles on the distal fragment distracts the fracture. Because most of these fractures are comminuted, the fragments are exposed and interosseous wires can be placed. Favorable fractures can be stabilized by placing one wire as seen in Fig. 13. Unfavorable fractures preferably require two wires placed through three or four holes (Fig. 14). Once the fragments are aligned, the site needs to be cleaned and the soft tissues sutured closed. The teeth are then manipulated into normal occlusion. When necessary, interdental wires

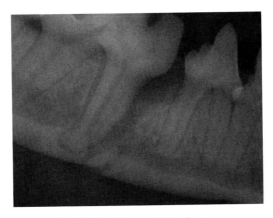

Fig. 10. Vertical mandibular fracture.

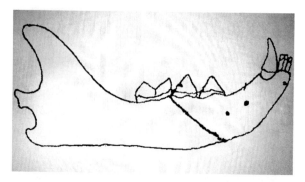

Fig. 11. Diagram depicting a favorable mandibular fracture. The fracture line runs ventrorostrally, and the pull of the masticatory muscles keeps the fragments together.

(24–26-gauge) are placed in a figure-of-eight or Stout loop arrangement around several of the teeth on either side of the fracture [4]. The repair is reinforced by applying composite resin to the etched lingual surface of the affected teeth. Wire-reinforced composite resin splints are much stronger than composite resin alone [4]. Once the composite resin is cured, the mouth is closed to ascertain that the splint is not interfering with occlusion. If it is, a "Goldie" burr, mounted on a slow handpiece, is used to remove surplus as well as to eliminate any spur or overhang that would irritate the patient or exacerbate plaque retention [10]. The patient is usually able to feed on gruel immediately. It is kept on a soft diet for the following 6 to 8 weeks until the splint is removed. These types of fractures respond well to acrylic and wire repairs [1,8,9,13], and the technique is easy [14]. At the time of removal, the jaw is palpated to confirm its stability, the patient is anesthetized, and a radiograph is obtained to demonstrate that signs of bony union are

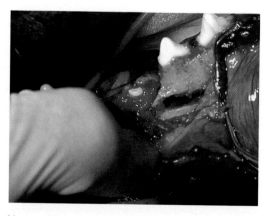

Fig. 12. Unfavorable mandibular fracture. The fracture line runs ventrocaudally; thus, the natural pull of the masticatory muscles distracts the fragments.

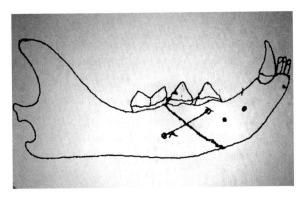

Fig. 13. This diagram shows how to stabilize a favorable mandibular fracture using only one wire. The wire is looped through two holes and is aligned perpendicular to the fracture line. Care is taken to avoid roots and neurovascular bundles when drilling the holes.

present [10]. If everything is satisfactory, the splint is taken off. A pair of cutting pliers is first used to crack chunks of resin (Fig. 15). As soon as the jaw is loose and the mouth can be opened, the patient is intubated (Fig. 16). Next, a finishing burr is gently run over the surface of the teeth to remove

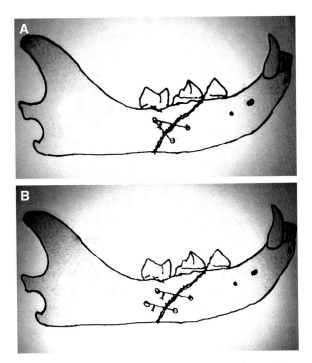

Fig. 14. The two diagrams show variations in the technique used to stabilize an unfavorable mandibular fracture: (A) two wires are passed through three holes, and (B) two wires are passed through four holes.

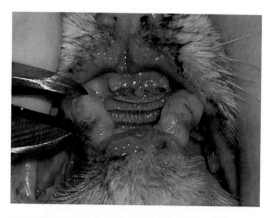

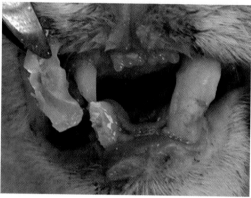

Fig. 15. The composite splint is cracked with a pair of pliers, taking care not to damage any enamel surface.

the remaining resin (Fig. 17). Remember not to put any pressure on this burr to avoid damaging the teeth. The teeth are finally polished with a fine prophylaxis paste, and the patient is allowed to recover. The splint usually causes a temporary gingivitis that resolves after its removal and professional cleaning.

Bilateral mandibular fracture

Rarer than unilateral fractures, bilateral mandibular fractures are much harder to repair. The mobility of the fragments is far greater, making proper alignment more difficult to attain. Luckily, the principles stay the same: use wires to stabilize the fragments, and then add rigidity by applying an acrylic splint on the lingual surface of the teeth (Fig. 18). If instability remains, bone loss at the fracture line may ensue, leading to nonunion. Correction may require a partial hemimandibulectomy [15]. Once the splint is in place,

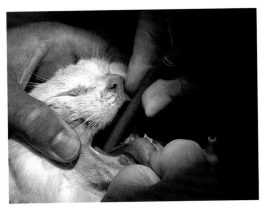

Fig. 16. The patient is intubated as soon as the mouth can be opened. The rest of the splint is removed once the endotracheal tube is in place and the patient is stable.

monitoring and postoperative care are the same as when dealing with unilateral fractures.

Mandibular ramus fracture

These fractures represent a small percentage of overall facial fractures [12,16]. They usually do not result in any displacement and are commonly managed conservatively using a tape muzzle and soft food for 2 to 4 weeks [17]. Avoiding hard food and hard objects for 8 weeks is also strongly recommended. If the coronoid fragment is preventing opening or closing of the jaw, it is surgically removed.

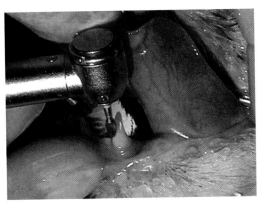

Fig. 17. The remaining pieces of composite are gently polished away using a finishing burr or a Roto-pro burr (Ellman International Inc., Oceanside, New York).

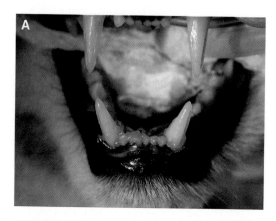

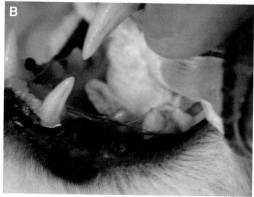

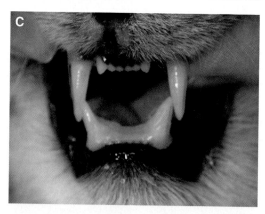

Fig. 18. (*A, B*) Placement of interdental wires to stabilize fracture fragments. Note that the blue gel on the teeth is phosphoric acid to etch the crown before applying the composite. (*C*) The composite splint is applied to the lingual surfaces of the mandibular teeth to minimize interference with proper occlusion.

Mandibular condylar or condylar neck fracture

Although more common than a mandibular ramus fracture, a mandibular condylar or condylar neck fracture is still a rare presentation [12,16]. Because it rarely results in malocclusion, conservative treatment is preferred. Mandibular condylar fractures may occur in conjunction with other fractures. The other fractures are stabilized, and the condylar damage is left untreated. Stabilization of the body of the mandible and restricted motion allow this fracture to heal on its own. Temporomandibular joint (TMJ) ankylosis is a rare sequela [18]. It is dealt with several weeks after the trauma when the patient is presented unable to open its mouth. Treatment of ankylosis consists of a condylectomy on the affected side [18]. Prednisone is administered after surgery to prevent fibrous adhesion at the condylectomy site [18]. Multiple small daily meals for several days after surgery encourage motion of the joint and prevent recurrence of ankylosis [18]. A unilateral condylectomy allows contralateral joint and muscles to adapt and prevents the formation of a malocclusion [18]. Continuation of TMJ pain and chronic crepitus may be signs of incomplete removal of the condyloid process [18].

Maxillary fracture

Maxilla fractures are rare, forming less than 2% of all fractures [19]. A large percentage of the time, fractures are present but the maxilla is not displaced. Some of these fractures may remain undetected. Displaced maxillary fractures are of more concern because they result in malocclusion. Because of its box shape, the maxilla breaks at more than one spot. An important sign of maxillary fracture is epistaxis. In severe cases, there may be gross facial deformity, oronasal communication, instability, malocclusion, and obstruction of the nasal passages (Fig. 19) [10]. It is wise to delay repair to allow stabilization of the patient, decreased swelling, and visualization of the demarcation between healthy and necrotic tissues [19]. The few days before surgery are best managed by applying a tape muzzle to support the nose (Fig. 20). The bones of the maxilla are thin except where teeth are anchored. This situation makes interosseous fixation difficult. It is best is to align the teeth, suture closed the soft tissue defects, and use composite resin interdental splints to stabilize the fractures. On the maxilla, composite splints are applied on the buccal surface of teeth to minimize interference with proper occlusion (Fig. 21) [10]. In cases, in which the maxilla is extremely mobile, the maxillary canine teeth, already included in the splint, can be bonded to the mandibular canine teeth (Fig. 22). This has two effects: it reinforces the stabilization of the fractured fragments, and it keeps the canine teeth properly occluded to each other while the maxilla is healing. The canine teeth are allowed to overlap by 1 or 2 mm so that the mouth is open wide enough to allow the patient to ingest a soft diet. The

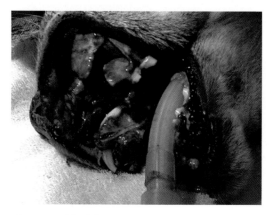

Fig. 19. Maxillary fracture with deformation, obstruction of nasal passages, mobility of fragments, and loss of occlusion.

composite resin is applied circumferentially around the canine teeth, creating two posts. If one canine is missing, a section of a syringe or a syringe casing is slipped over the remaining canine and the tube is filled with composite resin (Fig. 23). Another way to replace the missing tooth is to insert a wire in the maxillary gingiva above both canines or through the remaining tooth root of the broken canine. The wires are then inserted subgingivally on the buccal surfaces of the mandibular canine teeth to exit through one central hole below the chin (Fig. 24). This technique offers two further advantages: it prevents the patient from opening its mouth and trying to pull out the composite splint, and it serves as a guide for proper alignment of the canine teeth. As always, the splint is examined for the presence of spurs and overhangs. Monitoring consists of keeping the patient indoors and cleaning

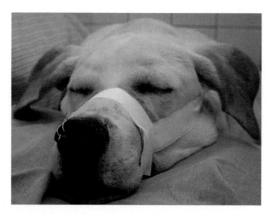

Fig. 20. Dog with multiple facial fractures and obvious mobility being supported with a tape muzzle while awaiting surgery.

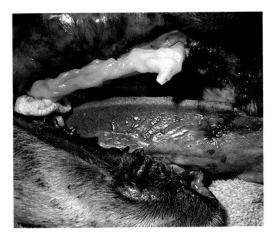

Fig. 21. Maxillary composite splint bonded to the buccal surfaces of the teeth so as not to interfere with occlusion.

the oral cavity daily to prevent buildup of food and inflammation of the oral mucosa. The splint is removed 6 to 8 weeks after surgery.

Maxillary and mandibular fracture

Because of its structure, it is easier to fix the mandible first, with wire and a composite resin splint. One then aligns the maxilla to the mandible and bonds the maxillary canines to the mandibular canines using composite resin (Fig. 25). This allows healing of both jaws in functional occlusion [20,21]. These animals have usually sustained severe trauma and often have trouble breathing properly because of damage to the nasal structures. Once their mouth is fixed in a semiopen position, it is difficult for them to eat. Nutritional support and the placement of an esophageal or a gastrotomy tube at the time of the repair are highly recommended (Fig. 26).

Edentulous patient

Intraoral composite resin splints work well to stabilize maxillofacial fractures. Their advantage is that they are bonded to teeth, negating the need to expose, drill, and fix the bones. When the patient is edentulous or nearly so, there is no surface onto which the splint can be bonded. The same type of repair can still be performed; the soft tissues defects are first sutured closed, and the bones are then manipulated in place. Before laying composite resin on top of the jaw, wires are introduced around the mesial and distal fragments. The wires are introduced through the ventral skin. They are pushed dorsally on the buccal surface of the damaged mandible, looped inside the mouth, and driven back ventrally on the lingual surface of the

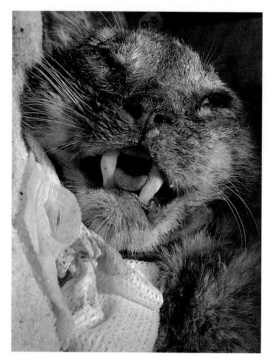

Fig. 22. The maxillary splint and the maxillary canine teeth are bonded to the mandibular canine teeth to stabilize the fractures better.

mandible to exit through the same hole. A ribbon of composite is then laid inside the mouth on top of the mandible. While the composite is setting, the ends of the wires are twisted and the loops are tightened on top of the ribbon of composite. More composite is laid down to cover the wires (Fig. 27).

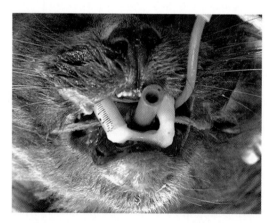

Fig. 23. The missing canine tooth is replaced by a post fabricated from a cut section of a 3-mL syringe. The tube is slipped over the remaining canine and filled with composite.

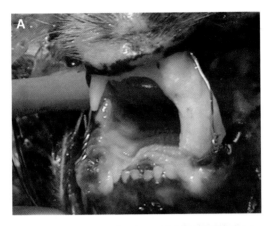

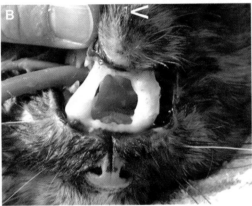

Fig. 24. A wire is threaded where the canine is missing. (*A, B*) Wire is placed on both sides of the maxilla and run along the buccal surfaces of the canine teeth to exit through one hole below the chin (*arrow in B*).

Those cerclage wires simply attach the splint to the jaw [22,23]. As before, the edges of the splint are palpated to make sure that they are smooth. Spurs and overhangs are removed. The patient is released on a soft diet and a mouthwash to keep the splint and the oral cavity clean. The splint is removed 8 to 10 weeks later. The longer period allows for slower healing in older patients.

Complications

Any type of maxillofacial fracture can be subject to the following complications. Some complications are attributable to the patient rather than to the fracture. For example, juvenile patients are more difficult to treat because they have unerupted adult teeth that are often in the line of fracture (Fig. 28) [24]. Dental buds are soft and easily destroyed. Another problem

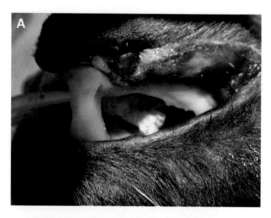

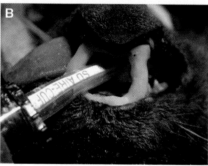

Fig. 25. The maxilla and mandible were fractured. After stabilization, they were bonded together to ensure that they would heal in functional occlusion. (*A, B*) Two views of the splint are shown.

that juvenile patients present the operator with is the fact that they are still growing. If the growth plates are damaged, the affected jaw heals but starts to deviate toward the injured side. The full extent of the deviation and the resulting malocclusion is not obvious until the patient is fully grown. Surgical or orthodontic work may be necessary months after the original insult to re-establish functional occlusion.

Geriatric patients present a separate set of possible complications; they heal slower, their bones are more brittle, they are often missing some teeth, and the teeth that are left may be suffering from advanced periodontal disease [24]. Periodontal disease means that teeth may have to be removed rather than serve as anchors for splints. They suffer from pathologic fractures secondary to neoplasms or severe periodontitis.

Patients also may present with concurrent injuries, such as shock, central nervous system (CNS) damage, airway trauma, other orthopedic injuries, nasal trauma, or an oronasal fistula [24,25]. The injuries may delay surgical repair to the point where fibrous adhesions have to be broken before proceeding with stabilization. The patient may also present with concurrent

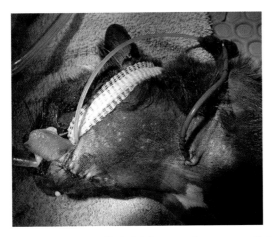

Fig. 26. This patient sustained 18 maxillofacial fractures. Its nose was flattened, and it was mouth breathing; thus, an esophageal feeding tube was placed for nutrition for the first few days.

illnesses, including diabetes, renal failure, heart disease, and other chronic internal disease. The concurrent problems may force the operator to choose repair methods that are quicker to perform rather than better for the patient.

Some complications are associated with the repair technique. For example, the use of a tape muzzle as the sole method of repair predisposes the patient to malunion or nonunion.

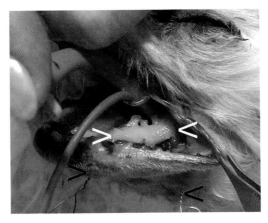

Fig. 27. While the splint is setting, the wires, looped over the composite (*white arrows*), are tightened by twisting the ends coming through the skin under the chin (*black arrows*). More composite is added to cover the wires, and the edges of the splint are smoothed out.

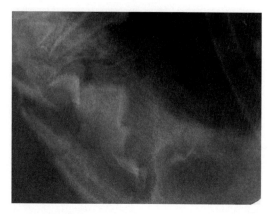

Fig. 28. This mandibular fracture also damaged the unerupted adult tooth. This tooth will probably have to be removed at a later date because of malformation.

Nonunion or delayed union can be repaired by using bone grafting [24,25]. Bone grafting is recommended even if the graft ends up communicating with the oral cavity [24]. Use of implants may lead to implant failure or migration.

An alveolar fracture causes loss of blood supply to the affected tooth. This results in pulpitis and pulp necrosis. Ultimately, the tooth has to be extracted or necessitates postponed endodontic treatment [26]. A follow-up radiograph 6 to 8 weeks after the accident may show a healed jaw with a periapical abscess around the root of the affected tooth (Fig. 29).

In some cases, hemimandibulectomy is chosen as the treatment for complicated, comminuted, or infected fractures. It is an economic radical procedure [24,27], but it causes further complications, such as dehiscence, shifting of the mandible, and drooping of the tongue [27]. The degree of dehiscence dictates the course to follow. If it represents a small section of the suture line, daily cleaning with a topical antiseptic, such as chlorhexidine, allows healing by secondary intention to take place. If a large section of the suture line dehisces, the dental surgeon needs to go back and repair the defect, taking care to eliminate any tension on the flaps sutured. Shifting of the mandible can disappear on its own with time. If not, placement of an incline plane to direct the canine tooth or teeth is possible. Shifting of the mandible and drooping of the tongue can be managed by performing a commissuroplasty and moving the commissure of the lips on the affected side up to the level of the first premolars (Fig. 30).

Of course, any maxillofacial fracture has to be considered to be infected; thus, antibiotic coverage is always a must. Complications from the infection include osteomyelitis and bony sequestra.

Discussion

Maxilla and mandible fractures do present the clinician with specific challenges: there is minimal soft tissue coverage, there are a lot of

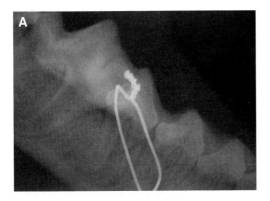

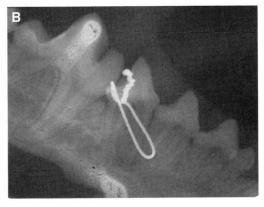

Fig. 29. (*A*) Fracture runs through the fourth premolar. The tooth is left in because it is serving as an anchor for stabilization of the fracture. (*B*) Same area 8 weeks after surgery; there is a good callus present, but there is also a periapical lucency around the mesial root of the fourth premolar that now has to be addressed.

neurovascular bundles in the area, and teeth are in the way of standard fixation techniques. Proponents of external fixators, pins, screws, and plates often do not even evaluate dental damage in their research [28]. Some even prefer to extract healthy teeth once healing has occurred rather than try to maintain occlusion during the repair process [29]. They also perform mandibular symphyseal realignment to re-establish functional occlusion rather than trying to re-establish occlusion during repair [29]. Using pins, plates, or screws not only causes damage to roots but results in bone resorption secondary to heat damage when pins are drilled in or secondary to stress protection as seen with plates [1,30]. The only argument for using plates and pins is that they provide the rigidity necessary for healing [3]. This is true, but the jaws do not bear weight and the amount of rigidity required is a lot less than in long bones and can be achieved using composite and wires. Plates are expensive and time-consuming [6]. Composite splints are

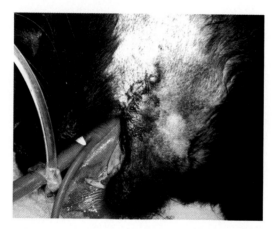

Fig. 30. A commissuroplasty was performed to control mandible deviation and tongue drooping after a hemimandibulectomy.

easier to work with and less expensive [1,11,14]. More importantly, they allow anatomic repositioning. Anatomic repositioning can result in complete periodontal repair [25]. As discussed in the previous sections, almost any type of fracture can be repaired using only wires and composite. Techniques and materials are changing; the time for pins and plates has come and gone. Today, wire and composite offer many advantages. Other things to consider in the future are the use of bone morphogenetic proteins. These compounds can induce new bone formation and may soon replace bone grafts. They can also be implanted directly at fracture sites to stimulate repair [31]. No matter which technique is selected, preservation of functional occlusion remains the prime goal. Bone healing alone is not enough; the patient has to continue to be able to feed itself.

References

[1] Kern DA, Smith MM, Stevenson S, et al. Evaluation of three fixation techniques for repair of mandibular fractures in dogs. J Am Vet Med Assoc 1995;206(12):1883–90.
[2] Maretta SM, Schrader SC, Matthiesen DT. Problems associated with the management and treatment of jaw fractures. In: Maretta SM, editor. Problems in veterinary medicine. Philadelphia: JB Lippincott; 1989. p. 220–47.
[3] Boudrieau RJ, Kudisch M. Miniplate fixation for repair of mandibular and maxillary fractures in 15 dogs and 3 cats. Vet Surg 1996;25(4):277–91.
[4] Verstraete FJM. Maxillofacial fractures. In: Slatter D, editor. Textbook of small animal surgery. 3rd edition. Philadelphia: WB Saunders; 1998. p. 2190–207.
[5] Nap RC, Meij BP, Hazewinkel HA. Mandibular and maxillary fractures in dogs and cats. Tijdschr Diergeneeskd 1994;119(16):456–62.
[6] Smith MM. Interdental wire and acrylic for oral fracture repair. In: Proceedings of the 13th Annual Veterinary Dental Forum. Nashville (TN): Annual Veterinary Dental Forum; 1999. p. 187–90.

[7] Maretta SM. Maxillofacial surgery. Vet Clin N Am Small Anim Pract 1998;28(5): 1285–96.

[8] O'Morrow C. Maxillary fracture fixation using interdental wire, and condylar neck fracture fixation using dental acrylic splinting. In: Proceedings of the 15th Annual Veterinary Dental Forum. Nashville (TN): Annual Veterinary Dental Forum; 2001. p. 140–1.

[9] Lyon KF. Treatment of a complicated mandibular fracture in a dog. In: Proceedings of the 14th Annual Veterinary Dental Forum. Nashville (TN): Annual Veterinary Dental Forum; 2000. p. 204.

[10] Legendre LFJ. Intraoral acrylic splints for maxillofacial fracture repair. J Vet Dent 2003; 20(2):70–8.

[11] Legendre LFJ. Use of maxillary and mandibular splints for restoration of normal occlusion following jaw trauma in a cat: a case report. J Vet Dent 1998;15(4):179–81.

[12] Umphlet RC, Johnson AL. Mandibular fractures in the dog: a retrospective study of 153 cases. Vet Surg 1990;19(4):272–5.

[13] Salisbury SK, Cantwell HD. Conservative management of fractures of the mandibular condyloid process in three cats and one dog. J Am Vet Med Assoc 1989;194(1):85–7.

[14] Bennett JW, Kapatkin AS, Manfra Maretta S. Dental composite for the fixation of mandibular fractures and luxations in 11 cats and 6 dogs. Vet Surg 1994;23(3):190–4.

[15] Orsini PG. Bilateral mandibular fracture in a 4 year old dog. In: Proceedings of the 11th Annual Veterinary Dental Forum. Nashville (TN): Annual Veterinary Dental Forum; 1997. p. 253.

[16] Weigel JP. Trauma of oral structures. In: Harvey CE, editor. Veterinary dentistry. Philadelphia: WB Saunders; 1985. p. 140–55.

[17] Harvey CE, Emily P. Oral surgery. In: Small animal dentistry. Philadelphia: Mosby; 1993. p. 312–77.

[18] Anderson MA, Orsini PG, Harvey CE. Temporomandibular ankylosis: treatment by unilateral condylectomy in two dogs and two cats. J Vet Dent 1996;13(1):23–5.

[19] Brown TR. Surgical repair of bilateral maxillary fracture and traumatic cleft palate in a dog. In: Proceedings of the 17th Annual Veterinary Dental Forum. Nashville (TN): Annual Veterinary Dental Forum; 2003. p. 257–9.

[20] Dumais Y. Stabilization of multiple fractures of the jaw of a cat. In: Proceedings of the 11th Annual Veterinary Dental Forum. Nashville (TN): Annual Veterinary Dental Forum; 1997. p. 264–5.

[21] Legendre LFJ. Bonding maxillary to mandibular canine teeth to repair jaw fractures in 4 cats. In: Proceedings of the 13th Annual Veterinary Dental Forum. Nashville (TN): Annual Veterinary Dental Forum; 1999. p. 156–7.

[22] Legendre LFJ. Non invasive techniques for maxillofacial fracture repairs. In: Proceedings of the 18th Annual Veterinary Dental Forum. Nashville (TN): Annual Veterinary Dental Forum; 2004.

[23] Hale FA. Management of a bilateral, pathologic, mandibular fracture in a dog. J Vet Dent 2002;19(1):22–4.

[24] Maretta SM. Maxillofacial fracture complications. In: Proceedings of the 17th Annual Veterinary Dental Forum. Nashville (TN): Annual Veterinary Dental Forum; 2003. p. 85–7.

[25] Smith MM. Complications associated with oral fracture repair. In: Proceedings of the 13th Annual Veterinary Dental Forum. Nashville (TN): Annual Veterinary Dental Forum; 1999. p. 104–7.

[26] Colmery B III. Orthopedic repair of oral cavity. In: Proceedings of the 13th Annual Veterinary Dental Forum. Nashville (TN): Annual Veterinary Dental Forum; 1999. p. 198–200.

[27] Lantz GC, Salisbury SK. Partial mandibulectomy for treatment of mandibular fractures in dogs: eight cases (1981–1984). J Am Vet Med Assoc 1987;191(2):243–5.

[28] Davidson JR, Bauer MS. Fractures of the mandible and maxilla. Vet Clin N Am Small Anim Pract 1992;22(1):109–19.

[29] Buchet M, Boudrieau RJ. Correction of malocclusion secondary to maxillary impaction fractures using a mandibular symphyseal realignment in eight cats. J Am Anim Hosp Assoc 1999;35(1):68–76.

[30] Eberhard TL. Mandibular fracture repair in a dog using a full splint external fixation device. In: Proceedings of the 12th Annual Veterinary Dental Forum. Nashville (TN): Annual Veterinary Dental Forum; 1998. p. 169–73.

[31] Kirker-Head CA. Potential applications and delivery strategies for bone morphogenetic proteins. Adv Drug Deliv Rev 2000;43(1):65–92.

ELSEVIER
SAUNDERS

Vet Clin Small Anim
35 (2005) 1009–1039

VETERINARY
CLINICS
Small Animal Practice

Mandibulectomy and Maxillectomy

Frank J.M. Verstraete, DrMedVet, MMedVet

*Department of Surgical and Radiological Sciences, School of Veterinary Medicine,
University of California, 2112 Tupper Hall, Davis, CA 95616, USA*

Malignant neoplasms of the oral cavity represent approximately 6% of all canine tumors [1], and the incidence is lower in cats [2]. A variety of neoplastic lesions occur, including odontogenic and nonodontogenic tumor types. Nonneoplastic masses, such as gingival hyperplasia and infectious conditions, may be confused with oral tumors. Conversely, oral neoplasms may present as nonhealing ulcerated lesions instead of "typical" prominent masses.

Oral tumors frequently go unnoticed by the animal's owner until the tumor reaches an advanced stage of development; it is therefore important to make an accurate assessment of the nature and extent of the condition at the first time of presentation [3]. The expected biologic behavior of an oral tumor depends on the species in which it occurs, the location in the oral cavity, the clinical stage, and the histopathologic nature of the tumor. Understanding the biologic behavior enables the clinician to select the method of treatment indicated and to inform the client correctly. For malignant oral tumors and benign but locally invasive lesions, surgical treatment by means of one of the mandibulectomy or maxillectomy techniques is most commonly indicated. Mandibulectomy and maxillectomy may also be indicated as salvage procedures for certain types of mandibular and maxillary fractures, and maxillectomy for oronasal fistula repair, but these applications are not discussed here [4–6].

Clinical staging

An accurate assessment requires a systematic approach and is achieved by using the "tumor node metastasis" (TNM) system [7,8]. The TNM system requires that the clinician sequentially evaluate the tumor, the regional lymph node, and any possible distant metastases.

E-mail address: fjverstraete@ucdavis.edu

First, the tumor is carefully inspected and palpated. The size and site of the tumor, the presence of any ulceration or necrosis, and any abnormal mobility of the teeth are important findings and should be recorded. Fixation of the tumor to underlying tissues suggests bone infiltration; this possibility should be further investigated radiologically. Second, the regional lymph nodes are palpated to evaluate their size, shape, consistency, and fixation to underlying tissues. Irregular enlargement and, especially, lack of mobility are highly suggestive of lymph node involvement. Finally, the patient is thoroughly examined by means of inspection, palpation, auscultation, thoracic radiographs, and abdominal ultrasound to detect any signs of distant metastasis.

Clinical staging enables the clinician to estimate the extent of the disease. The assessment should be complemented by obtaining a biopsy to determine the histopathologic nature of the lesion.

Diagnostic imaging of oral tumors

Radiography forms an integral part of assessing the tumor characteristics, particularly the extent of the tumor and the presence of bone involvement. Intraoral dental radiographs and extraoral skull radiographs are generally indicated in cases of suspected oral neoplasia. Other advanced diagnostic imaging techniques may be indicated in selected cases [6]. Tumors located in the maxilla often necessitate CT to visualize the intranasal or periorbital extent of the tumor. CT is also indicated with caudal mandibular lesions [9]. MRI and ultrasound can be useful for visualizing tumors with deep soft tissue infiltration and for lymph nodes.

The radiologic findings associated with oral tumors are often subtle and nonspecific. Careful and systematic evaluation of radiographs using specific radiologic descriptors may make it possible to associate different patterns with certain tumor types or may suggest a benign or malignant (aggressive) lesion [10–12]. Nevertheless, it cannot be overemphasized that the type of tumor usually cannot be determined radiologically and that a biopsy is always required. Equally important is to match the radiologic findings with the clinical features and location of the tumor and, after biopsy, with the histopathologic findings.

Bone involvement may be evidenced by varying degrees of bone resorption or new bone formation. It is generally accepted that bone lysis only becomes evident radiographically when more than 40% of the cortical bone has been demineralized; therefore, radiographs usually underestimate the extent of the tumor [1]. The presence of bone lysis is an indication of advanced bone infiltration, however, which influences the therapeutic plan. Good diagnostic imaging is especially important in correctly planning a mandibulectomy or maxillectomy.

Biopsy

The precise nature of an oral tumor is determined by the histopathologic examination of a biopsy; this is the mainstay of oncologic decision making [13]. Obtaining a biopsy is indicated for all oral masses and for any suspicious lesion. Various techniques are available. Fine-needle aspiration of oral and maxillofacial soft tissue lesions has been found to be valuable in human beings [14]. An incisional biopsy using a disposable biopsy punch is commonly performed in veterinary medicine (Fig. 1). For a particularly hard or bony tumor, a Michell trephine or Yamshidi needle is indicated. It is important to ensure that a representative specimen is obtained. Macroscopically normal tissue on the margin of the tumor should not necessarily be included in an incisional biopsy because this may violate previously unopened tissue planes, but it may also demonstrate the degree of tumor invasiveness [15]. The site of the biopsy should be chosen such that it falls within the boundaries of the tissue to be excised once the diagnosis is made

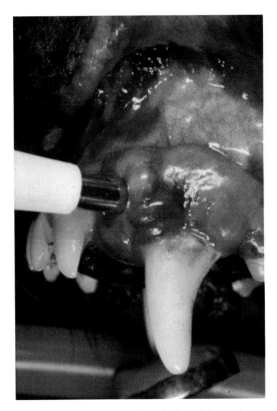

Fig. 1. Biopsy of a suspected oral tumor on the gingiva of the canine tooth is taken, using a disposable biopsy punch (*From* Verstraete FJM. Behandeling van orale tumoren bij de hond. Vlaams Diergeneesk Tijdschr 1993;62:145; with permission.)

[6,15]. In selected cases of small tumors on the gingival margin, an excisional biopsy may be indicated, where the tumor can easily be excised in toto.

Fine-needle aspiration of regional lymph nodes is routinely indicated and has been found to have a high sensitivity and specificity, contrary to palpation [6,16]. Excisional biopsy of any involved nodes is indicated, but their removal is unlikely to influence the outcome [17,18]. Excision of the ipsilateral parotid, mandibular, and medial retropharyngeal lymph nodes is invasive but provides a definitive assessment of regional lymph node metastasis [19–21].

A biopsy must be obtained as atraumatically as possible to minimize the exfoliation of neoplastic cells [15]. Although it has been shown that an incisional biopsy of oral squamous cell carcinoma in human beings results in neoplastic cells entering the bloodstream, a properly obtained biopsy is unlikely to enhance the occurrence of metastasis [13,22]. The biopsy should be adequately fixed and submitted to a pathologist with experience in oral pathology. The result of the histopathologic examination should be compatible with the clinical findings; if not, the matter should be discussed with the pathologist. If any doubt remains, an additional biopsy may be indicated. The biopsy result allows the clinician to select the most appropriate method of treatment scientifically.

Clinical presentation and biologic behavior of common oral nonodontogenic tumor types

Malignant melanoma

Malignant melanoma accounts for approximately 30% to 40% of malignant oral tumors and has been found to occur more commonly in old, male, and relatively small dogs [1]. Malignant melanoma is rare in the cat but seems to carry a grave prognosis in this species [23]. Oral melanoma has a site predilection for the buccal mucosa [1]. When it occurs on the gingiva, palate, or alveolar mucosa, bone involvement is variable and the radiologic features are atypical. Metastasis to the regional lymph nodes, lungs, and other organs takes place at an early stage, which accounts for the poor prognosis; the 1-year survival rate is on the order of 25%. The survival rate is negatively affected by the size and clinical stage of the tumor [1,24].

Melanomata may macroscopically and microscopically present as pigmented or unpigmented (not containing melanin). The absence of melanin may make the histopathologic diagnosis more difficult but has not been found to affect the prognosis [25].

Squamous cell carcinoma

Squamous cell carcinoma is diagnosed in 20% to 30% of oral tumors in the dog but is more common in the cat (61%–70% of oral tumors) [1,2].

There is no sex predilection in the dog, but older large-breed dogs are more commonly affected. Squamous cell carcinoma most often originates on the gingiva, especially on the rostral mandible, and infiltrates deeply. Bone invasion is usually evident on radiographs [26]. In the cat, the extent of bone involvement is often much greater than was anticipated from the clinical appearance of the lesion [27]. In the dog, regional lymph node and distant metastasis is rare, except for tonsillar and lingual squamous cell carcinomas. In the cat, regional lymph node metastasis is common but pulmonary metastasis occurs infrequently [27].

Papillary squamous cell carcinoma is a variant occasionally seen in young dogs (2–9 months of age) [28]. Metastasis does not seem to occur, and the prognosis after complete surgical excision is good.

Fibrosarcoma

Fibrosarcoma is less common in dogs (10%–20%), but it is the second most common oral tumor type in the cat (13%–17%) [1,2]. A predilection has been identified for large, male, and old dogs, although the average age is lower than that found in patients with squamous cell carcinoma or malignant melanoma. The palate is often involved, and this tumor is radiologically characterized by extensive bone resorption [26]. The regional lymph nodes are rarely involved, but lung metastasis occurs occasionally [1].

A common variant of this tumor type is histologically low-grade and biologically high-grade fibrosarcoma, which has been described in large-breed dogs (mostly Golden Retrievers) [29]. Clinically, this tumor presents as a rapidly enlarging swelling of the jaw covered by intact epithelium, contrary to the typical oral fibrosarcoma. The histopathologic findings are suggestive of a fibroma or a well-differentiated fibrosarcoma, which is in contrast to the tumor's rapid growth, invasion, and metastatic potential.

Osteosarcoma

Osteosarcoma of the mandible or maxilla presenting as an oral tumor is probably the fourth most common nonodontogenic tumor of the oral cavity in dogs, although reported incidences vary. Medium and large-sized breeds, middle-aged to older dogs, and female dogs seem to be more commonly affected [30–32]. Osteosarcoma of the jaw in the cat is much less common, only accounting for 2.4% of oral tumors [2]. The radiologic picture is usually atypical.

It has been suggested that the rate of metastasis of jaw osteosarcoma is lower than that of appendicular osteosarcoma [30]. In a recent study of mandibular osteosarcoma in dogs, it was found that the overall 1-year survival rate was 59% [33]. Dogs treated with surgery alone had a 1-year survival rate of 71%, which is higher than the 1-year survival rate for dogs with appendicular osteosarcoma.

Clinical presentation and biologic behavior of common odontogenic tumor types

Odontogenic tumors are generally considered to be rare in all species [34,35]. Precise epidemiologic data are not available for the dog and cat, however. One of the main reasons for this is the continuing confusion regarding the true nature of some of these lesions. In many surveys, the so-called "epulides," which are localized swellings on the gingival margin and which constitute a variety of pathologic entities, are either grouped together or excluded. Recent findings indicate that many epulides are odontogenic tumors [36,37]. Another reason is the fact that many clinicians do not routinely submit epulides for histopathologic examination, thereby introducing bias in the studies based on archival material [37].

Ameloblastoma

The central or intraosseous ameloblastoma is one of the most common odontogenic tumors, occasionally incorrectly referred to as adamantinoma. This tumor usually presents as a locally invasive neoplasm with osteolysis around the tooth roots and cystic changes [26]. Metastasis has not been described in dogs and cats.

The canine acanthomatous ameloblastoma is a benign odontogenic tumor with the same histologic characteristics as the centrally located ameloblastoma but appearing in the gingiva and mucosa of the tooth-bearing area of the jaws [37,38]. In one review of canine epulides, most lesions, which were originally classified as acanthomatous epulis, were found to be canine acanthomatous ameloblastoma [37]. Infiltration in the underlying bone is evident in most cases. The radiologic picture of canine acanthomatous ameloblastoma is dominated by discrete infiltration, alveolar bone resorption, and tooth displacement. Local recurrence is common after marginal excision, and wide or radical excision is therefore recommended [39].

Peripheral odontogenic fibroma

A large proportion of tumors previously described as fibromatous and ossifying epulides are peripheral odontogenic fibromas [37,40]. This is a slow-growing benign neoplasm characterized by the proliferation of fibrous tissue in which isolated islands or strands of odontogenic epithelium are present. A variety of bone, osteoid, dentinoid, or even cementum-like material may be found on histologic examination, and the radiologic features vary according to the presence and amount of these mineralized products. Peripheral odontogenic fibroma does not recur if adequately excised.

Odontoma

An odontoma is a tumor in which the epithelial and mesenchymal cells are well-differentiated, resulting in the formation of all dental tissue types [34]. An odontoma may also be considered a hamartoma rather than a well-differentiated neoplasm. The dental tissues may or may not exhibit a normal relation to each another. An odontoma in which tooth-like structures are present indicates advanced cellular differentiation and is referred to as a compound odontoma. Conversely, an odontoma in which the conglomerate of dental tissues bears no resemblance to a tooth is called a complex odontoma [34]. Odontomas have been diagnosed in young dogs and in the cat [34,35,41]. The radiologic appearance is typical and is a sharply defined mass of calcified material surrounded by a narrow radiolucent band or a variable number of tooth-like structures.

Feline inductive odontogenic tumor

This tumor type was originally described in young cats as inductive fibroameloblastoma [42]. The rostral maxilla is the most common site of occurrence. The tumor may be locally invasive, but metastasis has not been recorded.

Decision making

The choice of treatment is determined by the clinical stage and histopathologic nature of the tumor. A team approach to decision making involving a veterinary dentist, surgeon, medical oncologist, and radiation oncologist is ideal. Surgical excision remains the most frequently indicated and practical method of treatment. If surgical excision is impossible or not elected by the client, there remains the option of radiation treatment for radiosensitive and radiocurative tumors like squamous cell carcinoma. The necessary equipment is not readily available to most practitioners, however. In selected cases, preoperative radiation treatment may be indicated to reduce the size of the tumor. Postoperative radiation treatment should be anticipated if the size or location of the tumor makes it unlikely to achieve tumor-free margins.

Treatment options and associated expectations with regard to prognosis, possible complications, and postoperative appearance and function should be clearly discussed with the client.

Surgical principles

When contemplating surgical treatment, it is important to have a clear understanding of the procedure's objective [15,43]. In most cases, the surgical goal is to cure the patient; this is achieved by adequate excision, tumor-free margins, and the absence of metastatic disease. If the extent of the disease makes this impossible, palliative surgery can be performed. The objective of palliative surgery is not to cure the patient but to improve the quality of life and, if fortunate, achieve local control. A good example of this approach is the treatment of malignant melanoma. This tumor is known to spread at an early stage, but good local control can be achieved by wide excision of the primary tumor. Debulking is a third surgical objective; this entails removing most of the tumor before the application of other therapeutic modalities, such as radiation treatment.

Surgical excisions can be classified according to the width of the surgical margins [15,43,44]. Surrounding the tumor are a pseudocapsule and a reactive zone; the former is a macroscopically visible membrane consisting of normal and neoplastic cells, whereas the latter consists mainly of inflammatory cells. An intracapsular excision involves removing the tumor from within its pseudocapsule or the piecemeal removal of neoplastic tissue. This is rarely indicated but may be acceptable for a well-differentiated odontoma that can be curetted out of the jaw bone. A marginal excision involves a dissection plane located in the reactive zone around the tumor and its pseudocapsule. This type of excision is indicated for well-differentiated benign tumor types. Most of the odontogenic tumors fall into this category; the peripheral odontogenic fibroma is a good example [6]. Nonneoplastic growths, such as focal fibrous hyperplasia, can also be excised in this manner. Marginal excision is not indicated for malignant tumor types that are known to be infiltrative, however; not all the neoplastic tissue can be removed, and this almost invariably results in local tumor regrowth. These tumor types require at least wide excision [6]. This involves the en bloc removal of the tumor, pseudocapsule, reactive zone, and a wide margin of normal tissue. The macroscopically visible width of the surgical margin for oral squamous cell carcinoma in human beings has been extensively studied and is generally considered to be 10 mm [45,46]. The same guideline has been adopted in the veterinary literature, although specific studies are lacking [6,47]. For tumor types that are known to be relatively less invasive, a narrower margin can be used, whereas for tumor types that are known to be highly infiltrative, such as fibrosarcoma, a wider margin is indicated. These wide margins are achieved by performing a partial maxillectomy or mandibulectomy; these procedures are indicated for relatively small to medium-sized malignant tumors with or without bone infiltration.

A radical resection involves excision of the tumor together with its supporting tissue compartment (eg, a total mandibulectomy). This approach is appropriate and necessary for malignant tumors with considerable infiltration. This category includes most malignant nonodontogenic tumor types, such as squamous cell carcinoma and fibrosarcoma, that involve a major part of the jaw. The canine acanthomatous ameloblastoma can also be successfully managed using wide excision or radical resection, depending on tumor size and localization.

After a mandibulectomy or maxillectomy, the margins of the excised tissue should be examined for the completeness of the excision and the presence of neoplastic cells [48]. The borders of the specimen can be identified by means of sutures. The different margins of the specimen should preferably be marked with different dyes (Davidson Marking System; Bradley Products, Bloomington, MN) to enable accurate orientation.

Preoperative considerations

Prophylactic use of antibiotics

Wound healing in the oral cavity generally is rapid and uncomplicated because of the excellent blood supply. Hence, infectious complications are uncommon. Delayed wound healing and a higher incidence of wound infection should be anticipated in the presence of systemic diseases, after long-standing corticosteroid treatment, in animals undergoing chemotherapy, and if the surgical site has previously been irradiated.

Surgical technique plays an important role in preventing infectious complications. Care should be taken not to traumatize the oral soft tissues, including the wound edges and the more deeply situated tissues. Electrocoagulation should be used judiciously. During osteotomy, ostectomy, and osteoplasty, irrigation must be used to prevent thermal necrosis of bone.

Most oral tumor surgery procedures fall in the category of "clean-contaminated" surgical wounds [49]. These procedures are often extensive and traumatic, and most therefore warrant antibiotic prophylaxis. The choice of antibiotic and administration protocol remains controversial in human as well as veterinary oral surgery [49,50]. The principles of correct use of antibiotics apply [49]. A number of studies have shown that ampicillin, amoxicillin-clavulanic acid, certain cephalosporins, and clindamycin meet the requirements in dogs, cats, and people [51–55]. It is generally accepted that antibiotics must be administered within 2 hours before the procedure and not be continued for more than 4 hours after the procedure [49,51].

Anesthetic management

A detailed discussion of the anesthetic management of oral tumor surgery cases is beyond the scope of this article. Because considerable hemorrhage is possible, hemostasis should be assessed by means of the mucosal bleeding test, and further tests may be required [56]. Blood cross-matching is indicated, especially before a maxillectomy [57]. One or more regional nerve blocks are routinely performed to assist in achieving preemptive analgesia, except if the site for administering the block is involved in the tumorous process.

Positioning

Lateral recumbency is preferred by most veterinarians for mandibulectomy and maxillectomy procedures [6]. Lateral recumbency offers good exposure of the buccal surfaces of the uppermost teeth and jaws but only fair visualization of the palate and lingual surfaces of the opposite quadrants. Dorsal recumbency is recommended for a bilateral rostral maxillectomy [6,58]. The author prefers sternal recumbency, with the head elevated and the maxilla suspended between intravenous poles or secured to an anesthesia screen, for mandibulectomy procedures [59]. The main hazard of dorsal and sternal recumbency is fluid aspiration. The use of a cuffed endotracheal tube and pharyngeal pack is necessary to prevent aspiration. Having continuous suction available is helpful. In dorsal recumbency, the neck should be fully extended and the head end of the table slightly lowered.

Aseptic preparation

It is good practice to perform routine periodontal treatment during the anesthetic episode of the clinical staging, diagnostic imaging, and biopsy, especially if there is a large amount of plaque and calculus present [47]. By doing so, a cleaner surgical field and less inflamed gingival tissues are present when performing the major oral tumor surgery. This is also of benefit if radiation treatment is decided on after surgery.

Skin preparation is routine [6,60]. The mouth is rinsed with a suitable antiseptic solution before and during major oral surgery [61,62]. Chlorhexidine gluconate in an aqueous nonalcohol-containing solution is generally regarded to be the antiseptic of choice for the oral cavity in animals, whereas povidone-iodine is most commonly used in human beings [61,63]. Great care should be taken to avoid the eyes [62].

After positioning, draping, and aseptic preparation, the planned surgical margins and incisions are outlined using a sterile surgical skin marker (Secureline surgical skin marker; Precision Dynamics Corp., San Fernando, CA) (Fig. 2).

Mandibulectomy

A mandibulectomy is the en bloc excision of a mandible, or part of one or both mandibles, bearing an oral tumor. When performing a mandibulectomy, the soft tissues and bone are cut on both sides of the tumor without touching the actual tumor; other rules of oncologic surgery are also strictly adhered to [15]. The defect created is closed with soft tissues, and no attempt at reconstruction is generally performed [9,47].

The step-by-step technical details of these procedures are available in the standard surgical texts [6,47,59]. Only the salient features are discussed here.

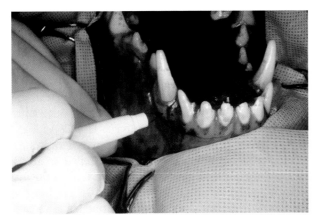

Fig. 2. The planned surgical margins and incisions are outlined using a sterile surgical skin marker.

Classification

Mandibulectomy procedures are classified according to the part of the mandible that is removed. A rim excision, with reference to mandibulectomy, is defined as a partial segmental excision leaving the ventral border of the mandible intact [64]. In a unilateral rostral mandibulectomy, only that part of the bone that carries the three incisors, canine, and first and second premolars is removed. This is indicated for a small tumor not crossing the mandibular symphysis. A bilateral rostral mandibulectomy is more commonly performed; here, the rostral parts of both mandibles are removed after an osteotomy between the second and third premolars. If necessary, the osteotomy can be performed as far caudally as between the fourth premolars and first molars [59]. In a segmental mandibulectomy, part of the body of the mandible is excised. The term *hemimandibulectomy* is often used in the veterinary literature to denote the complete excision of one of the two mandibles. The term *total* or *unilateral mandibulectomy* is therefore more appropriate. Similarly, when referring to the excision of one entire mandible and half of the other mandible, the term *one-and-one-half mandibulectomy* is preferred over *three-quarter mandibulectomy*. In a caudal mandibulectomy, the ramus of the mandible, including the condylar and coronoid processes, are removed.

Rim excision

A rim excision is a partial-thickness excision of the dorsal two thirds of the mandible, leaving the mandibular canal and its contents and the ventral cortex intact. This procedure has the advantage of maintaining the continuity of the mandible. This procedure is only indicated for wide excision of small and minimally invasive tumors on the alveolar margin [64] or for marginal excision of benign lesions, such as a small benign odontogenic tumor [6,57]. After mucoperiosteal incision, the soft tissues are subperiosteally elevated away from the planned ostectomy site. At the level of the attached gingiva, the soft tissue incision has to be narrower than the bony incision to be able to cover the bone tension-free with gingiva on completion of the procedure. The ostectomy is performed in an interdental space or on the mesial or distal line angle of teeth included in the fragment of bone to be removed. A surgical handpiece (INTRAsurge 300; KaVo America Corp., Lake Zurich, IL) designed for major oral surgery (no air insufflation, built-in sterile fluid irrigation) combined with an osteotomy burr (Lindemann burr; Hu-Friedy Mfg., Chicago, IL) are the instruments of choice for performing a precision ostectomy (Fig. 3). Cut bone margins may have to be smoothed using a round burr. The attached gingiva and alveolar mucosa are sutured over the bony defect.

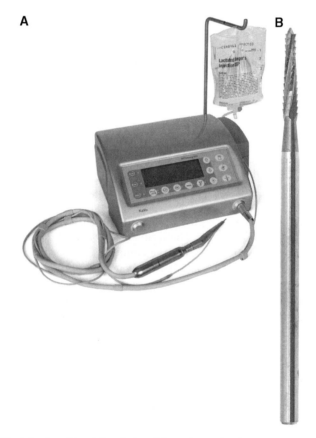

A   B

Fig. 3. (*A*) Dental unit and handpiece designed for major oral surgery (no air insufflation, built-in sterile fluid irrigation) (INTRAsurge 300; KaVo America Corp., Lake Zurich, IL). (*B*) Lindemann osteotomy burr (Lindemann burr; Hu-Friedy Mfg., Chicago, IL).

Unilateral rostral mandibulectomy

This procedure includes the removal of that part of one mandible that carries the incisors, canine, and first and second premolars in the dog; an osteotomy between the canine tooth and the first premolar or between the first and second premolar teeth is not indicated because this would transect the alveolus and root of the canine tooth. In the cat, the osteotomy is made just rostral to the third premolar. This procedure is rarely indicated if one applies the 10-mm surgical margin consistently because of the proximity of the mandibular symphysis.

The soft tissue incisions are determined by the surgical margins. When transecting the lower labial frenulum, the middle mental blood vessels are ligated to minimize blood loss. On the lingual aspect, care is taken to avoid the sublingual caruncle if the surgical margin allows it. The symphysis is split using a thin osteotome and mallet. An osteotomy interproximal at the second and third premolar teeth is preferably performed using an oral surgery handpiece, as described previously. This enables one to transect the ventral third of the mandible carefully, separating the two fragments without severing the inferior alveolar blood vessels; these can then be double-ligated and transected without hemorrhage. Alternatively, and more commonly, an oscillating or reciprocating bone saw is used, which is faster [6,47,59]. The inferior alveolar artery, which is transected during the osteotomy, is retrieved and ligated. The artery is inclined to retract into the mandibular canal; if this occurs, a hemostatic agent can be packed into the mandibular canal [6,47,59]. If necessary, the bone stump is smoothed using a round burr. A limited labial vestibular mucosal-submucosal flap is created by dissecting from the mandibulectomy site toward the lip margin between the submucosa and the skin. This largely prevents the hairy skin from being pulled into the oral cavity when closing the defect. The free edge of the flap is sutured to the attached gingiva at the symphysis in a single-interrupted pattern. Wedge excision of redundant skin is not required.

Bilateral rostral mandibulectomy

In a bilateral rostral mandibulectomy, both mandibles are amputated between the second and third premolars (Fig. 4), similar to the technique described previously. It is possible to go as far caudal as interproximal at the fourth premolar and first molar and still have adequate function and cosmesis [59]. In the latter case, the sublingual and mandibular salivary ducts are ligated. One variation is to taper the ostectomy at the alveolar margin; however, it may be necessary to remove the third premolar to achieve this [6,59]. The ventral margin can also be rounded.

The use of orthopedic implants to stabilize the remaining mandibles after a bilateral rostral mandibulectomy has been described, [65–68], although it is generally accepted that this is unnecessary and therefore rarely performed [6,47,59].

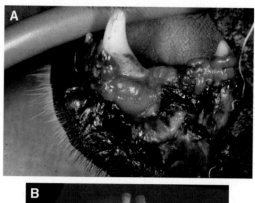

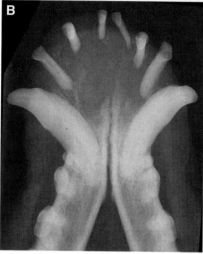

Fig. 4. (*A*) Squamous cell carcinoma of the rostral mandibles in a dog (*From* Verstraete FJM. Behandeling van orale tumoren bij de hond. Vlaams Diergeneesk Tijdschr 1993;62:145; with permission). (*B*) Corresponding radiograph. (*C*) Close-up view; no cheiloplasty was performed in this case. This is an example of surgery for cure. (*D*) Long-term follow-up clinical appearance after a bilateral rostral mandibulectomy; note the slight tongue protrusion.

Two techniques are available for the excision of the redundant skin (cheiloplasty) after a bilateral rostral mandibulectomy, and the choice may be dictated by the location of the tumor. For tumors occurring in the midline and extending facially, a single wedge of skin is excised on the facial aspect; this should preferably be done as part of the originally planned incision but can also be performed after the ostectomy. Alternatively, two wedges of skin may be excised at the level of the lower labial frenula. Wedge excision of skin should be conservative to ensure that tension-free closure is still possible. It is easier to evaluate the symmetry and cosmetic result of the wedge excision and closure when the patient is in sternal recumbency compared with dorsal recumbency. When repositioning the lip on the facial

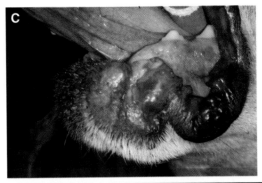

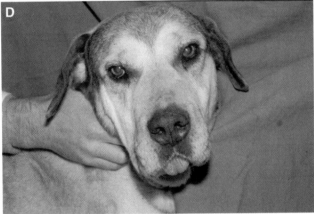

Fig. 4 (*continued*)

aspect, it is important to ensure that the lip margin is higher than the alveolar margin and the oral mucosa between the two mandibles, thereby creating a dam to help prevent drooling [59].

Segmental mandibulectomy

A segmental mandibulectomy involves a full-thickness ostectomy of a part of the body of the mandible caudal to the second premolar. This procedure is indicated for relatively small tumors in that area that are believed not to have infiltrated rostrally or caudally into the mandibular canal or caudally into the ramus of the mandible. An osteotomy and closure are performed as described previously. This procedure results in the devitalization of the teeth in the remaining rostral fragment of the mandible, which may require endodontic treatment.

Malocclusion is common after this type of mandibulectomy. Reconstruction using a free ulnar autograft, a microvascular coccygeal autograft, and a split-rib graft has been described in clinical case reports [69–71] as well as the use of a buttress plate and biodegradable mesh filled with cancellous bone in an experimental mandibular ostectomy model in dogs [72].

Caudal mandibulectomy

A caudal mandibulectomy involves the excision of the ramus of the mandible (including the coronoid, condylar, and angular processes) with or without part of the caudal aspect of the body of the mandible. It is occasionally indicated for relatively small tumors that are believed not to have infiltrated into the mandibular canal.

The standard approach includes a skin incision and osteotomy of the zygomatic arch [6,59]. In the author's experience, this is not always necessary, however, and the procedure can also be performed through an intraoral approach, especially in small patients. The osteotomy is performed as described previously, and the ramus is dissected similar to a total mandibulectomy.

Total unilateral mandibulectomy

This procedure entails removing one mandible and the surrounding soft tissues as dictated by the surgical margins (Fig. 5). It is indicated for relatively large and infiltrative tumors. Although this procedure can be performed through an intraoral approach alone with the patient in sternal recumbency, especially in small patients, it is generally recommended to perform the procedure with the patient in lateral recumbency and to incise the commissure to obtain better exposure of the ramus of the mandible [6,47,59]. After the intraoral incision, the dissection is started on the rostral aspect. The symphysis is split using an osteotome and mallet; this is done early in the procedure because it facilitates further dissection, especially on the lingual aspect of the mandible to be removed. The dissection of the ramus is done by subperiosteally elevating the muscles of mastication on the lateral and medial aspect, provided that the predetermined surgical margins allow this. Subperiosteal elevation is less traumatic and causes less hemorrhage than transection of the muscles. An early goal in the dissection process is to identify the mandibular foramen and ligate the inferior alveolar blood vessels before transection. The temporomandibular joint is located by palpation during manipulation of the mandible, and the lateral ligament and lateral aspect of the joint capsule are incised. As the dissection proceeds caudally on the medial aspect of the condylar process, it is important to remain as close to the bone as possible to avoid the inadvertent transection of the maxillary artery or one of its main branches, which lie in close proximity. Once the joint is disarticulated, the coronoid process is freed of its dorsal attachment to the temporal muscle, which is facilitated by manipulating the bone. The muscles of mastication are apposed with a few single-interrupted tacking sutures. The intraoral closure is routine. If the lip

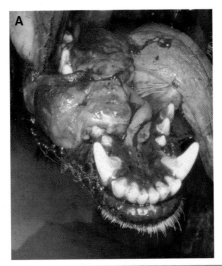

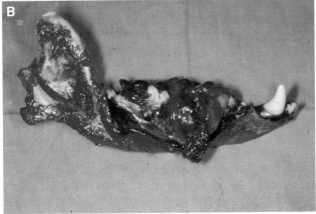

Fig. 5. (A) Malignant melanoma of the body of the mandible in a dog. (B) Mandibulectomy specimen. (C) Immediate follow-up clinical appearance after a total unilateral mandibulectomy; note the slight tongue protrusion, mild drooling, and the fact that no commissurorrhaphy was performed in this case. It was not possible to obtain adequate surgical margins in this case, and this is an example of surgery for palliation.

commissure was incised, a three-layer closure is performed, consisting of mucosa, muscularis, and skin.

A commissurorrhaphy, which is the surgical closure of the lips farther rostrally, is commonly performed at this stage to prevent protrusion of the tongue [6,47,59,66]. A full-thickness tangential excision of the mucocutaneous junctions of the upper and lower lips is performed up to the level of the maxillary first or second premolar, followed by a three-layer closure. This suture line may be subject to excessive extrinsic tension, and a vertical or

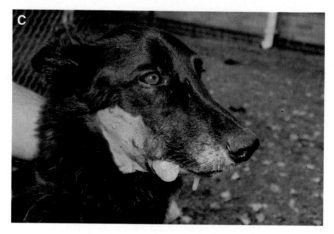

Fig. 5 (*continued*)

horizontal mattress suture tied over buttons on the rostral aspect of the new commissure may be used to prevent dehiscence.

A variation on this procedure is to perform an osteotomy at the level of the rostral edge of the masseter muscle, thereby leaving the most of the ramus behind [59]. This is less traumatic than a total mandibulectomy and may be indicated for tumors that are located relatively rostrally.

Maxillectomy

The term *maxillectomy* refers to the en bloc excision of a tumor on the upper jaw, which may involve parts the incisive, palatine, lacrimal, zygomatic, frontal, and vomer bones in addition to the maxilla proper. The principles of a maxillectomy are the same as for a mandibulectomy. During a maxillectomy, the nasal cavity is entered; this defect is closed using soft tissue flaps, particularly vestibular (ie, alveolar and buccal) mucosal-submucosal flaps with or without palatal mucoperiosteal flaps.

The step-by-step technical details of these procedures are available in standard surgical texts [6,58]. Only the salient features are discussed here.

Classification

The term *premaxillectomy* is often used in the veterinary literature to denote an excision confined to the incisive bone. The term *premaxilla* is not accepted veterinary anatomic nomenclature, however [73]; the term *incisivectomy* is therefore more appropriate. The term *hemimaxillectomy* is equally confusing if used to describe the surgical excision of one maxilla. Removing most of one maxillary bone (typically combined with the excision of all or parts of the incisive and palatine bones) is a complete or total unilateral maxillectomy. Various types of partial maxillectomy can be performed. With a unilateral rostral maxillectomy, the one incisive bone and the most rostral part of the maxillary bone are removed. Similarly, a bilateral rostral maxillectomy can be performed; this procedure can be combined with a nasal planectomy, which is the excision of the soft tissues and cartilages comprising the facial part of the nose [74,75]. A partial maxillectomy involving the midportion of the maxilla is known as a central maxillectomy, and one involving the caudal portion is known as a caudal maxillectomy [76]. A caudal maxillectomy can be combined with an orbitectomy, which entails removal of portions of bones that comprise the orbit, including the maxilla, palatine, zygomatic, lacrimal, and frontal bones [77].

Incisivectomy

This procedure is rarely indicated, given the need for 10-mm surgical margins for most oral tumor types. After the soft tissue incision and exposure of the bone, great care should be taken not to damage the canine teeth when performing an osteotomy on the distal line angle of the third incisors. An oral surgery handpiece with an osteotomy burr or a fine osteotome and mallet can be used for this purpose. Bleeding from the branches of the major palatine arteries at the palatine fissures should be anticipated. The nasal cavity is not entered in this procedure, but the ventrolateral nasal cartilages are exposed.

Surgical closure is achieved by means of a vestibular pedicle flap, created by making two vertical releasing incisions from the corners of the defect into the alveolar and buccal mucosa. The flap is raised to include mucosa and submucosa, advanced over the defect, and sutured to the palatal mucosa.

Unilateral and bilateral rostral maxillectomy

A unilateral rostral maxillectomy entails the removal of the incisive bone and the rostral aspect of the maxilla, generally including the incisors, canine, and first and second premolars in the dog and the incisors and canine in the cat. This procedure is occasionally indicated for small tumors on the buccal aspect of the canine tooth.

A bilateral rostral maxillectomy is more commonly performed (Fig. 6). The soft tissue incisions are made as dictated by the surgical margins and are designed to remove the incisors, canines, and first and second premolars in the dog and the incisors, canines, and second premolar in the cat. When making the palatal incision, the rugae pattern can be followed. Halfway between the midline and the alveolar margins, the major palatine arteries are encountered and must be ligated. The soft tissues are elevated a few millimeters away from the tumor at the planned osteotomy site. The classic oral surgery dictum is that the hard tissue incision should be smaller that the soft tissue incision so that the soft tissue suture line is supported by bone. Whether this is clinically important or influences the dehiscence rate is

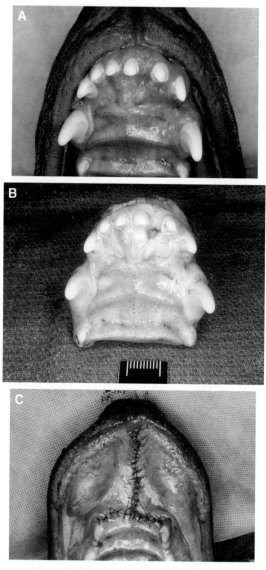

Fig. 6. (A) Histologically low-grade and biologically high-grade fibrosarcoma affecting the incisive bones and rostral maxillas in a dog. (B) Bilateral rostral maxillectomy specimen. (C) T-shaped wound closure. (D) Two-week follow-up clinical appearance; note the mild drooping of the nose.

unknown. The osteotomy can be made to coincide with the soft tissue incision [58]. In fact, even the opposite, namely, making the bony incision wider than the soft tissue incision, to facilitate suture placement has been advocated and has been found to be acceptable [6].

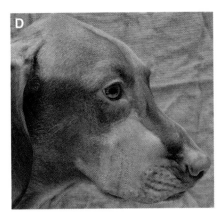

Fig. 6 (*continued*)

The osteotomy is performed as described previously. This results in exposure of the nasal cavity. Care should be taken when performing the palatal and lateral incisions not to cause unnecessary damage to the turbinates. The bony incision into the maxilla from the distal line angle of the second premolar can be angled and rounded to leave the nasal bone intact without transecting the alveolus of the canine tooth, provided that an adequate surgical margin is maintained. This preserves the dorsal attachment of the nasal cartilages and thereby prevents excessive drooping of the nose.

A unilateral or bilateral rostral maxillectomy is closed using a vestibular mucosal-submucosal flap. From the maxillectomy defect, the remaining alveolar mucosa and mainly the mucosa and submucosa of the upper lip are dissected toward the lip margin using Metzenbaum scissors. Sufficient tissue should be obtained to allow tension-free closure. The tissue plane at which the labial flap is dissected should be such that the mucosa, submucosa, and some subcutaneous tissue are included to ensure a flap of sufficient thickness [58]. Vertical releasing incisions may be used but are typically not necessary [6]. After a unilateral rostral maxillectomy, the vestibular flap is moved over the defect and sutured to the palatal mucosa in a single-layer or double-layer closure. With a bilateral rostral maxillectomy, tissues are moved from both sides, resulting in a T-shaped closure. If a two-layer closure is elected, the deep layer can consist of single-interrupted sutures between the deeper layers of the palatal mucosa and vestibular flap, with the knots on the nasal side [6,78]. Alternatively, the deep layer may consist of simple-interrupted sutures placed through holes drilled through the bony hard palate [58]; this may be prudent if wound healing complications are anticipated.

Central, caudal, and total unilateral maxillectomy

The surgical anatomy pertaining to a central maxillectomy and, especially, to a caudal or total unilateral maxillectomy is complicated by the presence of the infraorbital canal and associated neurovascular structures. The anatomy of the orbital aspect of the caudal maxilla is particularly complex. Although the infraorbital artery can easily be ligated at the infraorbital foramen, it is difficult, even with precision osteotomy instruments, to avoid transecting the infraorbital, sphenopalatine, and major palatine arteries when performing a caudal maxillary osteotomy, connecting the lateral maxillary, dorsal maxillary, and palatal osteotomies. The caudal maxillary osteotomy is therefore performed last [6,79].

Closure after a central, caudal, and total unilateral maxillectomy is performed using a vestibular mucosal-submucosal flap and a one-layer or two-layer closure, as described previously (Fig. 7). Tension-free closure of maxillectomy defects that extend beyond the midline of the hard palate is difficult to achieve.

As an alternative to the standard oral approach, a combined extraoral-dorsal and intraoral approach can be used for the resection of large maxillary tumors; this approach has been found to result in a lower recurrence rate, possibly because of the better exposure obtained [79].

Postoperative care

Pain management depends on the magnitude of the surgical procedure. A fentanyl patch applied 12 hours before surgery is routinely indicated [6,59]. This is supplemented with morphine or oxymorphone for the first 12 to 24 hours or longer, if needed [6].

Intravenous fluid therapy is continued until normal oral intake is ensured. Water is offered after 12 hours and soft food after 24 hours [6,47]. Nutritional support by means of an enteral feeding tube should be considered if the animal is not eating and drinking adequately within 3 days, which is unusual [47,58,59]. Soft food should be fed until the surgical wound has healed and the animal has functionally adapted to the absence of part of the jaw. Some hand-feeding may be necessary for the first few days. Patients should be prevented from chewing on sticks and hard chew toys.

Wound healing may be assessed 2 weeks after surgery. The surgical site should be evaluated for tumor recurrence every 3 to 6 months [47].

Outcome, appearance, and function

The success rate and prognosis depend on the tumor type. As a general rule, in the dog, the results obtained for odontogenic tumor types are excellent, good for squamous cell carcinoma, fair for fibrosarcoma and osteosarcoma, and poor for malignant melanoma. Outcome is also correlated with the presence or absence of tumor-free excision margins [32]. Failure occurs as local recurrence (eg, fibrosarcoma) or distant metastasis (eg, malignant melanoma) [1,6]. In the cat, again in general, the

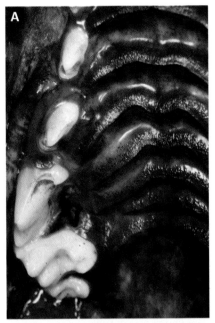

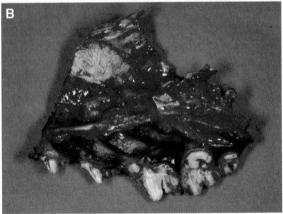

Fig. 7. (A) Osteosarcoma of the palatine process of the maxilla in a dog. (B) Unilateral caudal maxillectomy specimen. (C) Wound closure using a vestibular flap. (D) Two-week follow-up clinical appearance; note the slight facial concavity.

results obtained for malignant nonodontogenic tumors are poor, and cats do not seem to tolerate these procedures as well as dogs [47]. A detailed review of the success rates of the various techniques used on different tumor types and in different locations in dogs and cats with or without adjuvant therapy has recently been published [9].

The cosmetic and functional results of these procedures are surprisingly good (see Figs. 4–7). Some swelling may be present for the first few days

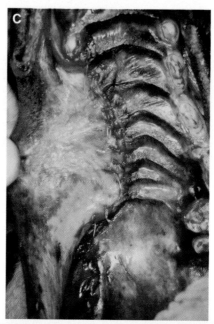

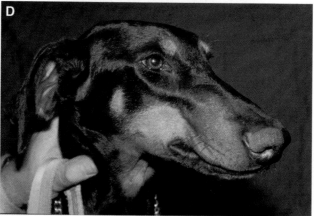

Fig. 7 (*continued*)

after the procedure. With a maxillectomy, subcutaneous emphysema is occasionally seen [6,57]; serohemorrhagic nasal discharge may be present for several days. Swelling and edema of the sublingual tissues may occur after a mandibulectomy [9,57].

The upper lips conceal most mandibulectomy defects when the mouth is closed. When the mouth is opened, the shortened jaws and protruding tongue are evident after a bilateral rostral mandibulectomy (see Fig. 4).

Mandibulectomy procedures resulting in the absence of one mandibular canine tooth cause the tongue to hang out from the affected side. Food prehension is usually temporarily impaired after a major mandibulectomy procedure, but dogs typically adapt well to the mandibular instability. Excessive drooling after a mandibulectomy is common but tends to improve with time (see Fig. 5D) [57]. Drooling after a bilateral rostral mandibulectomy can also be prevented to a certain extent by carefully reconstructing the lower lip in a raised position [59].

After a unilateral rostral maxillectomy, a slight facial concavity and lip elevation may be present. The lip should not be noticeably pulled inward if a large enough tension-free flap was created [58]. A bilateral rostral maxillectomy results in considerable deformity, caused by drooping of the nose (see Fig. 6); this does not seem to affect the breathing through the nostrils, however [58]. Lip elevation and tension on the flaps pulling the lips inward may result in the mandibular canines being lateral to the upper lips, which is not cosmetic [6,58]. A planectomy results in severe disfigurement, which may, however, be acceptable to the client [74]. The degree of facial concavity and lip distortion after a central, caudal, or total maxillectomy depends on the extent of the excision [6].

Client satisfaction after mandibulectomy and maxillectomy procedures in dogs has been studied and was found to be proportional to the postoperative survival time [80]. The postoperative cosmetic appearance was acceptable to most clients.

Complications

Hemorrhage

Hemorrhage is the main intraoperative complication, which typically occurs after the inadvertent transection of one of the main arteries (the inferior alveolar artery during a mandibulectomy and the infraorbital, sphenopalatine, and major palatine arteries during a maxillectomy) before ligation. Every attempt should be made to identify and ligate the arteries before transection. Excessive diffuse bleeding may also occur after trauma to the turbinates during a maxillectomy. Hemorrhage is controlled by pressure, blood vessel identification and ligation, absorbable hemostatic agents, or the focal use of electrocoagulation. The surgeon and the anesthetist should be adequately prepared and skilled to handle extensive blood loss. Preoperative bilateral temporary carotid artery ligation is occasionally indicated if severe hemorrhage is anticipated [47].

Hemorrhage may also occur after surgery if a ligature becomes undone or if hemostatic agents become dislodged as blood pressure rises. Careful monitoring for hemorrhage during the first 12 hours after surgery is therefore indicated.

Wound dehiscence

Wound dehiscence of the palatal closure after a maxillectomy (Fig. 8A) is a relatively common complication, with a reported incidence of 7% to 33%, 80% of which occurs caudal to the canine teeth [32,81,82]. This complication can largely be avoided by using correct technique [6,58]. In particular, vestibular mucosal-submucosal flaps should be tension-free and carefully sutured [6,58]. Electrocoagulation should be used judiciously [78]. Wound dehiscence may occur as a result of tumor recurrence; biopsy of the

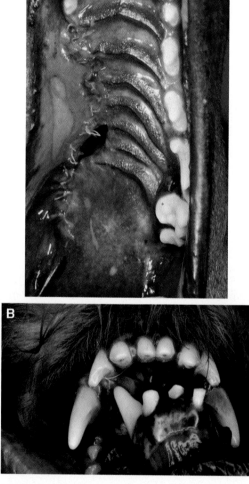

Fig. 8. Complications. (*A*) Dehiscence of the vestibular flap after a caudal maxillectomy in a dog. (*B*) Medial drift of the remaining mandible with palatal trauma after a unilateral total mandibulectomy in a dog. (*C*) Severe malocclusion after a caudal mandibulectomy in a cat.

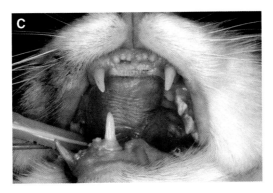

Fig. 8 (*continued*)

dehisced wound edges is therefore indicated when surgical repair is performed [58].

Wound dehiscence after a mandibulectomy is uncommon but may occur over the rostral end of the osteotomized mandible, especially at the alveolar margin, resulting in bone exposure [6,59]. Small areas of dehiscence may heal by second intention, whereas larger areas may have to be debrided and closed surgically. Dehiscence of the commissurorrhaphy performed on completion of a unilateral total mandibulectomy may also occur and is repaired by delayed primary closure.

Functional complications

It is common for the tongue to hang out laterally when a mandibular canine tooth is absent, as occurs after a unilateral rostral mandibulectomy or total mandibulectomy (see Figs. 4C and 5D). Ventral drooping of the tongue is evident after a bilateral rostral mandibulectomy. This is rarely a clinical problem, because motor function is not impaired. Performing a commissurorrhaphy after a total mandibulectomy helps to keep the tongue in the mouth and also reduces drooling. Loss of structural support of the tongue can occur with a bilateral rostral mandibulectomy performed farther caudally than the second premolar; in this case, a period of assisted feeding is necessary for the animal to adapt and the tongue to return to normal function [6,59].

Significant malocclusion can result from a segmental, caudal, or total mandibulectomy. An experimental study in dogs documented persistent instability after a partial mandibulectomy and microscopic degenerative changes in the temporomandibular joints, which were significantly more severe in the unoperated mandibles [83]. In clinical cases, the intact mandible and the rostral part of the operated mandible, if present, drift toward the side of the resection. If both mandibular canines are still present, some animals are unable to close their mouth with the canines in correct alignment, which then results in a significant malocclusion [71]. After a total mandibulectomy, this shift may result in the remaining mandibular canine traumatizing the hard palate (see Fig. 8B). This may be mild and transient or may cause ulceration [57]. In the latter case, crown reduction and endodontic treatment of the exposed pulp or extraction of the mandibular canine tooth is indicated to resolve and prevent further ulceration [57]. Malocclusion can be particularly severe in cats (see Fig. 8C), and temporary maxillomandibular fixation using interdental bonding has been suggested to prevent this complication [59].

The ability to retrieve toys and sticks and to pick up items may be impaired after a bilateral rostral maxillectomy [74]. After a maxillectomy, some mandibular teeth can occlude with the vestibular flap and cause mild and transient ulceration [57].

Maxillectomies and mandibulectomies involving the premolars and molars interfere with the natural cleaning action of mastication. Plaque and calculus tend to accumulate more rapidly on the remaining teeth of the opposing quadrant. Frequent routine periodontal treatment is therefore indicated [57].

References

[1] Withrow SJ. Cancer of the oral cavity. In: Withrow SJ, MacEwen EG, editors. Small animal clinical oncology. 3rd edition. Philadelphia: WB Saunders; 2001. p. 305–18.
[2] Stebbins KE, Morse CC, Goldschmidt MH. Feline oral neoplasia: a ten-year survey. Vet Pathol 1989;26(2):121–8.
[3] Oakes MG, Lewis DD, Hedlund CS, et al. Canine oral neoplasia. Compend Contin Educ Pract Vet 1993;15(1):90–104.
[4] Lantz GC, Salisbury SK. Partial mandibulectomy for treatment of mandibular fractures in dogs: eight cases (1981–1984). J Am Vet Med Assoc 1987;191(2):243–5.
[5] Manfra Marretta S. Maxillofacial surgery. Vet Clin N Am Small Anim Pract 1998;28(5): 1285–96.
[6] Salisbury SK. Maxillectomy and mandibulectomy. In: Slatter DH, editor. Textbook of small animal surgery. 3rd edition. Philadelphia: WB Saunders; 2003. p. 561–72.
[7] Owen LN. TNM classification of tumours in domestic animals. Geneva: World Health Organization; 1980.
[8] White RAS, Jefferies AR, Freedman LS. Clinical staging for oropharyngeal malignancies in the dog. J Small Anim Pract 1985;26:581–94.
[9] Séguin B. Tumors of the mandible, maxilla, and calvarium. In: Slatter DH, editor. Textbook of small animal surgery. 3rd edition. Philadelphia: WB Saunders; 2003. p. 2488–502.
[10] Miles D. The interpretive method. In: Miles DA, Kaugars GE, Van Dis M, et al, editors. Oral and maxillofacial radiology: radiologic/pathologic correlations. 1st edition. Philadelphia: WB Saunders; 1991. p. 1–5.
[11] White SC, Pharoah MJ. Benign tumors of the jaws. In: Oral radiology—principles and interpretation. 5th edition. St. Louis: Mosby; 2004. p. 410–57.
[12] Wood RE. Malignant diseases of the jaws. In: White SC, Pharoah MJ, editors. Oral radiology—principles and interpretation. 5th edition. St. Louis: Mosby; 2004. p. 458–84.

[13] Withrow SJ. The 3 rules of good oncology—biopsy, biopsy, biopsy. J Am Anim Hosp Assoc 1991;27(3):311–4.

[14] Daskalopoulou D, Rapidis AD, Maounis N, et al. Fine-needle aspiration cytology in tumors and tumor-like conditions of the oral and maxillofacial region: diagnostic reliability and limitations. Cancer 1997;81(4):238–52.

[15] Gilson SD, Stone EA. Principles of oncologic surgery. Compend Contin Educ Pract Vet 1990;12(6):827–38.

[16] Langenbach A, McManus PM, Hendrick MJ, et al. Sensitivity and specificity of methods of assessing the regional lymph nodes for evidence of metastasis in dogs and cats with solid tumors. J Am Vet Med Assoc 2001;218(9):1424–8.

[17] Gilson SD. Clinical management of the regional lymph node. Vet Clin N Am Small Anim Pract 1995;25(1):149–67.

[18] Cady B. Lymph node metastases. Indicators, but not governors of survival. Arch Surg 1984;119(9):1067–72.

[19] Smith MM. Surgical approach for lymph node staging of oral and maxillofacial neoplasms in dogs. J Am Anim Hosp Assoc 1995;31(6):514–8.

[20] Smith MM. Surgical approach for lymph node staging of oral and maxillofacial neoplasms in dogs. J Vet Dent 2002;19(3):170–4.

[21] Herring ES, Smith MM, Robertson JL. Lymph node staging of oral and maxillofacial neoplasms in 31 dogs and cats. J Vet Dent 2002;19(3):122–6.

[22] Kusukawa J, Suefuji Y, Ryu F, et al. Dissemination of cancer cells into circulation occurs by incisional biopsy of oral squamous cell carcinoma. J Oral Pathol Med 2000;29(7):303–7.

[23] Patnaik AK, Mooney S. Feline melanoma: a comparative study of ocular, oral, and dermal neoplasms. Vet Pathol 1988;25(2):105–12.

[24] Harvey HJ, MacEwen EG, Braun D, et al. Prognostic criteria for dogs with oral melanoma. J Am Vet Med Assoc 1981;178(6):580–2.

[25] Bostock DE. Prognosis after surgical excision of canine melanomas. Vet Pathol 1979;16(1):32–40.

[26] Frew DG, Dobson JM. Radiological assessment of 50 cases of incisive or maxillary neoplasia in the dog. J Small Anim Pract 1992;33(1):11–8.

[27] Postorino Reeves NC, Turrel JM, Withrow SJ. Oral squamous cell carcinoma in the cat. J Am Anim Hosp Assoc 1993;29(5):438–41.

[28] Ogilvie GK, Sundberg JP, O'Banion MK, et al. Papillary squamous cell carcinoma in three young dogs. J Am Vet Med Assoc 1988;192(7):933–6.

[29] Ciekot PA, Powers BE, Withrow SJ, et al. Histologically low-grade, yet biologically high-grade, fibrosarcomas of the mandible and maxilla in dogs: 25 cases (1982–1991). J Am Vet Med Assoc 1994;204(4):610–5.

[30] Heyman SJ, Diefenderfer DL, Goldschmidt MH, et al. Canine axial skeletal osteosarcoma. A retrospective study of 116 cases (1986 to 1989). Vet Surg 1992;21(4):304–10.

[31] Schwarz PD, Withrow SJ, Curtis CR, et al. Mandibular resection as a treatment for oral cancer in 81 dogs. J Am Anim Hosp Assoc 1991;27(6):601–10.

[32] Schwarz PD, Withrow SJ, Curtis CR, et al. Partial maxillary resection as a treatment for oral cancer in 61 dogs. J Am Anim Hosp Assoc 1991;27(6):617–24.

[33] Straw RC, Powers BE, Klausner J, et al. Canine mandibular osteosarcoma: 51 cases (1980–1992). J Am Anim Hosp Assoc 1996;32(3):257–62.

[34] Verstraete FJM. Oral pathology. In: Slatter DH, editor. Textbook of small animal surgery. 3rd edition. Philadelphia: WB Saunders; 2003. p. 2638–51.

[35] Gardner DG. An orderly approach to the study of odontogenic tumours in animals. J Comp Pathol 1992;107(4):427–38.

[36] Gardner DG. Epulides in the dog: a review. J Oral Pathol Med 1996;25(1):32–7.

[37] Verstraete FJM, Ligthelm AJ, Weber A. The histological nature of epulides in dogs. J Comp Pathol 1992;106(2):169–82.

[38] Gardner DG, Baker DC. The relationship of the canine acanthomatous epulis to ameloblastoma. J Comp Pathol 1993;108(1):47–55.

[39] Bostock DE, White RAS. Classification and behaviour after surgery of canine 'epulides.' J Comp Pathol 1987;97(2):197–206.

[40] Gardner DG, Baker DC. Fibromatous epulis in dogs and peripheral odontogenic fibroma in human beings: two equivalent lesions. Oral Surg Oral Med Oral Pathol 1991;71(3):317–21.

[41] Poulet FM, Valentine BA, Summers BA. A survey of epithelial odontogenic tumors and cysts in dogs and cats. Vet Pathol 1992;29(5):369–80.

[42] Gardner DG, Dubielzig RR. Feline inductive odontogenic tumor (inductive fibroamelo-blastoma)—a tumor unique to cats. J Oral Pathol Med 1995;24(4):185–90.

[43] Soderstrom MJ, Gilson SD. Principles of surgical oncology. Vet Clin N Am Small Anim Pract 1995;25(1):97–110.

[44] Enneking WF. Surgical procedures. In: Musculoskeletal tumor surgery. 1st edition. New York: Churchill Livingstone; 1983. p. 89–122.

[45] McMahon J, O'Brien CJ, Pathak I, et al. Influence of condition of surgical margins on local recurrence and disease-specific survival in oral and oropharyngeal cancer. Br J Oral Maxillofac Surg 2003;41(4):224–31.

[46] Batsakis JG. Surgical excision margins: a pathologist's perspective. Adv Anat Pathol 1999; 6(3):140–8.

[47] Hedlund CS. Surgery of the oral cavity and oropharynx. In: Fossum TW, editor. Small animal surgery. 2nd ed. St. Louis: Mosby; 2002. p. 274–306.

[48] Mann FA, Pace LW. Marking margins of tumorectomies and excisional biopsies to facilitate histological assessment of excision completeness. Semin Vet Med Surg (Small Anim) 1993; 8(4):279–83.

[49] Peterson LJ. Principles of antibiotic therapy. In: Topazian RG, Goldberg MH, editors. Oral and maxillofacial infections. 3rd edition. Philadelphia: WB Saunders; 1994. p. 160–97.

[50] Norris LH, Doku HC. Antimicrobial prophylaxis in oral surgery. Curr Opin Dent 1992;2: 85–92.

[51] Callender DL. Antibiotic prophylaxis in head and neck oncologic surgery: the role of gram-negative coverage. Int J Antimicrob Agents 1999;12(Suppl 1):S21–7.

[52] Johnson JT, Kachman K, Wagner RL, et al. Comparison of ampicillin/sulbactam versus clindamycin in the prevention of infection in patients undergoing head and neck surgery. Head Neck 1997;19(5):367–71.

[53] Harvey CE, Thornsberry C, Miller BR, et al. Antimicrobial susceptibility of subgingival bacterial flora in dogs with gingivitis. J Vet Dent 1995;12(4):151–5.

[54] Harvey CE, Thornsberry C, Miller BR, et al. Antimicrobial susceptibility of subgingival bacterial flora in cats with gingivitis. J Vet Dent 1995;12(4):157–60.

[55] Mueller SC, Henkel KO, Neumann J, et al. Perioperative antibiotic prophylaxis in maxillofacial surgery: penetration of clindamycin into various tissues. J Craniomaxillofac Surg 1999;27(3):172–6.

[56] Marks SL. The buccal mucosal bleeding time. J Am Anim Hosp Assoc 2000;36(4):289–90.

[57] Salisbury SK. Aggressive cancer surgery and aftercare. In: Morrison WB, editor. Cancer in dogs and cats—medical and surgical management. 2nd edition. Jackson, WY: Teton NewMedia; 2002. p. 249–301.

[58] Dernell WS, Schwarz PD, Withrow SJ. Maxillectomy and premaxillectomy. In: Bojrab MJ, editor. Current techniques in small animal surgery. 4th edition. Baltimore: Williams & Wilkins; 1998. p. 124–32.

[59] Dernell WS, Schwarz PD, Withrow SJ. Mandibulectomy. In: Bojrab MJ, editor. Current techniques in small animal surgery. 4th edition. Baltimore: Williams & Wilkins; 1998. p. 132–42.

[60] Cockshutt J. Principles of surgical asepsis. In: Slatter DH, editor. Textbook of small animal surgery. 3rd edition. Philadelphia: WB Saunders; 2003. p. 149–55.

[61] Summers AN, Larson DL, Edmiston CE, et al. Efficacy of preoperative decontamination of the oral cavity. Plast Reconstr Surg 2000;106(4):895–900.

[62] Morgan JP, Haug RH, Kosman JW. Antimicrobial skin preparations for the maxillofacial region. J Oral Maxillofac Surg 1996;54(1):89–94.

[63] Verstraete FJM. Self-assessment color review of veterinary dentistry. Ames: Iowa State University Press; 1999.

[64] Brown JS, Kalavrezos N, D'Souza J, et al. Factors that influence the method of mandibular resection in the management of oral squamous cell carcinoma. Br J Oral Maxillofac Surg 2002;40(4):275–84.

[65] Vernon FF, Helphrey M. Rostral mandibulectomy. Three case reports in dogs. Vet Surg 1983;12(1):26–9.

[66] Withrow SJ, Holmberg DL. Mandibulectomy in the treatment of oral cancer. J Am Anim Hosp Assoc 1983;19(3):273–86.

[67] Penwick RC, Nunamaker DM. Rostral mandibulectomy: a treatment for oral neoplasia in the dog and cat. J Am Anim Hosp Assoc 1987;23(1):19–25.

[68] Bradney IW, Hobson HP, Stromberg PC. Rostral mandibulectomy combined with intermandibular bone graft in treatment of oral neoplasia. J Am Anim Hosp Assoc 1987; 23(6):611–5.

[69] Bracker KE, Trout NJ. Use of a free cortical ulnar autograft following en bloc resection of a mandibular tumor. J Am Anim Hosp Assoc 2000;36(1):76–9.

[70] Yeh L-S, Hou S-M. Repair of a mandibular defect with a free vascularized coccygeal vertebra transfer in a dog. Vet Surg 1994;23(4):281–5.

[71] Boudrieau RJ, Mitchell SL, Seeherman H. Mandibular reconstruction of a partial hemimandibulectomy in a dog with severe malocclusion. Vet Surg 2004;33(2):119–30.

[72] Strong EB, Rubinstein B, Pahlavan N, et al. Mandibular reconstruction with an alloplastic bone tray in dogs. Otolaryngol Head Neck Surg 2003;129(4):417–26.

[73] Anonymous. Nomina Anatomica Veterinaria. 4th edition. Zurich and Ithaca: World Association of Veterinary Anatomists; 1994.

[74] Lascelles BD, Henderson RA, Seguin B, et al. Bilateral rostral maxillectomy and nasal planectomy for large rostral maxillofacial neoplasms in six dogs and one cat. J Am Anim Hosp Assoc 2004;40(2):137–46.

[75] Kirpensteijn J, Withrow SJ, Straw RC. Combined resection of the nasal planum and premaxilla in three dogs. Vet Surg 1994;23(5):341–6.

[76] Salisbury SK, Richardson DC, Lantz GC. Partial maxillectomy and premaxillectomy in the treatment of oral neoplasia in the dog and cat. Vet Surg 1986;15(1):16–26.

[77] O'Brien MG, Withrow SJ, Straw RC, et al. Total and partial orbitectomy for the treatment of periorbital tumors in 24 dogs and 6 cats: a retrospective study. Vet Surg 1996;25(6):471–9.

[78] Salisbury SK, Thacker HL, Pantzer EE, et al. Partial maxillectomy in the dog. Comparison of suture material and closure techniques. Vet Surg 1985;14(4):265–76.

[79] Lascelles BD, Thomson MJ, Dernell WS, et al. Combined dorsolateral and intraoral approach for the resection of tumors of the maxilla in the dog. J Am Anim Hosp Assoc 2003; 39(3):294–305.

[80] Fox LE, Geoghegan SL, Davis LH, et al. Owner satisfaction with partial mandibulectomy or maxillectomy for treatment of oral tumors in 27 dogs. J Am Anim Hosp Assoc 1997;33(1): 25–31.

[81] Wallace J, Matthiesen DT, Patnaik AK. Hemimaxillectomy for the treatment of oral tumors in 69 dogs. Vet Surg 1992;21(5):337–41.

[82] Harvey CE. Oral surgery. Radical resection of maxillary and mandibular lesions. Vet Clin N Am Small Anim Pract 1986;16(5):983–93.

[83] Umphlet RC, Johnson AL, Eurell JC, et al. The effect of partial rostral hemimandibulectomy on mandibular mobility and temporomandibular joint morphology in the dog. Vet Surg 1988;17(4):186–93.

ELSEVIER
SAUNDERS

Vet Clin Small Anim
35 (2005) 1041–1058

VETERINARY
CLINICS
Small Animal Practice

Regional Anesthesia and Analgesia for Oral and Dental Procedures

Judy Rochette, DVM

220 North Sea Avenue, Burnaby, British Columbia, Canada V5B 1K5

Rationale for using multimodal analgesia

We have come a long way in our treatment of animal pain, especially within the last decade. Research has extended to veterinary medicine many of the practices and products previously used in the human field. Incorporating local anesthetic nerve blocks and multimodal analgesia into daily practice is beneficial for the client, the patient, the veterinarian, and the practice.

Pets are becoming members of society's definition of a nuclear family, and as such, clients are looking for the same level of care for their pet as they would expect for themselves. Concern for their pet's comfort or safety may cause a client to decline a necessary procedure or to have the procedure done elsewhere. Veterinarians who emphasize analgesic care are perceived as sensitive, caring, and more competent, which reassures the client. A pet that is appropriately managed should be comfortable at home and should need smaller quantities of analgesics and less frequent dosing. This means cost savings and less stress for the client. All these benefits translate to a satisfied client.

The patient benefits from nerve blocks and preemptive analgesics because they lead to a decrease in intraoperative and postoperative pain. Less pain means that a lighter anesthetic plane can be used, which translates to more stable vital organ function, a smoother recovery, and earlier discharge from the hospital. Preemptive analgesia means that less potent and smaller amounts of analgesics are needed in the postoperative period, which means less "work" for the animal's system and lower risk of toxicity. A comfortable recovery, hospital stay, and recuperation mean that the animal is less likely to self-traumatize and that pain-induced immune suppression,

E-mail address: i.caven@ieee.org

cardiac rhythm disturbances, hypertension, inappetence, and cachexia are avoided, which translates to better healing. A less stressful experience at the veterinary clinic means that the animal is also less distressed about visiting the clinic in future, a fact that the client certainly notices.

Your business should benefit from offering this service, because clients are more willing to allow current and future procedures to be performed on their pet if they perceive such procedures to be pain-free. The equipment needed to perform nerve blocks is already available in a veterinary hospital, and only one type of regional anesthetic agent is needed for all species of all sizes. Using analgesics leads to saving on anesthetic injectables and gases and, if billed out appropriately, can actually generate revenue. A decrease in the dosing frequency of postoperative analgesics translates to savings of your technician's time. A comfortable patient is also significantly safer to work with because such patients have calmer recoveries and are less likely to show aggression when they are handled after surgery. This all translates to increased revenue for the clinic.

The benefits to you, the practitioner, include a safer working environment, expansion of your skill base, and the comfort of knowing that you are offering humane medicine.

Process of pain generation

Effective treatment of clinical pain depends on understanding the mechanisms involved in the formation and maintenance of a pain experience. Noxious stimuli are converted into electrical activity at sensory nerve endings. The neural impulses are then transmitted via the dorsal root ganglia to the dorsal horn of the spinal cord. The electrical signals are sent on to the cerebral cortex. Once the impulses reach the cortex, perception occurs in the conscious patient.

The noxious stimuli that begin the pain process can arise in two phases. The first phase is the sensory input, which arises directly from oral manipulations. The second and more prolonged phase of noxious stimulation is the result of inflammation caused by the surgery. Inflammatory mediators cause the impulse threshold in the sensory nerve endings to decrease, resulting in a state of hyperalgesia and peripheral sensitization. Disproportionate numbers of impulses are sent on to the dorsal horn, where N-methyl-D-aspartate (NMDA) receptors respond to this repeated exposure by accelerating their own rate of pulse discharge, further amplifying the signal. This increased NMDA receptor activity is known as central stimulation or "wind-up." Dorsal horn neurons stay "wound up" even after the original noxious stimuli stop [1], causing non–pain-related signals to be interpreted as painful. Research has found that central sensitization can last days, weeks, or possibly a lifetime, such that a single painful insult early in life may have such long-lasting effects as to lower a patient's pain threshold permanently [2]. The purpose of preemptive analgesia is thus to prevent the transmission of noxious impulses to the brain and to stop central sensitization from developing.

The pain experience can be modulated in several ways. A local anesthetic block shuts down the formation of a painful sensation by preventing neural impulses from reaching the spinal cord. All other medications modulate or ameliorate a pain impulse that has been allowed to form or the conscious perception of that pain. Acute pain impulses are well controlled with opioids because these agents modulate wind-up and conscious perception of pain. Chronic pain requires aggressive multimodal therapy as soon as it is diagnosed, because physiologic changes in neuronal nociceptive processing occur and may lead to "resistance to treatment" [3] or opioid tolerance [4]. The degree of pain and its source (eg, somatic, neuropathic) combined with duration, species of interest, and country of residence determine the most appropriate therapeutics to add to the opioid.

There are many grading systems for determining how much pain an animal is in; however, mild to moderate or moderate pain should be expected with most dental procedures. For stomatitis, multiple extractions, fracture repair, head trauma, cancer, and mucositis after radiation therapy, expect moderate to severe or severe pain. Severe to excruciating pain should be anticipated with bone cancer, especially after a biopsy [5]. The World Health Organization (WHO) has a recommended analgesia ladder (Table 1) [4].

Most dental pain is somatic (ie, arising from diseased tissues), but cancer or trauma, for example, may cause neurogenic distress by directly insulting the nervous tissues. Therapeutics, such as tramadol (Ultram; Ortho-McNeil Pharmaceutical, Raritan, NJ) or gabapentin (Neurontine; Park-David Division of Pfizer, New York, NY) may be useful in these cases. Most dental cases have some degree of chronicity to them by the time the patient is presented for treatment. The actual dental manipulations cause acute stimulation, but chronic pain should be expected with odontoclastic resorptive lesions, stomatitis, and cancer, for example. NMDA receptor blockers are helpful. Species of interest can be a factor in choosing medications, because cats react poorly to many drugs that are used safely in dogs and many products are not labeled for use in cats. Country of residence can affect access to drugs, such as buprenorphine (Buprenex; Reckitt

Table 1
The World Health Organization recommended analgesia ladder

Mild pain	Treat with NSAIDs, acetaminophen
Moderate pain	Treat with NSAIDs + mild opioids
Severe pain	Use a stronger opioid, perhaps added to NSAID
Refractory pain	Control may require alternative routes of delivery, interventions, blocks, neural stimulations, neurolysis.

Adapted from Veterinary Information Network. Pain management in cancer patients. Available at: www.vin.com/Members/Proceedings/Proceedings.plx?CID=WVC2004&PID=pr05460&O=VIN. Accessed September 2004.

Benckiser Pharmaceuticals, Richmond, VA), which is not available in Canada.

Local anesthetic agents

Local anesthetic agents prevent or retard the conduction of afferent pain impulses by entering and occupying ion channels in a nerve cell membrane, preventing depolarization. Uptake into the membrane is improved with a higher concentration of agent or a larger volume. Blood flow through the area decreases the quantity and concentration of agent situated around the nerve. Duration of effect is thus improved if vasoconstrictors are added to the injectable product. Cell membrane uptake is poor; therefore, blockade is decreased in an infection or in an acid environment.

The most commonly used local anesthetic agents are mepivacaine, lidocaine, and bupivacaine. Time to onset of sensory blockage is fastest for mepivacaine (Carbocaine; AstraZeneca, Wayne, PA) and slowest for bupivacaine (Marcaine; AstraZeneca, Wayne, PA). Mepivacaine is effective for 1.5 to 2.0 hours, whereas bupivacaine begins to attenuate after 6 hours. Lidocaine (Xylocaine; AstraZeneca, Wayne, PA) produces onset of analgesia in 2 to 5 minutes and lasts 20 minutes (without epinephrine) to 2 hours (with epinephrine). These products can be purchased in ampules that contain 1.8 mL or in larger multidose bottles.

The maximum safe dose of local anesthetic agent for a dog or cat is 2 mg/kg divided between the necessary sites. If the patient is small, the total volume allowed could be quite limited. In these animals, lidocaine can be diluted with saline [6] or the 0.25% solution of bupivacaine can be used, because larger volumes can be infused without reaching toxic doses. In practice, bupivacaine 0.5% at a rate of 0.25 mL per site is adequate to achieve full desensitization in a cat. Even in large dogs, 1 mL per site is sufficient to achieve complete analgesia. A 1- or 3-mL syringe with a 0.625- to 1.5-inch, 25-gauge needle is usually adequate for placing the blocks.

Facial innervation

The pain receptors in the dental hard and soft tissues are free nerve endings. A-δ fibers transmit sharp localized pain; A-β fibers conduct touch and pressure; and C fibers provide the sensations of burning, aching, and throbbing [7]. These fibers are incorporated into nerves that form the sensory branches of the trigeminal (fifth cranial) nerve. The branches of concern to oral and dental surgeons are the maxillary and mandibular divisions.

The maxillary division leaves the trigeminal ganglion and exits the brain case through the foramen rotundum, courses through the periorbita, and enters the infraorbital canal. Just before entering the caudal limit of the infraorbital canal, the nerve sends off branches that become the major and minor palatine nerves. These nerves innervate the hard and soft palates, their mucosa, and the nasopharynx. These branches are desensitized with the maxillary nerve block. The maxillary division also gives off the caudal maxillary alveolar nerve, which supplies the maxillary molars and their associated soft tissues and is blocked with the caudal infraorbital nerve block. After giving off the caudal maxillary alveolar nerve, the maxillary nerve enters the infraorbital canal and is now called the infraorbital nerve. While the infraorbital nerve is traversing the infraorbital canal, it gives off two more branches that exit ventrally from the canal. The middle maxillary alveolar nerve innervates the premolars and associated buccal gingiva. The rostral maxillary alveolar nerve supplies the canine, incisors, and associated buccal gingiva. The remaining fibers of the infraorbital nerve then exit the cranial extent of the infraorbital canal to innervate the lateral and dorsal cutaneous structures of the rostral maxilla and upper lip. The middle maxillary alveolar, rostral maxillary alveolar, and infraorbital nerves are blocked by the cranial infraorbital nerve block.

The mandibular division of the trigeminal nerve arises from the trigeminal ganglion, exits the cranium via the foramen ovale, and divides into multiple branches. One such branch is the mandibular, or alveolar, nerve. The mandibular nerve enters the mandible on the lingual side via the mandibular foramen. The nerve then courses rostrally within the bone to innervate the mandibular teeth to the mesial midline; this nerve can be blocked with the mandibular nerve block. At the level of the second premolar (dogs) or rostral to the third premolar (cats), the mandibular nerve gives off mental nerve branches. These branches exit through the mental foramina and serve the cutaneous areas of the chin, lip, and rostral buccal gingiva and mucosa. These nerves, and possibly the mesial portion of the mandibular nerve, can be blocked with the mental nerve block.

Sites for regional anesthetic placement

Cranial and caudal infraorbital nerve blocks

The cranial end of the infraorbital foramen is located apical to the distal root of the third premolar just ventrorostral to where the zygomatic arch meets the maxillary bone. The anesthetic needle should be directed slightly dorsal to horizontal and slightly mesiad to the long axis of the maxilla. The block anesthetizes the ipsilateral premolar, canine, and incisor teeth as well as associated soft tissues. If the needle is advanced deep into the foramen or if digital pressure is placed over the cranial end of the infraorbital canal after injection, a caudal infraorbital nerve block has been accomplished, and the caudal maxillary nerve is also desensitized. This block anesthetizes all ipsilateral dentition and soft tissues, including the molars (Figs. 1B, 2B, and 3).

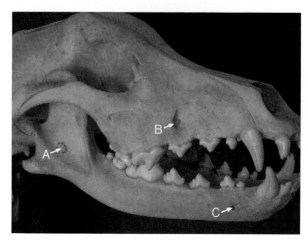

Fig. 1. Foramina of interest in the canine skull. The arrow next to A points to the position of the mandibular foramen on the lingual side of the mandible. The arrow next to B points to the infraorbital foramen. The arrow next to C points to the middle mental foramen.

Maxillary nerve block

The maxillary nerve block desensitizes the complete hemimaxilla, including the soft tissues, dentition, and palate. If an approach is made as though for a caudal infraorbital nerve block but is carried slightly further, the needle should approximate the orbital end of the infraorbital canal. The major and minor palatine nerves are in the immediate vicinity; thus, depositing anesthetic agent to diffuse throughout the area is likely to

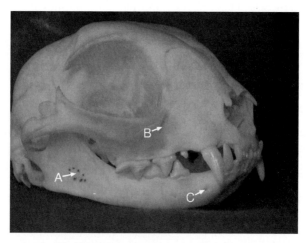

Fig. 2. Foramina of interest in the feline skull. The arrow next to A points to the position of the mandibular foramen on the lingual side of the mandible. The arrow next to B points to the infraorbital foramen. The arrow next to C points to the middle mental foramen.

desensitize these nerves as well (see Fig. 3). Alternatively, there is an extraoral technique by which the needle is inserted through the skin perpendicular to the long axis of the head, under the rostroventral limit of the zygomatic arch, at the dorsocaudal limit of the hard palate (Figs. 4 and 5).

Mental nerve block

In the dog, the middle mental foramen is palpated ventral to the mesial root of the second premolar. In the cat, the foramen is located under the lip frenulum approximately equidistant between the third premolar and the canine. If the needle enters the foramen, the block should anesthetize the ipsilateral soft tissues, the canine and incisor teeth, and possibly the premolars. If the anesthetic is deposited outside the foramen, only the buccal soft tissues from the canine forward to the midline receive analgesia (Figs. 1C and 2C; Fig. 6).

There is concern that penetration of a foramen with a needle may cause trauma to the nerve. This is especially possible when attempting to block the mental nerve in a small animal. For this reason, it is recommended to use the mandibular nerve block in cats and small dogs, which should provide blockade for the area while avoiding iatrogenic trauma (Fig. 7).

Mandibular (alveolar) nerve block

The mandibular nerve block can be done intraorally or extraorally. The foramen is a depression located on the medial side of the ramus of the mandible. It is approximately equidistant between the mesial and distal borders of the ramus and at a height midway between the dorsal and ventral

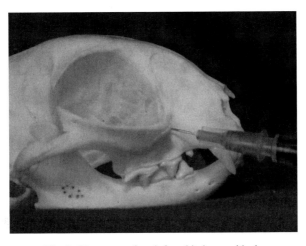

Fig. 3. Placement of an infraorbital nerve block.

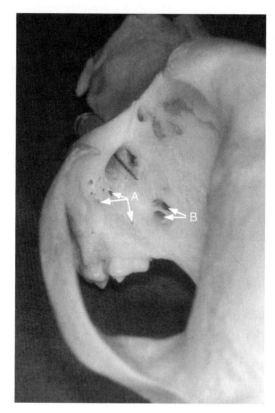

Fig. 4. Maxillary nerve block via the infraorbital foramen. The needle is placed deep into the infraorbital canal. The arrows next to A point to foramina leading to the distal premolars and molars. The arrows next to B point to the foramina for the major and minor palatine nerves.

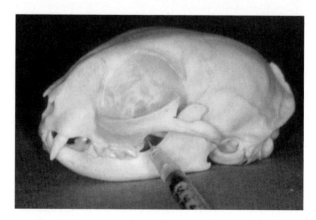

Fig. 5. Extraoral approach for a maxillary nerve block.

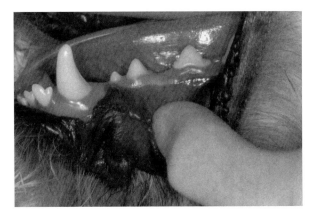

Fig. 6. Location of the middle mental foramen in the dog.

edges of the body of the mandible. The nerve is anesthetized before it enters the mandible and blocks all the soft tissues and dentition on that side of the mouth. The intraoral approach involves directing the syringe across the tongue from the opposite side of the mouth and placing the anesthetic agent in proximity to the foramen. In the extraoral approach, the needle is inserted through the skin at right angles to the ventral border of the mandible. The foramen is on a line drawn from the lateral canthus of the eye, through the midpoint of the zygomatic arch, to the ventral aspect of the mandible. In the dog, this contact point should be approximately 0.5 to 1.0 cm mesial to the angular process. With a finger inserted into the animal's mouth and palpating the foramen, the needle should be walked off the medial edge of the mandible and advanced dorsally until it can be felt in proximity to the foramen. Anesthetic agent is deposited around the nerve as it enters the foramen (see Figs. 1A and 2A; Fig. 8).

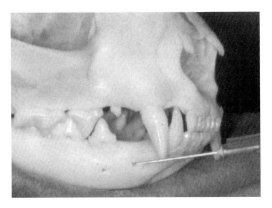

Fig. 7. A 25-gauge needle and the middle mental foramen in the cat. Iatrogenic trauma may occur from trying to place a mental nerve block in cats and small dogs.

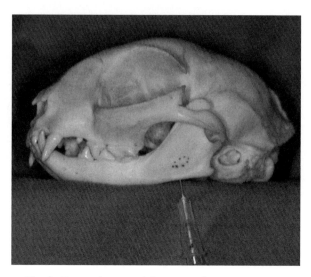

Fig. 8. Extraoral approach for a mandibular nerve block.

A less technique-sensitive method for blockading a limited area is with infiltration of that area. Anesthetic agent is placed under the soft tissues on the buccal and medial sides of the tooth adjacent to the bone. The agent diffuses into the bone and desensitizes the tooth. This technique only works for maxillary teeth, because the cortical bone is too dense in the mandible for infusion to occur. Intraosseous anesthesia does not have this latter limitation. A specially designed intraosseous needle (Dentsply Canada Ltd., Woodbridge, Ontario, Canada) is placed directly into the interproximal bone without predrilling, and agent is delivered. Analgesia is immediate, and an injection port stays available should additional anesthetic agent be needed.

A third method of desensitizing a single tooth uses intraligamentary anesthesia. Anesthetic agent at a maximum dose of 0.2 mL per root is injected into the periodontal ligament space using a special syringe. Onset of analgesia takes 10 to 15 minutes. This injection provides periodontal ligament, gingival, and apical afferent sensory nerve analgesia [7]. This technique does not work in the presence of infection or severe periodontal disease. For these cases, intraosseous anesthesia or a specific nerve block should be considered.

Opioids

Opioids are appropriate for controlling short-term pain. Pharmaceuticals with μ-agonist activity provide excellent analgesia for moderate to severe pain. Combined with nonsteroidal anti-inflammatory drugs (NSAIDs) or NMDA receptor antagonists, for example, opioids can also treat chronic or refractive conditions.

The response to narcotics is species dependent. The feline reaction is possibly the result of a different opiate receptor population. Dogs show central nervous system (CNS) depression, hypothermia, and miosis, whereas cats may develop CNS excitation, hyperthermia, and mydriasis. Cases of "morphine mania" are usually the result of giving excessive quantities of a pure μ-agonist to a nonpainful cat. Coadministration of a tranquilizer, such as acepromazine (PromAce, Fort Dodge Animal Health, Madison, NJ; 0.05 mg/kg administered subcutaneously or intramuscularly) [8] can reduce this side effect, as does giving smaller quantities of μ-opioid.

Commonly used narcotics are listed in the following sections, including their salient features.

Morphine

Morphine (Morphine; AstraZeneca, Wayne, PA) is the standard by which all opioids are measured, but it has variable intensity and duration of effect in the cat. Given intravenously, morphine causes histamine release and frequently causes vomiting if given to a nonpainful animal. Nausea does not occur if pain is present.

Methadone

Methadone (Methadone; AAIPharma, LLC, Wilmington, NC) is similar to morphine in duration and degree of analgesia but is less likely to induce vomiting. Methadone also affects NMDA receptors by means of a noncompetitive mechanism [9]. It is a relatively expensive drug.

Oxymorphone

Oxymorphone (Numorphane; Endo Labs, Chadds Ford, PA) is also an expensive opioid and has recently been a victim to supply problems. It can be used intravenously without histamine release and can be absorbed across mucous membranes. This latter characteristic means that oxymorphone can be sent home for intranasal application at a dose of 0.05 to 0.1 mg/kg administered every 4 to 6 hours. Oxymorphone is not effectively antagonized by naloxone in cats; thus, overly narcotized patients are difficult to reverse.

Fentanyl

Fentanyl (Duragesic; Janssen Pharmaceuticals, Titusville, NJ) has a short duration when given systemically, usually lasting only 30 to 60 minutes. It is most useful as a constant rate infusion (CRI) or in a transdermal patch.

Transdermal patches are useful for control of significant pain of longer duration. Uptake of fentanyl through the skin varies between species, even within a species, but seems to be faster in cats [8]. The time required to reach steady-state plasma concentrations fluctuates, but comfort seems to begin between 6 and 12 hours after application, and analgesia can last for 4 to 5 days. Because of the variation in absorption, all patients with a transdermal patch should be observed for breakthrough pain. Animals weighing less than 2.5 kg may absorb too high a dose even from the smallest patch; thus, an alternative analgesic protocol should be considered.

The use of a fentanyl patch is off-label for a veterinary patient. If sending an animal home with an active patch, ensure that the pet is going to a "safe" household (eg, the clients are trustworthy, children and other pets do not have access to the patch).

Hydromorphone

Hydromorphone (Dilaudid; Abbott Laboratories, Abbot Park, IL) does not have a ceiling to its analgesic effects [10]. Animals demonstrating severe pain that is refractory to a single dose of hydromorphone may experience relief when the dose is increased. Analgesia can last for up to 6 hours [8]. Hydromorphone is not licensed for use in animals but is an economic alternative to oxymorphone. It often induces vomiting when given to a non-painful animal (ie, as premedication before surgery).

Butorphanol

Butorphanol is useful for mild to moderate pain. It has a ceiling effect for its analgesia, meaning that higher doses do not produce better analgesia. It is not appropriate for significant somatic pain [11], and some researchers question whether it is analgesic in animals at all [12].

Buprenorphine

Buprenorphine is a partial μ-agonist that is good for mild to moderate pain. It has a tremendous affinity for the μ-receptor and competitively inhibits other μ-agonists from binding [13]. Buprenorphine can be used to antagonize morphine or fentanyl without loss of analgesia but is difficult to reverse and may cause residual blockade even after it is no longer systemically active. Residual blockade may be a concern if buprenorphine is used after surgery while waiting for a fentanyl patch to take effect.

Buprenorphine is 100% bioavailable via the transmucosal route. Combined with an acceptable taste and a small dose volume (0.02 mg/kg = 0.066 mL/kg), these properties make it an excellent option for feline use. A 3-day transdermal [3] buprenorphine patch is available in human medicine, and a 7-day patch is under development.

Codeine

Historically, codeine has been more useful for home therapy than for in-hospital treatment. Codeine is metabolized to morphine, but cats can only convert less than 10% of a given dose, [14] and a rare animal may show excitation after treatment.

Codeine has an unpleasant taste and is only 60% bioavailable by the oral route [14]. Flavoring makes syrups more acceptable. A transdermal paste has been formulated that can be applied to the pinnae, which seems to be effective, is easier to use, and does not require oral manipulation, making it ideal for postdental patients.

Tramadol

Tramadol is a synthetic derivative of codeine and is one of the most useful drugs available to veterinarians for treating chronic and neuropathic pain. It is not technically an opioid; therefore, it is not controlled. Tramadol does cause μ-receptor stimulation, but it is also a monoamine (ie, serotonin) reuptake inhibitor. This inhibition enhances dorsal horn downregulation of pain impulses and produces mild antianxiety effects [13]. Tramadol has been used short term in cats, but the safety of long-term use is unknown. It should not be used with other tricyclic antidepressants (TCAs), selective serotonin reuptake inhibitors (SSRIs), or monoamine oxidase (MAO) inhibitors, and, [13,15] because it may lower seizure thresholds, caution is advised with epileptics.

Naloxone

Naloxone is a μ-antagonist used to correct overzealous opioid use. Cats do not react predictably to this agent [14,16]. It has a short duration of effect, which may necessitate retreatment.

α_2-Agonists

The α_2-agonists can be ideal adjuncts to general anesthetics. They provide sedation, analgesia, and muscle relaxation and significantly reduce the quantities of injectable and inhalant anesthetic agents needed to induce and maintain anesthesia. Xylazine, medetomidine, and romifidine are in this class. Studies have been completed with medetomidine, which, although off-label for use in cats, can work synergistically with opioids in the perioperative period [17–19]. Preoperative sedation and preemptive analgesia are achieved with drastically less volume than label recommendations. In the postoperative period, ultralow doses, alone or with opioids, can enhance and prolong the analgesic effects of the opioids, with limited effect on cardiovascular function. Synergy means the dose of opioid needed is also reduced, usually by half. Because of possible side effects, all α_2-agonist use should be limited to healthy animals. Atipamezole reverses the sedative and analgesic effects of medetomidine.

Nonsteroidal anti-inflammatory drugs

Opioids are effective before and after surgery when surgical inflammation has not fully developed. After the initial period of insult or in cases of chronic disease, NSAIDs may prove to be advantageous for pain control via their combined anti-inflammatory and analgesic actions.

The principal mode of action of all NSAIDs is to block prostaglandin production by binding and inhibiting cyclooxygenase (COX). Although the result of this effect is mainly a reduction in inflammation and peripheral nociceptor sensitization, wind-up is also reduced or prevented. There is some evidence that certain NSAIDs, such as acetaminophen, have a central analgesic action [13], possibly against a new variant of COX enzyme [20]. Acetaminophen can be used in dogs as a first-line therapy when NSAIDs cannot be used.

NSAIDs should only be used in healthy, young, normotensive, normo-volemic animals without evidence of gastric ulceration, bleeding diathesis, or compromised renal function. Ulcer prophylaxis can be used in a high-risk animal. Of interest, misoprostol, a synthetic prostaglandin analogue that prevents and helps to heal gastrointestinal ulceration caused by NSAIDs also enhances the anti-inflammatory and analgesic effects of NSAIDs [14]. Caution should be exercised when using NSAIDs in cats because of the drugs' prolonged half-life and the potential for toxicity. Few studies have been performed to examine the feline response to these compounds; thus, close monitoring should accompany long-term therapy. Before using an NSAID for cats, it should be checked for labeled use in this species.

N-methyl-D-aspartate receptor blockers

Blocking NMDA receptors impairs the wind-up phenomenon; therefore, acute and chronic pain is better managed [8]. Controlling central sensitization allows other analgesics to be more effective, but NMDA receptor antagonists also act to increase opioid receptor sensitivity, reduce opioid tolerance, and minimize rebound hyperalgesia (the phenomenon of markedly increased pain that occurs when an opioid wears off) [13].

Ketamine is the best-known NMDA receptor blocker. It is most effective as a CRI. The antiviral agent amantadine is also included in this category of agents [20]. It is most effective when used as an adjunctive therapy to an NSAID. A less frequently referenced NMDA receptor antagonist is dextromethorphan [21]. Commercial dextromethorphan products are only cost-effective in a smaller dog or cat. Compounding is necessary for use in a larger animal.

Analgesic adjuncts

Gabapentin

Gabapentin is an anticonvulsant with purported analgesic activity. Its mechanism of action is unclear; it may act on NMDA receptors [20], or it may inhibit postsynaptic neuron firing in general [13]. It has been used for

Table 2
Analgesic agents for use in dogs and cats

Drug	Dosages
Acetaminophen	C: Contraindicated D: 10–15 mg/kg PO q 8–12 h
Amantadine	C: 3 mg/kg PO SID D: 3–5 mg/kg PO SID or 1–2 mg/kg BID
Amitriptyline	C: 0.5–2.0 mg/kg PO SID D: 3–5 mg/kg PO SID
Bupivacaine	1–2 mg/kg q 6–8 h
Buprenorphine	C: 0.01–0.02 mg/kg SQ, IM, IV, sublingual q 4–6 h D: 0.005–0.02 mg/kg SQ, IM, IV q 4–8 h
Butorphanol	0.2–0.4 mg/kg SQ, IM, IV q 1–2 h 0.5–1 mg/kg PO q 4–8 h
Carprofen	C: 1–2 mg/kg SQ q 12–18 h D: 2 mg/kg PO BID or 4 mg/kg PO SID
Codeine	0.5–1.0 mg/kg PO TID
Deracoxib	D: 3–4 mg/kg PO SID × 7 days, then 1–2 mg/kg SID
Dextromethorphan	0.5–2 mg/kg PO TID–QID
Etodolac	C: Not recommended D: 5–15 mg/kg PO 24 h
Fentanyl	2–5 µg/kg/h transdermal C: Loading dose: 1–2 µg/kg IV, then CRI: 1–4 µg/kg/h IV D: Loading dose: 1–2 µg/kg IV, then CRI: 5–10 µg/kg/h IV
Gabapentin	C: 2–10 mg/kg PO SID–BID D: 3–10 mg/kg PO SID–BID
Hydromorphone	C: 0.02–0.1 mg/kg SQ, IM, IV q 4–6 h D: 0.05–0.2 mg/kg SQ, IM, IV q 4–6 h
Imipramine	C: 2.5–5.0 mg PO BID D: 1–2 mg/kg q 8–12 h
Ketamine	Loading dose: 0.2–0.5 mg/kg IV, then CRI: 2–10 µg/kg/min IV during surgery, then 2 µg/kg/min after surgery for up to 18 hours (this works out to 60 mg of ketamine in 1000 mL of LRS given at 2 mL/kg/h)
Ketoprofen	C: 2 mg/kg SQ once, then 1 mg/kg SID D: 2 mg/kg SQ, IM, IV once, then 1 mg/kg SID
	C: 2 mg/kg PO once, then 1 mg/kg SID, maximum 5 days D: 2 mg/kg PO once, then 1 mg/kg SID
Lidocaine	C: 2–6 mg/kg, maximum 2 mL total D: 2–6 mg/kg
Medetomidine	1.0 µg/kg, with equal volume of butorphanol, IV (this produce's heavy sedation and is not recommended if planning on going on to a GA) Before surgery with atropine + opiate C: 5–10 µg/kg IM D: 2–5 µg/kg IM After surgery alone C: 4–8 µg/kg IM D: 2–4 µg/kg IM

(continued on next page)

Table 2 (*continued*)

Drug	Dosages
	After surgery with opiate C: 2–4 μg/kg IM D: 1–2 μg/kg IM (After surgery, opiate is given at one half the dose used in premedication (eg, butorphanol at 0.2–0.4 mg/kg in premedication is 0.1–0.2 mg/kg after surgery)
Meloxicam	0.2 mg/kg SQ once C: 0.2 mg/kg PO SID × 1 day, then 0.1 mg/cat PO q 1–3 days D: 0.2 mg/kg PO SID × 1 day, then 0.1 mg/kg q 24 h
Meperidine	C: 5–10 mg/kg IM q 2–3 h D: 3–5 mg/kg IM q 2–3 h
Methadone	C: 0.05–0.5 mg/kg SQ, IM, IV q 4–6 h D: 0.1–1.0 mg/kg SQ, IM, IV q 4–6 h
Misoprostol	C: 1–3 μg/kg PO q 8 h D: 1–5 μg/kg PO q 8 h
Morphine	C: 0.1–0.5 mg/kg SQ, IM q 4–6 h D: 0.5–1.0 mg/kg SQ, IM q 4–6 h C: 0.02–0.05 mg/kg IV q 1–2 h D: 0.05–0.1 mg/kg IV q 1–2 h
Morphine oral	C: 0.2–0.5 TID–QID D: 0.5–2.0 TID–QID
Morphine oral (sustained release)	C: Not available D: 0.5–1.0 PO BID–TID
Naloxone	0.04 mg/kg diluted with 10 mL saline, give 1 mL/min IV until symptoms resolve, then q 45–180 min
Oxymorphone	C: 0.05–0.1 mg/kg SQ, IM q 2–4 h D: 0.05–0.2 mg/kg SQ, IM q 2–4 h C: 0.03 mg/kg IV q 45–60 min D: 0.06 mg/kg IV q 45–60 min
Piroxicam	C: 1 mg/cat PO SID maximum 7 days[a] D: 0.3 mg/kg PO q 48 h
Tolfenamic acid	4 mg/kg SQ, IM once C: 4 mg/kg PO SID for 3–5 days D: 4 mg/kg PO SID for 5 consecutive days per week
Tramadol	C: 2–4 mg/kg PO BID D: 1–2 mg/kg PO BID to QID, maximum 10 mg/kg/d
Vedaprofen	D: 0.5 mg/kg PO 24 h, maximum 28 days

All doses and labelling for use should be verified by the practitioner before use.

Abbreviations: BID, twice daily; C, cat; CRI, continuous rate infusion; D, dog; GA, general anesthetic; h, hours; IM, intramuscular; IV, intravenous; LRS, lactated Ringer's solution; min, minutes; PO, orally; q, every; QID, four times daily; SID, once daily; SQ, subcutaneous; TID, three times daily.

[a] After compounding, drug is only stable for 10 days.

REGIONAL ANESTHESIA AND ANALGESIA

chronic and neuropathic pain. It is an expensive drug; therefore, it is not suggested as a first choice for chronic pain [8,13]. Once pain is controlled, the patient should be weaned off the drug slowly [8].

Tricyclic antidepressants

Anxiety lowers pain thresholds [16], which is why TCAs have been used in human beings and animals as adjuncts to other analgesics (especially opioids) for chronic pain [3]. TCAs act to inhibit serotonin and norepinephrine reuptake, part of the biochemistry of wind-up. They may have other analgesic effects as well, including possible actions at opioid receptors and on nerve transmission [13]. Amitriptyline and imipramine are the most commonly used drugs in this class.

Other adjuncts

Acupuncture, physiotherapy, and nutraceutical agents may also be used to provide comfort, especially in chronic pain cases.

Summary

It is beneficial to provide local anesthetic nerve blocks and multimodal analgesia. Nerve blocks arrest a pain impulse before it is formed. The most commonly used blocks for oral and dental surgery are the infraorbital, maxillary, mental, and mandibular blocks. Source of pain, duration, and subject species, for example, can all be factors in determining the therapeutics used for acute and chronic pain control. Opioids, NSAIDs, NMDA receptor blockers, TCAs, and other adjuncts can all be used (Table 2).

References

[1] VIN Web site. Safe and effective acute pain relief for cats. Available at: www.vin.com/ Members/Proceedings/Proceedings.plx?CID = PAIN2003&PID = 5814&O = VIN. Accessed September 2004.
[2] Taddio A, Katz J, Ilersich A, Koren G. Effect of neonatal circumcision on pain response during subsequent routine vaccination. Lancet 1997;349:599–603.
[3] VIN Web site. Can chronic pain in cats be managed? Yes! Available at: www.vin.com/ Members/Proceedings/Proceedings.plx?CID = PAIN2003&PID = 5816&O = VIN. Accessed September 2004.
[4] VIN Web site. Pain management in cancer patients. Available at: www.vin.com/Members/ Proceedings/Proceedings.plx?CID = WVC2004&PID = pr05460&O = VIN. Accessed September 2004.
[5] VIN Web site. Pain management alternatives for common surgeries. Available at: www.vin.com/Members/Proceedings/Proceedings.plx?CIN = PAIN2003&PID = 5815&O = VIN. Accessed August 2004.
[6] Duke T. Local and regional anesthetic and analgesic techniques in the dog and cat: Part II, infiltration and nerve blocks. Can Vet J 2000;41:949–52.

[7] VIN Web site. Pain management. Available at: www.vin.com/Members/Proceedings/Proceedings.plx?CID = WVC2004PID = 585&O = Generic. Accessed August 10, 2004.

[8] VIN Web site. Anesthesia and analgesia for cats. Available at: www.vin.com/Members/Proceedings/Proceedings.plx?CID = WVC2004&PID = pr05479&O = VIN. Accessed August 10, 2004.

[9] Callahan RJ, Au JD, Paul M, et al. Functional inhibition by methadone of N-methyl-D-aspartate receptors expressed in Xenopus oocytes: stereospecific and subunit effects. Anesth Analg 2004;98(3):653–9.

[10] Pettifer G, Dyson D. Hydromorphone: a cost-effective alternative to the use of oxymorphone. Can Vet J 2000;41:135–7.

[11] Sawyer D, Rech R. Analgesia and behavioural effects of butorphanol, nalbuphine, and pentazocine in the cat. J Am Anim Hosp Assoc 1987;23:438–46.

[12] Wagner AE. Is butorphanol analgesic in dogs and cats? Veterinary Medicine 1999;94:346–50.

[13] Veterinary Anesthesia Support Group Web site. Chronic pain management. Available at: www.vasg.org/chronic_pain_management.htm. Accessed September 18, 2004.

[14] Boothe DM. Control of pain in cats. In: Proceedings of the Fifth Continuing Education Feline Symposium. Mercer, WA, 2002. p. 29–43.

[15] VIN Web site. Tramadol dose for dogs; methadone vs. morphine. Available at: www.vin.com/Members/SearchDB/Boards/B0320000/B0317987.htm. Accessed July 24, 2004.

[16] VIN Web site. Animal pain: figuring out what is going on. Available at: www.vin.com/Members/Proceedings/Proceedings.plx?CID = PAIN2003&PID = 5813&O = VIN. Accessed July 24, 2004.

[17] Lemke KA. Perioperative use of selective alpha-2 agonists and antagonists in small animals. Can Vet J 2004;45:475–80.

[18] Muir WW III, Ford JL, Karpa GE, et al. Effects of intramuscular administration of low doses of medetomidine and medetomidine-butorphanol in middle-aged and old dogs. J Am Vet Med Assoc 1999;215:1116–20.

[19] Ansah OB, Vainio O, Hellsten C, et al. Postoperative pain control in cats: clinical trials with medetomidine and butorphanol. Vet Surg 2002;31:99–103.

[20] VIN Web site. Managing chronic pain in dogs: the next level. Available at: www.vin.com/Members/Proceedings/Proceedings.plx?CID = PAIN2003&PID = 5817&O = VIN. Accessed July 24, 2004.

[21] VIN Web site. Oral analgesics for cats and dogs. Available at: www.vin.com/Members/SearchDB/boards/B0290000/B0285795.htm. Accessed July 24, 2004.

ELSEVIER
SAUNDERS

Vet Clin Small Anim
35 (2005) 1059–1063

VETERINARY
CLINICS
Small Animal Practice

Appendix

American Veterinary Dental College Approved Case-Log Abbreviations

Steven E. Holmstrom, DVM

Animal Dental Clinic, 987 Laurel Street, San Carlos, CA 94070, USA

The American Veterinary Dental College has established the following list of abbreviations. They can be used on dental charts or in case records. This version is current for the 2005 Credentials and TSC cycles. Abbreviations for use in the Diagnosis column are shown in bold text. Abbreviations for use in the Procedure column are shown in normal text.

Tooth Identification

Use of the Triadan tooth numbering system or anatomical description L (left), R (right), MN (mandibular), MX (maxillary), C (canine), I1-3 (incisor), M1-3 (molar), PM1-4 (premolar) is permitted in case logs.

	Definition
AB	**abrasion**
APG	apexogenesis
APX	apexification
AT	**attrition**
B	biopsy
B/E	biopsy excisional
B/I	biopsy incisional
BG	bone graft (includes placement of bone substitute or bone stimulant material)
C	**canine**
CA	**caries**
CBU	core build up
CFL	**cleft lip**
CFL/R	cleft lip repair
CFP	**cleft palate**
CFP/R	cleft palate repair

(continued on next page)

0195-5616/05/$ - see front matter © 2005 Elsevier Inc. All rights reserved.
doi:10.1016/j.cvsm.2005.03.007

vetsmall.theclinics.com

	Definition
CMO	**cranio-mandibular osteopathy**
CR	crown
CRA	crown amputation
CR/M	crown metal
CRL	crown lengthening
CR/PFM	crown porcelain fused to metal
CR/P	crown preparation
CRR	crown reduction
CS	culture/susceptibility
DT	**deciduous (primary) tooth**
DTC	**dentigerous cyst**
E	**enamel**
E/D	**enamel defect**
E/H	**enamel hypocalcification or hypoplasia**
FB	**foreign body**
F	flap
F/AR	apically repositioned periodontal flap
F/CR	coronally repositioned periodontal flap
F/L	lateral sliding periodontal flap
FGG	free gingival graft
FRE	frenoplasty (frenotomy, frenectomy)
FX	**fracture (tooth or jaw)**
FX/R	repair of jaw fracture
FX/R/P	pin repair of jaw fracture
FX/R/PL	plate repair of jaw fracture
FX/R/S	screw repair of jaw fracture
FX/R/WIR	wire repair of jaw fracture
FX/R/WIR/C	cerclage wire repair of jaw fracture
FX/R/WIR/ID	interdental wire repair of jaw fracture
FX/R/WIR/OS	osseous wire repair of jaw fracture
G	**granuloma**
G/B	**buccal granuloma (cheek chewing lesion)**
G/L	**sublingual granuloma (tongue chewing lesion)**
G/E/L	**eosinophilic granuloma—lip**
G/E/P	**eosinophilic granuloma—palate**
G/E/T	**eosinophilic granuloma—tongue**
GH	**gingival hyperplasia/hypertrophy**
GR	**gingival recession**
GTR	guided tissue regeneration
GV	gingivoplasty (gingivectomy)
IM	impression and model
IMP	implant
I1,2,3	**Incisor teeth**
IO	interceptive (extraction) orthodontics
IO/D	deciduous (primary) tooth interceptive orthodontics
IO/P	permanent (secondary) tooth interceptive orthodontics
IP	inclined plane
IP/AC	acrylic inclined plane
IP/C	composite inclined plane
IP/M	metal (ie, lab produced) inclined plane

(continued on next page)

	Definition
LAC	laceration
LAC/B	laceration buccal (cheek)
LAC/L	laceration lip
LAC/T	laceration tongue
M1,2,3	molar teeth
MAL	malocclusion
MAL/1	class I malocclusion (normal jaw relationship, specific teeth are incorrectly positioned)
MAL/2	class II malocclusion (mandible shorter than maxilla)
MAL/3	class III malocclusion (maxilla shorter than mandible)
MAL/BN	base narrow mandibular canine tooth
MAL/AXB	anterior crossbite
MAL/PXB	posterior crossbite
MAL/WRY	wry bite
MN	mandible or mandibular
MN/FX	mandibular fracture
MX	maxilla or maxillary
MX/FX	maxillary fracture
OA	orthodontic appliance
OAA	adjust orthodontic appliance
OA/BKT	bracket orthodontic appliance
OA/BU	button orthodontic appliance
OA/EC	elastic (power chain) orthodontic appliance
OA/WIR	wire orthodontic appliance
OAI	install orthodontic appliance
OAR	remove orthodontic appliance
OC	orthodontic/genetic consultation
OM	oral mass
OM/AD	adenocarcinoma
OM/EPA	acanthomatous ameloblastoma (epulis)
OM/EPF	fibromatous epulis
OM/EPO	osseifying epulis
OM/FS	fibrosarcoma
OM/LS	lymphosarcoma
OM/MM	malignant melanoma
OM/OS	osteosarcoma
OM/PAP	papillomatosis
OM/SCC	squamous cell carcinoma
ONF	oronasal fistula
ONF/R	oronasal fistula repair
OR	orthodontic recheck
OST	osteomyelitis
PC	pulp capping
PC/D	direct pulp capping
PC/I	indirect pulp capping
PDI	periodontal disease index
PD0	normal periodontium
PD1	gingivitis only
PD2	<25% attachment loss
PD3	25%–50% attachment loss

(continued on next page)

	Definition
PD4	**>50% attachment loss**
PE	**pulp exposure**
PM1,2,3,4	**premolar teeth**
PRO	periodontal prophylaxis (examination, scaling, polishing, irrigation)
R	restoration of tooth
R/A	restoration with amalgam
R/C	restoration with composite
R/CP	restoration with compomer
R/I	restoration with glass ionomer
RAD	**radiograph**
RC	root canal therapy
RC/S	surgical root canal therapy
RD	**retained deciduous (primary) tooth**
RL	**root resorption lesion**
RL1	**RL into enamel only**
RL2	**RL into dentin**
RL3	**RL into pulp or root canal**
RL4	**RL3 + extensive structural damage**
RL5	**RL crown lost, root tips remain**
RPC	root planning—closed
RPO	root planning—open
RRX	root resection (crown left intact)
RR	**internal root resorption**
RRT	**retained root tip**
RTR	**retained tooth root**
S	surgery
S/M	mandibulectomy
S/P	Palate surgery
S/X	maxillectomy
SC	subgingival curettage
SN	**supernumerary**
SPL	splint
SPL/AC	acrylic splint
SPL/C	composite splint
SPL/WIR	wire reinforced splint
ST	**stomatitis**
ST/CU	**stomatitis—contact ulcers**
ST/FFS	**stomatitis—feline faucitis-stomatitis**
SYM	**symphysis**
SYM/S	**symphyseal separation**
SYM/WIR	wire repair of symphyseal separation
T	**tooth**
T/A	**avulsed tooth**
T/FX	**fractured tooth**
T/I	**impacted tooth**
T/LUX	**luxated tooth**
T/NE	**near pulp exposure**
T/NV	**non-vital tooth**
T/PE	**pulp exposure**

(*continued on next page*)

	Definition
T/V	**vital tooth**
TMJ	**temporomandibular joint**
TMJ/C	temporomandibular joint condylectomy
TMJ/D	**TMJ dysplasia**
TMJ/FX	**TMJ fracture**
TMJ/LUX	**TMJ luxation**
TMJ/R	reduction of TMJ luxation
TP	**treatment plan**
TRX	tooth partial resection (e.g. hemisection)
VP	vital pulp therapy
X	simple closed extraction of a tooth
XS	extraction with tooth sectioning, non-surgical
XSS	surgical (open) extraction of a tooth

ELSEVIER
SAUNDERS

Vet Clin Small Anim
35 (2005) 1065–1072

VETERINARY
CLINICS
Small Animal Practice

Index

Note: Page numbers of article titles are in **boldface** type.

doi:10.1016/S0195-5616(05)00079-3
vetsmall.theclinics.com

Tooth eruption
  timing of, 789

Tooth extraction
  canine teeth, 981–982
  complications of, 982–983
  coronal gingiva incised from tooth in,
    973
  described, 972–973
  elevating, luxating, and removing
    tooth in, 979–980
  flaps in, 974
  home care follow-up, 984
  in cats, 982
  in dogs, 981–982
  precautions in, 982–983
  radiographs in, 973
  roots and root pieces, 982
  sectioning tooth and alveolar bone
    removal in, 975–978
  smoothing alveolar bone in, 980
  steps in, 973–981
  suturing flap in, 981

Tooth resorption
  in domestic cats
    causes of
      update on, **913–942.** See
        also *Feline
        odontoclastic resorptive
        lesions (FORL).*

Total unilateral mandibulectomy,
  1024–1026

Total unilateral maxillectomy, 1029–1030

Tramadol
  for oral and dental procedures, 1053

Trauma
  local
    FORL and, 929–932

Tricyclic antidepressants
  for oral and dental procedures, 1057

Tumor(s)
  oral, **1009–1039.** See also *Oral tumors.*

U

Unilateral rostral mandibulectomy, 1021

Unilateral rostral maxillectomy, 1027–1029

V

Vascular system
  in dogs and cats, 776–779

Veterinary dentistry
  juvenile, **789–817**
    cleft palates, 791–792
    conditions that occur at
      any time, 814–815
    deep occlusal pits, 811
    deformed teeth, 808–809
    delayed eruption of primary
      teeth, 796–798
    dental crowding, 802–804
    dentigerous cysts, 800–801
    first visits (8-week and 12-week
      checkups), 792–798
    fracture of immature permanent
      teeth, 813–814
    malocclusions, 792–795,
      804–808
    maxillofacial fractures,
      814–815
    microglossia, 790–791
    odontomas, 809–811
    oral tumors, 815
    persistent primary teeth,
      798–800
    problems recognized in first
      weeks of life, 790–792
    six months to 1 year, 811–814
    six-month spaying or neutering
      visit, 800–811
    soft tissue impaction, 801–802
    supernumerary teeth, 802
    third visit (4-month checkup),
      798–800

Veterinary oral health care
  gold standard of, **781–787**
    anesthesia and preoperative
      workup in, 782–783
    periodontics in, 784–786
    radiology in, 783–784
    rechecks in, 787

Vital pulp therapy
  for endodontic disease, 844–850

Vitamin D
  activity of
    FORL effects on, 921–929
  for FORL, 933–936

Vitamin D metabolites
  for FORL, 933–936

W

Wound dehiscence
  after oral tumor excision, 1034–1035

Changing Your Address?

Make sure your subscription changes too! When you notify us of your new address, you can help make our job easier by including an exact copy of your Clinics label number with your old address (see illustration below.) This number identifies you to our computer system and will speed the processing of your address change. Please be sure this label number accompanies your old address and your corrected address—you can send an old Clinics label with your number on it or just copy it exactly and send it to the address listed below.

We appreciate your help in our attempt to give you continuous coverage. Thank you.

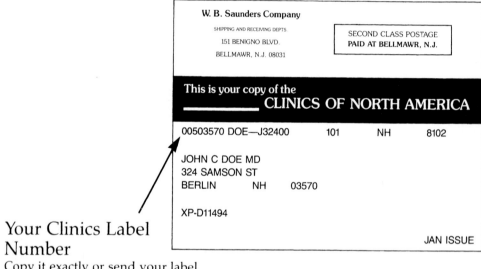

Your Clinics Label Number

Copy it exactly or send your label
along with your address to:
W.B. Saunders Company, Customer Service
Orlando, FL 32887-4800
Call Toll Free 1-800-654-2452

Please allow four to six weeks for delivery of new subscriptions and for processing address changes.

8 Ways To Expand Your Practice
Step 1: Return this card.

Elsevier Clinics and Journals offer you that rare combination of up-to-date scholarly data, step-by-step techniques and authoritative insights...information you can easily apply to the situations you encounter in daily practice. You'll be better able to diagnose and treat a wider range of veterinary problems and broaden your client base.

Just indicate your choice(s) on the card below, fill out the rest of the card and drop it in the mail.

Your satisfaction is guaranteed. If you do not find that the periodical meets your expectations, write *cancel* on the invoice and return it within 30 days. You are under no further obligation.

SUBSCRIBE TODAY!
DETACH AND MAIL THIS NO-RISK CARD TODAY!

YES! Please start my subscription to the periodicals checked below with the ❑ first issue of the calendar year or ❑ current issues. If not completely satisfied with my first issue, I may write "cancel" on the invoice and return it within 30 days at no further obligation

Please Print:

Name_____

Address_____

_____

City_____ State _____

ZIP _____

Method of Payment

❑ Check (payable to **Elsevier**; add the applicable sales tax for your area)

❑ VISA   ❑ MasterCard   ❑ AmEx   ❑ Bill me

Card number _____

Exp. date _____

Signature _____

Staple this to your purchase order to expedite delivery

*To receive in-training rate, orders must be accompanied by the name of affiliated institution, dates of residency and signature of coordinator on institution letterhead. Orders will be billed at the individual rate until proof of resident status is received.

This is not a renewal notice. Professional references may be tax-deductible. © **Elsevier 2005.** Offer valid in U.S. only. Prices subject to change without notice. **MO 10806 DF4169**

❑ **Clinical Techniques in Equine Practice**
Volume 4 (4 issues)
Individuals $124; Institutions $209; In-training $62*

❑ **Clinical Techniques in Small Animal Practice**
Volume 10 (4 issues)
Individuals $134; Institutions $220; In-training $67*

❑ **Journal of Equine Veterinary Science**
Volume 22 (12 issues)
Individuals $171; Institutions $242; In-training $54*

❑ **Seminars in Avian and Exotic Pet Medicine**
Volume 4 (4 issues)
Individuals $116; Institutions $220; In-training $54*

❑ **Veterinary Clinics-Equine Practice**
Volume 21 (3 issues)
Individuals $145; Institutions $230

❑ **Veterinary Clinics-Exotic Animal Practice**
Volume 8 (3 issues)
Individuals $130; Institutions $215

❑ **Veterinary Clinics-Food Animal Practice**
Volume 21 (3 issues)
Individuals $115; Institutions $182

❑ **Veterinary Clinics-Small Animal Practice**
Volume 35 (6 issues)
Individuals $170; Institutions $260

Elsevier, the premier publisher in veterinary medicine, keeps you current with the latest developments in your field to help you achieve optimal patient care. Subscribe today to any of the publications listed below and save considerably over the single issue price.

Clinical Techniques in Equine Practice
Clinical Techniques in Small Animal Practice
Journal of Equine Veterinary Science
Seminars in Avian and Exotic Pet Medicine
Veterinary Clinics – Equine Practice
Veterinary Clinics – Exotic Animal Practice
Veterinary Clinics – Food Animal Practice
Veterinary Clinics – Small Animal Practice

Just fill out the card on the reverse and drop it in the mail.
YOUR SATISFACTION IS GUARANTEED.

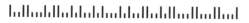